METHODS IN MOLECULAR BIOLOGY

For further volumes:
http://www.springer.com/series/7651

Molecular Typing of Blood Cell Antigens

Edited by

Peter Bugert

*Institute of Transfusion Medicine and Immunology,
Medical Faculty Mannheim, German Red Cross Blood Service Baden-Wurttemberg – Hessen,
Heidelberg University, Mannheim, Germany*

Humana Press

Editor
Peter Bugert
Institute of Transfusion Medicine and Immunology
Medical Faculty Mannheim, German Red Cross
Blood Service Baden-Wurttemberg – Hessen
Heidelberg University
Mannheim, Germany

ISSN 1064-3745 ISSN 1940-6029 (electronic)
Methods in Molecular Biology
ISBN 978-1-4939-2689-3 ISBN 978-1-4939-2690-9 (eBook)
DOI 10.1007/978-1-4939-2690-9

Library of Congress Control Number: 2015938771

Springer New York Heidelberg Dordrecht London

Printed on acid-free paper

Humana Press is a brand of Springer
Springer Science+Business Media LLC New York is part of Springer Science+Business Media (www.springer.com)

Preface

Blood cells are characterized by the surface expression of a variety of antigens that are defined by their capacity to induce an immune response in the autologous or allogenic setting. Antigens on red blood cells are designated as blood groups, and the more than 300 blood group antigens are assigned to currently 35 blood group systems by the International Society for Blood Transfusion (ISBT). In 1990, the ABO blood group system was the first that was characterized on the molecular level. Since then the molecular basis of all blood group systems has been discovered. In clinical diagnosis of blood group antigens and antibodies, serological methods are still the gold standard widely used all over the world. However, molecular blood grouping is an upcoming field with increasing portion of commercialized techniques and methods. In contrast to blood groups, molecular typing is more advanced in the area of human leukocyte antigens (HLA). This rapid progress was driven by the fact that serological HLA phenotyping had a much lower diagnostic value compared to genotyping. Nowadays, low to high resolution HLA genotyping is the gold standard in matched organ or stem cell transplantation. In addition to red and white cell antigens blood platelets represent another cellular component carrying a variety of antigens. The molecular basis of the clinically most relevant human platelet antigens (HPA) is known. Genotyping is straightforward since the antigens are defined by diallelic single nucleotide polymorphisms (SNPs) in glycoprotein genes. Very similar is true for the human neutrophil antigens (HNA). Thus, SNP typing is also an important topic of this book.

The majority of molecular antigen typing methods and techniques are performed on genomic DNA involving PCR-based amplification of the target genes. Many of the methods have been developed for diagnostic use with particular requirements for robustness and quality control. The detailed protocols described in this book can be applied to introduce the methods in the lab. The validation of such a new method or the ongoing quality control is important for the diagnostic use. The first chapter of this book gives a short overview of the minimal demands with regard to first time or ongoing validation. Such diagnostic systems have a great relevance in blood transfusion and organ transplantation.

The aim of this volume about Molecular Typing of Blood Cell Antigens is to bring together a variety of protocols useful for the DNA-based typing of blood cell antigens. The methodological spectrum ranges from rather simple approaches with low technical complexity to highly sophisticated modern developments. In transfusion medicine the blood group genotyping methods need to be flexible for the individual diagnosis of patients on one side. On the other side techniques are required that allow a high-throughput and complex analysis of multiple blood group systems in large numbers of blood donors. The HLA genetics is characterized by a limited number of gene loci, however, each with a remarkably high number of gene variants mostly based on exonic SNPs. This kind of molecular genetic complexity is challenging for genotyping techniques. Therefore, many technical and methodological developments can be observed in the HLA field including in silico methods to deduce HLA types from RNA sequencing data. The review about novel approaches and technologies in molecular HLA typing (*see* Chapter 18) is highly recommended.

This book summarizes contributions from leading international experts in the field of DNA typing for blood cell antigens. As editor of this volume I am very grateful indeed to them for their willingness to provide an insight into their knowledge and to provide the detailed step-by-step protocols. I also wish to thank my colleagues Karin Janetzko and Erwin Scharberg for many fruitful discussions and their considerable input.

Mannheim, Germany ***Peter Bugert***

Contents

Contributors

MARCO ANDREANI • *Laboratory of Immunogenetics and Transplant Biology – IME Foundation, Polyclinic of Tor Vergata University, Rome, Italy*
JOHN BAECH • *Department of Clinical Immunology, Aalborg Hospital, Aalborg, Denmark*
GERALD BERTRAND • *Histocompatibilty and Immunogenetics Laboratory, Etablissement Français du Sang (EFS) Bretagne, Rennes, France*
LOÏC J. BLUM • *Institut de Chimie et Biochimie Moléculaires et Supramoléculaires, Equipe Génie Enzymatique, Membranes Biomimétiques et Assemblages Supramoléculaires (GEMBAS) UMR 5246 ICBMS, Université Lyon1 - CNRS, Villeurbanne, France*
STEPHANIE A. BOCCOZ • *AXO Science SAS, Villeurbanne, France*
SEBASTIAN BOEGEL • *TRON gGmbH – Translational Oncology at Johannes Gutenberg-University Medical Center gGmbH, Mainz, Germany; University Medical Center of the Johannes Gutenberg-University, Mainz, Germany*
CAROL M. BRUZZONE • *Department of Medicine, University of Minnesota Medical School, Minneapolis, MN, USA*
PETER BUGERT • *Institute of Transfusion Medicine and Immunology, Medical Faculty Mannheim, German Red Cross Blood Service Baden-Württemberg – Hessen, Heidelberg University, Mannheim, Germany*
JÜRGEN BUX • *German Red Cross Blood Service West, Hagen, Germany*
JOHN C. CASTLE • *4-Antibody AG, Basel, Switzerland; TRON gGmbH – Translational Oncology at Johannes Gutenberg-University Medical Center gGmbH, Mainz, Germany*
FREDERIK BANCH CLAUSEN • *Department of Clinical Immunology, Rigshospitalet, Copenhagen University Hospital, Copenhagen, Denmark*
FABIANA CONTI • *Section of Transfusion Medicine and Cellular Therapy, Department of Hemotherapy, Hospital Albert Einstein, São Paulo, Brazil*
MARCIN CZERWIŃSKI • *Ludwik Hirszfeld Institute of Immunology and Experimental Therapy, Polish Academy of Sciences, Wrocław, Poland; Faculty of Physical Education and Physiotherapy, Opole University of Technology, Opole, Poland*
ANDREA DOESCHER • *German Red Cross Blood Transfusion Service NSTOB, Oldenburg, Germany*
PAUL P.J. DUNN • *University Hospitals Leicester NHS Trust, Leicester General Hospital, Leicester, UK*
MORTEN HANEFELD DZIEGIEL • *Department of Clinical Immunology, Rigshospitalet, Copenhagen University Hospital, Copenhagen, Denmark*
CLAUDE FÉREC • *Etablissement Français du Sang (EFS) – Bretagne, Brest, France; Institut National de la Santé et de la Recherche Médicale (INSERM), UMR 1078, Brest, France; Faculté de Médecine et des Sciences de la Santé, Université de Bretagne Occidentale, Brest, France; Laboratoire de Génétique Moléculaire et d'Histocompatibilité, Centre Hospitalier Régional Universitaire (CHRU), Hôpital Morvan, Brest, France*
YANN FICHOU • *Etablissement Français du Sang (EFS) – Bretagne, Brest, France; Institut National de la Santé et de la Recherche Médicale (INSERM), UMR 1078, Brest, France*
BEAT M. FREY • *Department of Molecular Diagnostics and Research (MOC), Blood Transfusion Service Zurich, Swiss Red Cross, Schlieren, Switzerland*

CHRISTOPH GASSNER • *Department of Molecular Diagnostics and Research (MOC), Blood Transfusion Service Zurich, Swiss Red Cross, Schlieren, Switzerland*
GAËLLE LE GOFF • *AXO Science SAS, Villeurbanne, France*
MAGDALENA GRODECKA • *Ludwik Hirszfeld Institute of Immunology and Experimental Therapy, Polish Academy of Sciences, Wrocław, Poland*
TAKAYUKI HONDA • *Department of Laboratory Medicine, Shinshu University, Matsumoto, Japan*
LIANG-IN LIN • *Department of Clinical Laboratory Sciences and Medical Biotechnology, College of Medicine, National Taiwan University, Taipei, Taiwan; Department of Laboratory Medicine, National Taiwan University Hospital, Taipei, Taiwan*
MARTIN LÖWER • *TRON gGmbH – Translational Oncology at Johannes Gutenberg-University Medical Center gGmbH, Mainz, Germany*
EWA ŁUKASIK • *Ludwik Hirszfeld Institute of Immunology and Experimental Therapy, Polish Academy of Sciences, Wrocław, Poland*
EDYTA MAJORCZYK • *Ludwik Hirszfeld Institute of Immunology and Experimental Therapy, Polish Academy of Sciences, Wrocław, Poland; Faculty of Physical Education and Physiotherapy, Opole University of Technology, Opole, Poland*
DAMMIKA P. MANAGE • *Department of Oncology, University of Alberta and Cross Cancer Institute, Edmonton, Canada*
CHRISTOPHE A. MARQUETTE • *Institut de Chimie et Biochimie Moléculaires et Supramoléculaires, Equipe Génie Enzymatique, Membranes Biomimétiques et Assemblages Supramoléculaires (GEMBAS) UMR 5246 ICBMS, Université Lyon1 - CNRS, Villeurbanne, France*
KAZUYUKI MATSUDA • *Department of Laboratory Medicine, Shinshu University, Matsumoto, Japan*
PAUL METCALFE • *National Institute for Biological Standards and Control, Herts, UK*
STEFAN MEYER • *Department of Molecular Diagnostics and Research (MOC), Blood Transfusion Service Zurich, Swiss Red Cross, Schlieren, Switzerland*
THOMAS H. MÜLLER • *German Red Cross Blood Transfusion Service NSTOB, Oldenburg, Germany*
KASPAR R. NIELSEN • *Department of Clinical Immunology, Aalborg Hospital, Aalborg, Denmark*
SHUN-CHUNG PAI • *Taiwan Blood Services Foundation, Taipei, Taiwan*
LINDA M. PILARSKI • *Department of Oncology, University of Alberta and Cross Cancer Institute, Edmonton, Canada*
ANGELIKA REIL • *German Red Cross Blood Service West, Hagen, Germany; DRK-Blutspendedienst West, Hagen, Germany*
KLAUS RIENECK • *Department of Clinical Immunology, Rigshospitalet, Copenhagen University Hospital, Copenhagen, Denmark*
GABRIELE RINK • *Institute of Transfusion Medicine and Immunology, Medical Faculty Mannheim, German Red Cross Blood Service Baden-Württemberg – Hessen, Heidelberg University, Mannheim, Germany*
UGUR SAHIN • *TRON gGmbH – Translational Oncology at Johannes Gutenberg-University Medical Center gGmbH, Mainz, Germany; University Medical Center of the Johannes Gutenberg-University, Mainz, Germany; BioNTech AG, Mainz, Germany*
ERWIN A. SCHARBERG • *Institute of Transfusion Medicine and Immunohematology, German Red Cross Blood Service Baden-Württemberg – Hessen, Baden-Baden, Germany*

JELLE SCHOLTALBERS • *European Molecular Biology Laboratory, Heidelberg, Germany; TRON gGmbH – Translational Oncology at Johannes Gutenberg-University Medical Center gGmbH, Mainz, Germany*
ANA MARIA SELL • *Laboratório de Imunogenética, Departamento de Ciências Básicas da Saúde, Universidade Estadual de Maringá, Maringá, Paraná, Brazil*
CLIFFORD J. STEER • *Department of Medicine, University of Minnesota Medical School, Minneapolis, MN, USA*
RUDI STEFFENSEN • *Department of Clinical Immunology, Aalborg Hospital, Aalborg, Denmark*
MANUELA TESTI • *Laboratory of Immunogenetics and Transplant Biology – IME Foundation, Polyclinic of Tor Vergata University, Rome, Italy*
NADINE TROST • *Department of Molecular Diagnostics and Research (MOC), Blood Transfusion Service Zurich, Swiss Red Cross, Schlieren, Switzerland*
JEANE ELIETE LAGUILA VISENTAINER • *Laboratório de Imunogenética, Departamento de Ciências Básicas da Saúde, Universidade Estadual de Maringá, Maringá, Paraná, Brazil*
KAZIMIERA WAŚNIOWSKA • *Ludwik Hirszfeld Institute of Immunology and Experimental Therapy, Polish Academy of Sciences, Wrocław, Poland; Faculty of Physical Education and Physiotherapy, Opole University of Technology, Opole, Poland*
CAROLA WIECKHUSEN • *Institute of Transfusion Medicine and Immunology, Medical Faculty Mannheim, German Red Cross Blood Service Baden-Württemberg – Hessen, Heidelberg University, Mannheim, Germany*

Chapter 1

Validation of Genotyping Protocols for Diagnostic Use

Paul Metcalfe

Abstract

This chapter contains some advice for first validating a new genotyping method and then continuing to ensure that it performs well when adopted for routine use. It should be applicable to most of the genotyping methods described in this volume; however, because the range of techniques is so wide and these recommendations have been written with PCR amplification in mind, the reader may need to adapt some of the recommendations for non-PCR based tests.

It does not include any advice on how to handle unscreened human samples within the laboratory, and it assumes that the laboratory already has established good practice for DNA amplification and the avoidance of contamination.

Key words Genotyping, Protocol, Validation

1 Initial Validation of a New Genotyping Method

1. It is essential to start with a small panel (4–6) of DNA samples which have been prepared recently by a routine method. They should be available in bulk so that the same samples can be used repeatedly for the initial runs; thus any differences observed from run to run can be assumed to be related to varying conditions rather than variations in sample quality or differing genotypes.
2. Samples from the same donors should have been phenotyped as far as possible and genotyped by a technique already established in the same laboratory or by an external laboratory if this is a new area for the developing lab. The panel should include as wide a range of genotypes as possible in such a small panel.
3. If the genotyping technique involves oligonucleotide primers or probes, then the sequences should be checked carefully to see if their function could be affected by underlying SNPs (other than the one which may be the target of the genotyping test). Additional SNPs that are situated several bases from the

Peter Bugert (ed.), *Molecular Typing of Blood Cell Antigens*, Methods in Molecular Biology, vol. 1310,
DOI 10.1007/978-1-4939-2690-9_1, © Springer Science+Business Media New York 2015

3′ end of primer sequences have been shown to have significant effects on efficiency of amplification.

4. The small panel of samples should be used in all initial tests carried out to get the technique working. For example, if the genotyping assay involves PCR, then this stage will involve multiple experiments where concentrations of primers and template (and possibly buffer and dNTPs) are varied, usually one at a time. PCR conditions will be established primarily by varying annealing temperature(s) and cycle number. If the new genotyping assay is required to run under the same conditions as an existing technique (i.e., "multiplexed"), then possibly both sets of conditions will have to be varied in order to achieve a common protocol.
5. When the new technique appears to work and the expected results can be reliably obtained from the small panel, then the same samples can be tested in dilution to define a working range for acceptable DNA concentration in subsequent patient samples. Degraded DNA is not the same problem as low DNA concentration and another measure of DNA quality should be integrated if degradation is suspected.
6. For techniques involving PCR, users could explore aliquoting and freezing of primer mixes at this stage. If they can be stored ready for use in individual tubes, either in strips or plates, then time will be saved and mistakes made whilst setting up the test will be less likely.
7. When all parameters have been explored and a robust set of conditions have been adopted, then a large-scale validation study should be carried out and documented. At least 200 blinded samples, including at least five examples of each common genotype, should be tested and compared with results previously obtained by another method (internal or external). The panel should include as many heterozygotes as possible as these are more prone to error than homozygotes. Rare genotypes should also be included in the panel if possible. The racial mix in the intended patient population should be considered and if necessary additional samples of rare genotypes should be obtained from an external laboratory.
8. If either CE-marked or WHO endorsed DNA reference materials are available, then these should also be tested at this stage.

2 Ongoing Validation of an Established Genotyping Method

Continuing validation of a method depends on the frequency of testing and the scale of the change being made and the following is only a guide. There are no specific recommendations made for the number of samples required for **steps 1** and **2** because this depends on the total number of possible genotypes; for example, a small panel would be required to control the reactions detecting only one SNP but if the method simultaneously detects multiple SNPs, then more controls would be required.

1. A small set of controls, incorporating a range of genotypes with as many heterozygotes as possible, should be included in each assay if reasonably practicable.
2. A larger panel, incorporating each genotype at least once, should be used to validate new batches of primers, new bulk preparations of primer mixes, or new batches of Taq, dNTPs, or PCR reaction buffer.
3. If a major change is made, for example an alteration to the cycling parameters or a new PCR machine, then the technique should be revalidated using a panel similar to that described in Subheading 1, **step 7**.
4. It is important to record the batch numbers of all reagents used in each genotyping run and to keep a log of the dates when critical reagents are changed. It is also important to carry out regular temperature calibration of any thermocycler block after consultation with the manufacturer concerning the recommended interval for such testing.
5. If possible automated reading, interpretation, and recording of results should be incorporated into the method rather than operator-dependent steps, in order to lower the operator error rate. However, it is important to store documentary evidence of the actual test result (e.g., photo of gel, screenshot of trace) rather than just the interpreted genotype result. In this way results can be checked and subtle changes in performance can be detected.
6. The laboratory should join an external QA scheme if one is available for the genotypes involved.

Chapter 2

High-Resolution Melting Analysis of Single Nucleotide Polymorphisms

Carol M. Bruzzone and Clifford J. Steer

Abstract

The technology of Single Nucleotide Polymorphism (SNP) detection has evolved steadily through mobility shift studies, mass cleavage product evaluations, heterodimer differences in chemical, conformational, and enzymatic properties, mass spectroscopy and sequencing, to allele-specific hybridization probe methods. Each method presented challenges of labor intensity, unreliable efficiencies, complicated optimizations, and issues of sample quantity and quality. Concurrently the value of SNP detection in basic research and personalized medicine has continued to grow. Accessing the secrets of genetic individuality is the next frontier in moving medicine from the description of very low frequency and highly deleterious nucleotide changes to the study of very low frequency polymorphisms, lower penetrance polymorphisms, and polymorphisms with public health importance. High-Resolution Melting (HRM) analysis of SNP status became an option for high throughput settings with the development of double-stranded dyes that do not interfere with PCR amplification in saturation, eliminate dye jumping, and nearest neighbor sequence changes influence melt temperature via amplicon strand locking chemistry. This method is able to distinguish transitions, transversions, and identify novel changes at or near the SNP of interest rapidly, inexpensively, and without post-amplification assay techniques or extensive technical interpretation of data. For probe or solid matrix based assays, the investigator initially defines a set of target sequences for binding. These assays are not only difficult due to the optimization of binding conditions but are unable to detect sequences that were not included in the design, often have marginalized binding due to a "one size fits all" reaction, and are not distinct in the case of heterozygotes.

Key words Single nucleotide polymorphism, High-resolution melting, Personalized medicine, Dye chemistry, Transition, Transversion, Minor allele, Major allele, Ancestral allele

1 Introduction

Single Nucleotide Polymorphisms (SNPs) are the result of genomic variation or changes of a single nucleotide in the genomic DNA. Each person is heterozygous (HTZ) for approximately three million bases, has about one SNP every 1,000 bases or about 3.2 million differences in our diploid genome [1]. Nucleotide changes can occur anywhere in the genome. Many occur outside of protein

Peter Bugert (ed.), *Molecular Typing of Blood Cell Antigens*, Methods in Molecular Biology, vol. 1310,
DOI 10.1007/978-1-4939-2690-9_2, © Springer Science+Business Media New York 2015

coding regions and sense and antisense conventional naming do not apply. Naming of genomic DNA following current database convention is "top strand and bottom strand." The prevalent or first reported sequence is referred to as the major allele (MJA) or ancestral allele. Any rare allele is referred to as a minor allele (MIA). The changed sequences are classified as transitions, where a double ring nucleotide or a single ring nucleotide is replaced with other nucleotides of the same number rings or, a transversion where a nucleotide is replaced with either of the two nucleotides with a different ring number. Transversions are also described as strand swaps if the minor allele top strand demonstrates the nucleotide of the bottom strand from the major allele. SNPs can be detected through the melting properties of the PCR products due to the gain or loss of inter-strand hydrogen bond pair, the absence of dye at mismatch sites, and the conformational distortion at mismatch sites [2–4]. Since melting temperature is not dependent on quantity of PCR product, this method is efficiency independent. Homozygous MJA and Homozygous MIA status can be observed in the peak melt temperature (PTm) difference. Heterozygous samples generate a melt profile that is complex and broadened.

Developments in double-stranded dyes have resolved the issues of dye jumping, dye saturation, and dye locked strand pairs allowing the detection of nearest neighbor changes [5]. High-resolution melting failed to differentiate longer, 208 *versus* 319, base pair (bp) amplicons by melting temperature [6] but is capable of detecting genotype status in amplicons of ~100 bp [7]. Genotype detection employing HRM does not require the investigator to predict the population of outcomes. HRM of short amplicons, optimized for melt differences, rapidly and clearly categorizes samples into one of three expected outcomes or identifies samples with unexpected outcomes for further study.

1.1 Prepare, Cycle, Report: The PCR for HRM Analysis of SNPs

Preparing to distinguish SNP status by HRM requires that the vocabulary and mathematical basis of PCR be understood in advance of the physical preparation of an experiment. Vendor specific and historical terms describe the components and process of PCR in publications and vendor documents. These are largely a result of patent considerations and historical process. To understand the process of PCR and create a document for publication that will have transparency and portability, we should follow the Minimum Information for Publication of Quantitative Real-Time PCR Experiments (MIQE) standardized nomenclature [8]. In this document we use Quantification cycle (Cq) terminology instead of crossing point (Roche).

Limitations in the availability and archival goals of any sample require that assays be developed using the smallest quantity of precious starting material. The functional availability of any gDNA target must be assessed to create the optimal reaction. Although we discuss PCR as capable of detecting a single copy, we usually initiate gDNA PCR reactions with template concentrations of about 20 ng of DNA in 15 μl reactions.

The size of the human diploid genome is around 6×10^9 bp. The average molecular weight a nucleotide bp is approximately 660 g per mole: 6×10^9 bp times 660 g/mole = 3.96 pico grams (pg) DNA per genome, and a single genome has two copies of the target SNP. Thus, 20 ng DNA contain approximately 10,100 targets: (20,000 pg/3.96 pg/genome) × two copies/genome = 10,100 copies (*see* **Note 1**).

The candidate SNP will be selected based on the needs of the study or the clinical application. Evaluation of a candidate SNP, design of the synthetic target, and that of the primers all begin with retrieval of the genomic sequence of interest from an appropriate registry source such as NCBI (http://NCBI.nlm.nih.gov). The sequence for a few hundred bp on each side of the SNP sequence needs to be retrieved and the documentation of the SNP should be read. Observations that are critical immediately are the number of minor alleles at the location of interest, and the presence of other variations in the candidate amplicon or primer areas. This assay is applicable to single minor alleles present in conserved sequences with flanking regions appropriate for primer placement.

Most SNPs are candidates for this method. However, SNPs with multiple minor alleles or have flanking sequence areas that are highly repetitious making it difficult to locate a primer, are not candidates for this protocol (*see* **Note 2**). Double or triple nucleotide polymorphisms are extremely rare due to the combined effects of how rare the genomic change event would be and the potentially highly deleterious effect of changing one or two amino acids in an exon [9]. We do not have experience with detecting double or triple nucleotide polymorphisms but suggest that this method would be likely to detect this as a novel profile (*see* **Note 3**).

Primers that will generate a product of ~500 bp amplicon should be designed using standard primer selecting software or from basic principles for sequence validation. A synthetic target is ordered to include the outer boundaries of all the primers or ~1 kbp. DNA synthesis sources such as Integrated DNA Technologies (Coralville, IA, USA) provide nanogram amounts of synthetic template that can provide an unlimited amount of target.

Three or four primers for each side of the SNP but not including the SNP itself need to be designed to create an amplicon of ~100 bp. The melting behavior of the amplicon is dependent on the length, composition, and location of the SNP within the amplicon. In our experience there are no software options that will substitute for the real evaluation of amplicon melt studies using a panel of primers. A Cq analysis of serial dilutions of the synthetic template, gDNA, and control samples to determine the best primer pair, salt concentration and gDNA quantity is a critical prerequisite to sample analysis (*see* **Note 4**).

Cycling involves the accurate binding of the primers to their targets, the procession of the polymerase enzyme, and the incorporation of the dye or detection molecule. Setting the cycling parameters will depend upon the machine and software version being used. Supplies, equipment, and software will depend upon the user situation. Operators should convert the terminology of their equipment and consumable product vendor to follow MIQE standards and create in-house standard operating protocols utilizing MIQE terminology to enhance the transparency of the protocol and results. However, classical PCR concepts remain relevant in this modernized setting.

Cycling to detect SNPs is possible due to the advances in equipment and supplies, and most notably in dye chemistry. When SYBR green binds to the double-stranded DNA of the PCR products, it will emit light upon excitation; and the intensity of fluorescence increases as the PCR products accumulate. SYBR green chemistry was quick to be accepted for quantitative PCR applications [10, 11]. Although it is accurate and inexpensive, there have been issues of polymerase inhibition, dye jumping, and strand rearrangements in its application. Contemporary dyes such as Roche Applied Sciences Resolight Dye have been perfected to not interfere with polymerase activity in saturation and lock strands during the melt and annealing process of HRM. The dye does not discriminate the various types of double-stranded DNA, gDNA, SNP amplicon PCR products, or primer-dimers. However, the large melt temperature difference between any primer-dimer and the 100 bp amplicon clearly separate these outcomes. In addition, Cq analysis prior to sample testing insures that the correct quantity of gDNA or synthetic template is used to offset these effects. Dilution studies of each SNP must be completed to determine the correct starting gDNA template concentration and the Cq matching of the synthetic control.

The modern polymerase enzyme does not amplify at temperatures below 75 °C. A hot start and touchdown protocol greatly enhance pure amplicon generation. Similarly, advances in the heat transfer capabilities of the thermal blocks and light transmission of the plastic plates have made this work much more accurate. Software that allows data acquisition at 25 data points per degree for every well makes creation of the differential profiles possible. However, software has not been developed that designs the primers needed for this study or sorts the data. Contamination amplification inhibition (CAI) is a concern of HRM, as in real time quantification PCR [12] and must be considered. In a study of eight SNP analyses, CAI varied between SNPs using the same gDNA sample set [7].

Reporting is the classification of the melt profiles into one of the three expected, or in rare cases, a unique outcome. A critical component of MIQE is that the data have a transparency that enables interpretation. HRM analysis based on melt profiles clearly separates the data into predicted outcomes and identifies those that are unique [3, 13]. Much in the style of relative quantification of PCR, this assay uses outcomes against controls or each other to classify the sample outcomes as a relative melt temperature and relative melt peak width assay. Observing the loss of fluorescence for the population of amplicons during melt cycle, the homozygous samples generate a sharp profile consistent with a pure sample. Homozygous samples differ by PTm due to the different chemistry at the SNP. The PCR product of a homozygous sample will contain a single top and bottom strands. Post melt and rapid reannealing of the sample will be pure and the amplicons will have dye saturation. A wide melt profile is generated from the HTZ samples since it is a population of amplicons. Half of the amplicons in an HTZ sample will have a mismatch site that does not have a locking dye. One fourth of the amplicons will be each of the homozygous amplicons with dye saturation.

The raw data shown here was generated with Roche LightCycler® 480 System. The X-axis temperature will vary according to the target SNP and optimization by the user. The Y-axis will vary due to efficiency and will be affected by the same optimization factors and reflect efficiency of amplification. In all cases, it is best to refer to the manual for the equipment and the supplies kit as these are nonstandard and will continue to change.

1.2 Homozygous Samples

The MJA and MIA homozygotes will have melt profiles that differ by PTm (Fig. 1). Although it is often possible to deduce which genotype will have higher melt temperatures based on the presence of hydrogen bonds, it is important to follow an assay design and protocol to optimize the difference and confirm the assay ability to detect and differentiate MJA from MIA. The MIA may be at a very low frequency in the sample set and the laboratory must know that the assay is able to detect rare events.

1.3 Enhanced Separation of Homozygous Samples: Spiked Samples

Optimized assays sometimes produce PTm profiles that are distinct but have close temperatures. Furthermore, inter-sample variation will produce a slight range of PTm for the MIA and the MJA. It may be advantageous or necessary to maximize the difference in PTm between MIA and MJA through a process called spiking to ensure the PTms do not merge.

Maximizing the PTm difference can be accomplished by spiking the samples with a small amount of the hottest melt template [14]. The amount to add is based on the quantification cycle (Cq) of the synthetic template and the sample gDNA. The spike will destabilize the colder melting homozygous samples to slightly

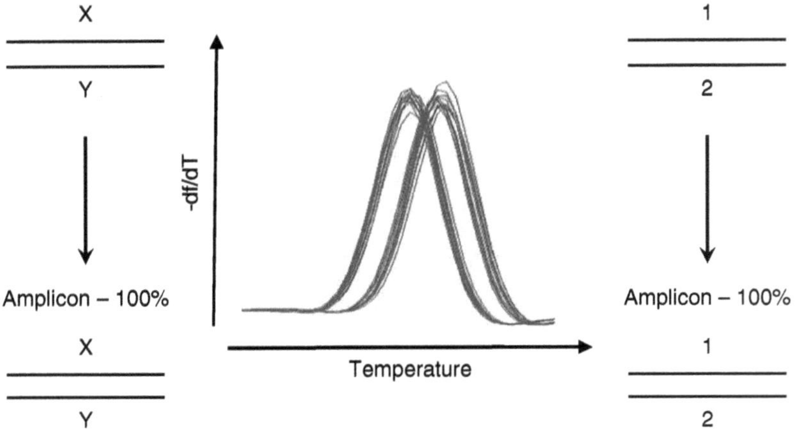

Fig. 1 Homozygous Melt Profiles. The melt profiles of homozygous samples demonstrate a sharp profile and can be differentiated by the peak melt temperature difference. The complete melting and rapid cooling process in the presence of the locking dye creates a pure population of amplicons in homozygous samples

colder and not affect the hotter melting samples or the HTZ samples. A range of spike concentrations should be generated with control samples to determine an optimal outcome that differentiates the homozygous temperatures while maintaining peak shape difference integrity and the smallest amount of spike that effects a statistically significant difference in the PTm. In general a 20 % of target spike will make a good starting point.

Three genotypes of a spiked assay are shown in Fig. 2, in which the MJA and MIA are separated and the three profiles are retained. The homozygous pure outcome for the colder amplicon is converted to a destabilized mix of four amplicon pairings of the Cold Top Strand (CTS), Cold Bottom Strand (CBS), Hot Top Strand (HTS), and Hot Bottom Strand (HBS). In a 20 % spike scenario nearly two thirds of the amplicons are identical to the non-spiked outcome and about a third of the amplicons now melt cooler. A very small portion of higher melt temperature amplicon pairings (≤4 %) contributes to the widened PTm. Without a spike the hotter melt allele would also have produced 100 % hot melt amplicon.

1.4 Heterozygous Samples

The PCR product of an HTZ sample will contain two top strands and two bottom strand species. Complete melting and cooling in the presence of the locking dye produces a heterogenous population of either top and bottom strand amplicons present in approximately equal (25 %) per possible strand pairing. The shape and width of the HTZ sample is distinctive and statistically differs from the width of a homozygous peak (Fig. 3.). The area under any curve is proportional to efficiency.

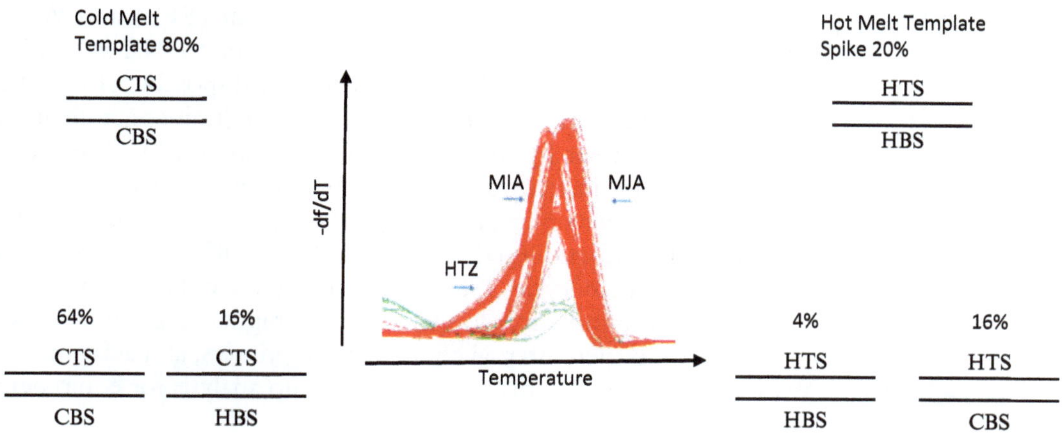

Fig. 2 Spiked Reaction Melt Profiles. The two homozygous profiles and the heterozygous profile for a SNP are shown in a 20 % spiked assay. The colder melting homozygous profile is produced from the mixed population of four possible amplicon pairings in very unequal concentrations. The low level destabilizing mix of the amplicons produced from the spike shift the PTm slightly colder but the higher concentration of the pure cold melt amplicon preserves the shape and height characteristic of a homozygous sample. The hotter PTm amplicon is unchanged by the addition of hot amplicon target. The heterozygous amplicon remains distinctive and differentiated. *CTS* cold top strand, *CBS* cold bottom strand, *HTS* hot top strand, *HBS* hot bottom strand, *MIA* minor allele, *MJA* major allele, *HTZ* heterozygous

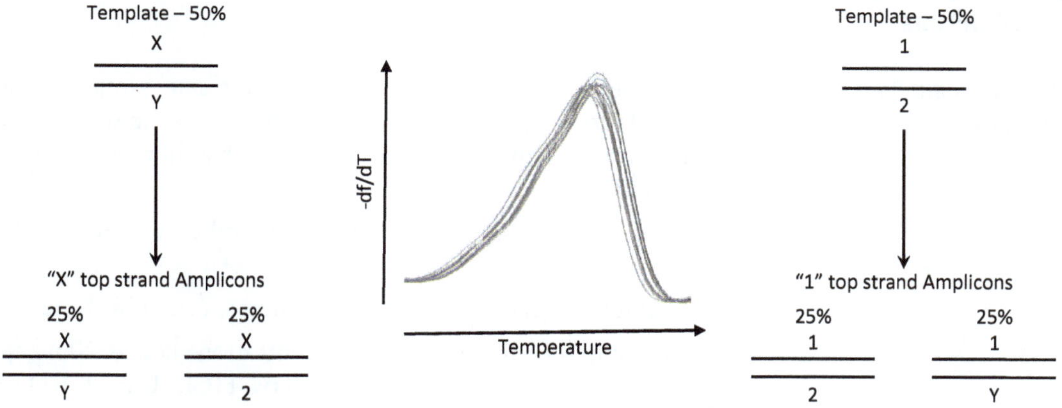

Fig. 3 Components of the Heterozygous Melt Profile. A heterozygous genotype sample produces two upper strands and two lower strands during PCR. The dye locks either top strand with either bottom strand producing a population of four amplicon pairings. Each pairing has a separate PTm and melting the mixture produces a wide and shortened pattern that is the overlapping results of these reactions. Heterozygous melt begins with the coldest temperature melting mismatch unsaturated amplicon pair and ends with the hottest temperature matched and dye saturated amplicon pair

Two strand pairings are missing a dye molecule and have a conformational distortion at the single nucleotide mismatch. The lack of dye and the conformational distortion lowers the start melt. Melting progresses through the population of melt temperatures and terminates at the highest melt temperature of the homozygous samples.

Follow all Personal Protective Equipment (PPE) and Waste Disposal Regulations (WDR). Human genomic DNA is considered a biosafety level 1 (BSL1) hazard. Wear disposable gloves and face mask and work in a setting and manner to limit contamination of the experiment by the user or from extraneous DNA sources. Follow vendor instructions for storing all reagents. Maintain master mix solutions on ice; and limit light exposure to solutions that contain dye. Store diluted plates of gDNA at −80 °C until use; and limit freeze thaw cycles. Store plates ready for cycling at 4 °C for brief periods, and never longer than overnight. Maintain supplies such as TE buffer, internal control DNA, primers, and assay master mix in aliquots. Practice worst-case backup analysis for equipment and sample storage.

Commercially available locking dye amplification kits, optical cover films and plates matched to the device, and DNase free low retention disposable pipet tips, 96 well plates, and tubes are used throughout. No products need preparation by the operator laboratory. The required equipment includes, vortex mixer, pipets, microvolume spectrophotometer, LED plate loading guide (*see* **Note 5**) plate spinner, refrigerator, −80 °C freezer, and appropriate qPCR machine with computer.

2 Materials

2.1 Genomic DNA Samples

1. Collect starting material (i.e., blood or tissue samples) and process following guidelines and regulations of the sponsoring institution and funding agency with strict adherence to PPE and WDR.
2. Isolate gDNA using standardized approved commercial isolation kit.
3. Quantitate the gDNA with microvolume spectrophotometer.
4. Dilute the gDNA to a standard concentration such as 20 ng/μl in commercially available 10 mM Tris–HCl, 1 mM EDTA pH 8.0 buffer.
5. Store experimental samples in aliquots in 96-well plates or other airtight low nucleic acid retention container as appropriate. Cover with foil, wrap and label as biohazard and store in −80 °C until use.
6. Purchase commercial grade high purity large quantity gDNA from the same species of interest (*see* **Note 6**).
7. Collect and process identical control samples from sources, which are distinct from the study samples. These control samples should be from normal or, non-disease state individuals, of the same tissue source and population demographics (*see* **Note 7**).

2.2 Primers

1. Standard HPLC purification primers are ordered through overnight processing supplier.
2. Dilute primers using vendor stated yield to 100 μM with TE buffer.
3. Aliquot enough primer for a few (2–5) assays, label, and store in a dark box at 4 °C.

2.3 Synthetic Targets

1. Determine the sequence of the area, 500–1,000 bp vicinity, of the SNP using a database resource such as NCBI (http://NCBI.nlm.nih.gov), research center specific resource, or primary sequencing.
2. Order commercial DNA for SNP vicinity with SNP of interest having 250–500 bp of flank sequence on each side (Integrated DNA Technologies). Order both the major allele target and the minor allele target (*see* **Note 8**).
3. Dilute synthetic target using vendor stated yield to 100 μM with TE buffer.
4. Aliquot into 3–5 tubes, label, and store in a dark box at 4 °C.
5. Quantification of the synthetic targets, Cq measurement, is done through standard PCR such as Expand HiFi (Roche). Serial dilutions of the synthetic target and purification method control samples need to be compared for functional amplification equality.

2.4 High-Resolution Melt Supplies

1. High-Resolution Melt kit purchased from commercial supplier contains the fluorescent locking dye, assay buffer, and polymerase (LightCycler® 480 High Resolution Melting Master, Roche).
2. 384-well optical white plates with matched optical foils (Roche).

3 Methods

3.1 Assay Development

1. Target Selection: HRM detection of SNP is dependent on a single nucleotide difference imbedded in an area of DNA that is expected to be very highly conserved. Additional variations in sequence within the amplicon are not acceptable. Targets must have areas flanking the SNP that are amenable to primer creation (*see* **Note 9**). Targets will be defined by the project. The sequence of the target and the flanking DNA is retrieved from a database such as NCBI (http://NCBI.nlm.nih.gov). The SNP and the flanking DNA are evaluated for suitability to this assay (*see* **Note 3**). Both genotype synthetic control targets are designed, synthesized, and included in assay development as they establish the melt temperature relationship for strand swap SNPs, ensure the assay is optimized to differentiate MIA and MJA, and may be used in spiked assays.

2. Primer Design: several software tools exist to design primers. A primer pair for each SNP should be designed using traditional primer tools to generate an amplicon of ~500 bp. Evaluate this pair by standard PCR (Expand HiFi Roche) and agarose gel electrophoretic sizing criteria. This pair of primers will be used for sequencing studies if the data requires. However, none of the tools available at this writing are concerned with the issues of HRM differentiation of short amplicons. Hand design three or four primers for the melt analysis protocol from each side of the SNP, not including the SNP site to make final PCR amplicons of ~100 bp (*see* **Note 10**). These primers are designed using basic primer theory of G/C composition and length.

3. Primer Pair Selection: Each left primer for the melt analysis protocol is tested against each right primer for each SNP using the synthetic target diluted to ~10 copies per reaction as target. Amplicon melt performance is evaluated and the best pair or pairs are considered. The primer pair with the best performance against the synthetic template should next be tested for off-target priming using the commercial gDNA (*see* **Note 11**). Any primer pair that generates off-target annealing can be modified to higher specificity through additional 3′ nucleotides and touchdown annealing. Finally, any primer pair that has demonstrated ability to differentiate the homozygous states based on the synthetic template and does not create an off-target product with commercial gDNA is tested with samples created with the same purification protocol. A set of 10–20 control gDNA samples should be prepared in serial dilutions to test sample CAI effects. A starting concentration of 20 ng of gDNA/15 μl reaction (*see* **Note 12**) contains ~10,000 copies of the target of interest and is often the correct amount of starting material, but lesser quantities such as 10 ng/15 μl and 2 ng/15 μl should also be tested. Include both homozygous synthetic targets samples and prepare a HTZ control sample with half of each synthetic target and compare the diluted samples to the three expected outcomes (*see* **Note 13**). Keep in mind that with a small set of control samples the observed melt profiles are likely to be only the most common SNP sequences. If there are CAI effects, a more dilute sample will usually reduce the errors in amplification. SNP locations where a primer cannot be designed (*see* **Note 2**), and SNPs with more than one minor allele required alternative assay methods. Some SNPs demonstrate different but close Tms and additional assay design steps may be necessary (*see* **Note 14**).

4. Quantification Cycle Analysis: To use the synthetic template as a spike or as an in range homozygous control for the assay, it is necessary to have a measurement of the functional concentration of the synthetic target and gDNA purified by the same

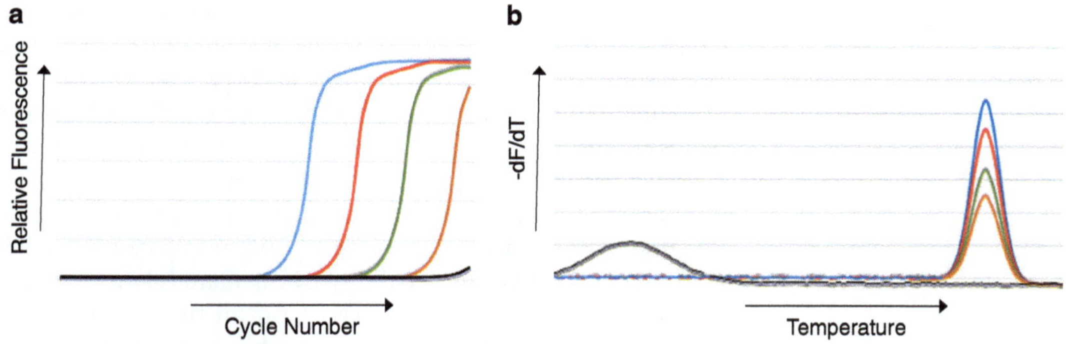

Fig. 4 Hypothetical Basic Principles of Fluorescence. (**a**) The accumulation of fluorescence as double-stranded amplicon is shown. Fluorescence is initially below detectable levels, progresses through linear phase where, at perfect efficiency, the quantity of amplicon DNA doubles each cycle to plateau, and amplification efficiency has dropped off due to product interference. (**b**) The melting of a PCR product post amplification results in the liberation of the dye and loss of fluorescence. The change in fluorescence with that in temperature is commonly expressed as the negative derivative (-dF/dT) and generates a peak melt temperature determination. The area under the -dF/dT curve is proportional to the quantity of melted amplicon. The shape of the -dF/dT curve and the number of peaks reflects purity of the amplicon sample. The most efficacious reactions demonstrate the earliest linear phase (panel (**a**)) and the highest peak -dF/dT (panel (**b**)), represented here in blue tracings. Differing quantities in the synthesis of amplicon DNA is reflected by cycle number in the linear phase. Differing quantities of melted DNA is reflected by differences in area under the -dF/dT curves but has no effect on peak melt temperature. No template controls or failed samples can create off target products in late cycle and lack a discrete -dF/dT curve (*black tracings*)

method as the samples. To measure Cq, create a dilution series of the synthetic template and the control gDNA. Set up the PCR reaction as intended for sample analysis. Perform the PCR reaction as per the sample analysis or a standard PCR reaction such as an Expand HiFi assay (Roche). Most thermal cycler current software tools have an option to determine Cq but will name it by their product line patent naming system. The Cq measurement is based on the concept that in PCR each cycle during log phase will double the quantity of amplicon. Therefore, any two templates that demonstrate an equal fluorescence differ in concentration by the square of difference in cycle number to achieve this fluorescence. For example two samples with equal fluorescence that required two additional cycles in one sample would show a concentration difference of four fold. The more concentrated sample would, of course, be first to achieve the selected fluorescence. As demonstrated over a decade ago the basic principle of logarithmic expansion of amplicon number by PCR follows fluorescence accumulation by cycle number in a pattern that allows the determination of relative concentration. Figure 4 demonstrates the two basic principles of PCR. Panel A is the accumulation of double-stranded DNA as increased fluorescence with cycle number on the X-axis and fluorescence on the Y-axis. This curve is used to determine the relative concentrations of the synthetic template and gDNA, and is recorded as Cq. The Cq is used to compare functional concentration of different samples. Panel B shows the loss of double-stranded DNA as the negative second derivative of fluorescence when the temperature is increased. The number, shape, and height of the peak(s) reveals the purity of the amplicon(s), and the efficiency of amplification. Each instrument will have the capability to calculate relative quantification and create a melting curve. Consult the owner's manual or technical support to determine how to generate these data outputs. To calculate concentration without software support, inspect the amplification curves for typical sigmoid shape of below detectable fluorescence, log phase, and product priming flattening. This is based on the normal plot of fluorescence on the Y-axis and cycle number on the X-axis. Select a fluorescence level in which the reactions to be compared are in log phase. Produce a new X-axis at this fluorescence. Interpret the cycle number by creating a vertical line from the point that the curve and the new X-axis intersect. Use the dilution series and the cycle number difference to estimate the functional concentration of the synthetic template.

5. Triplicate Samples: Polymerase enzymes currently available are highly accurate and expectations are that the industry will continue to improve. The efficiencies are such that DNA Polymerase in the HotStart HiFidelity Polymerase Kit (Qiagen FAQ 2013–2014) is ~2.3×10^{-6} (per base, per cycle), meaning, one error may occur every $4.5–5 \times 10^{5}$ bases. Establishing an assay for a large number of samples derived from a precious and limited stock leads to a recommendation that all samples be assayed in triplicate to guard against the very rare, albeit possible, early cycle copy error. Early cycle copy error would establish a different amplicon template for all subsequent cycles. This rare event would be extremely unlikely in more than one replicate. Late cycle errors would not affect the outcome in this assay due to dilution effects. Triplicate samples further validate unique observations through their distinctive profile. In our very large study, a few samples had individual replicate failures with the remaining duplicates matching a predicted profile and Sanger sequence validated unique profiles that were observed as triplicate outcomes [7].

6. Spiking an Assay: An assay that demonstrates close homozygous state PTms can benefit from spiking. A spiked assay has a small amount of the hotter melt target added to all samples in the master mix. Samples with the homozygous hot allele genotype are unchanged by the addition of the same target.

Heterozygous genotype samples are identified by distinctive peak shapes rather than PTm. Heterozygous genotype samples in spiked assays will retain a broad lower peak fluorescence bumpy profile. Heterozygous spiked amplicon pairs will be approximately 36 % HTS-HBS, 24 % HTS-CBS and 24 % CTS-HBS and 16 % CTS-CBS instead of the 25 %, each possible pairing due to the addition of hot amplicon spike. The colder PTm homozygous genotype samples are destabilized to a slightly colder PTm and slightly shorter and broader profile by the low concentration of amplicons from the spike. The spike template concentration is kept small enough that the cold melt samples are not converted to a HTZ-like outcome as the majority of amplicons (~64 %) remain CTS-CBS. *See* Figs. 2 and 3 to contrast the relative presence of the four amplicons in a cold melt spiked sample versus a heterozygous sample.

3.2 Sample Analysis

1. Set up a work space including waste receptacle. Make a small temporary desktop biohazard waste receptacle to make waste collection easier. Wear appropriate PPE for BSL1 work. Have reserve disposable products available. Use as much automation as possible for all pipetting steps. Open fresh boxes of pipet tips and have extras available. Set out 96-well plates for the triplicate replica plates for each SNP to be pipetted. Cover plates except while they are being used. Prepare any equipment that is not stored ready to use such as the LED loading guide and reserve instrument time on the thermal cycler if applicable.
2. Prepare master mix for the SNP(s) to be pipetted. Thoroughly mix master reagents in a low retention disposable container. A 384-well plate with 15 μl per well will require ~6 ml of master mix depending upon pipetting error. Wrap the master mix container in foil to protect it from light. Maintain the master mix in an ice bucket.
3. Defrost gDNA samples, vortex briefly, and centrifuge the sample tubes or multi well plate to drive samples to the bottom of the wells. Use an automated pipet programmed for a dilution protocol to pick up a volume adequate for the triplicate master mix plus pipetting error and loss, i.e., 3.2× master mix then 3.2× DNA from the 96-well plate of gDNA samples. The pipetting step for many automated pipets would be: pick up clean tip, pick up master mix, add air barrier, pick up gDNA, dispense into triplicate replica plate, and discard pipet tip in biohazard waste container. Dispense, with pipet mixing if available, into the same location in a second 96-well plate. Repeat until all samples have master mix added and are in Triplicate Replica Plate (Fig. 5).

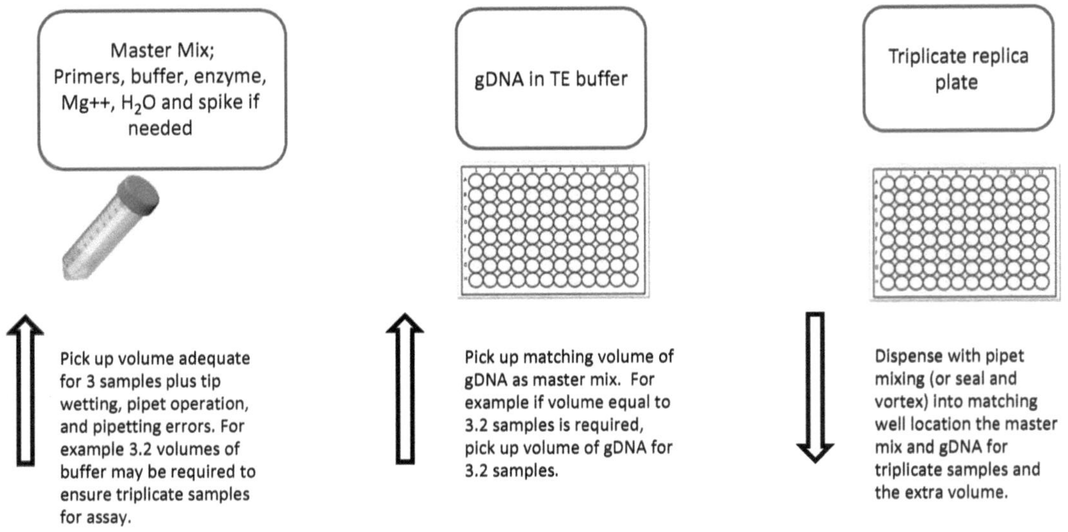

Fig. 5 Work Flow to Create the Triplicate Replica Plate. Master mix is dilution pipetted with each gDNA sample into the same location on a triplicate replica plate. Dilution pipetting allows two solutions of unequal volumes to be aspirated serially and dispensed into a single final location. With dilution pipetting the Master Mix must be pipetted first to eliminate contamination of the master mix with gDNA

4. Cover both plates with foil. Return the DNA plate to storage or refrigerate if setting up more than one assay in this thawing. Pipet mix while dispensing or seal and vortex the triplicate replica plate. Centrifuge the triplicate replica plate for 5 min in a plate spinner to consolidate the template and master mix in each well.
5. Set up the loading guide with a fresh 384-well white plate. Turn the guide on to advance in triplicates, left to right, top to bottom. Rotate the triplicate replica plate with master mix and DNA quarter (¼) turn clockwise. The samples in the 96-well plate will become the triplicates in the 384-well plate following the pattern shown in Fig. 6. A 96-well plate turned ¼ clockwise will match in triplicate a 384-well plate.
6. Set an automatic pipet to dispense the HRM assay volume (i.e., 15 μl) three times. Open a fresh box of 96 pipet tips and orient it the same pattern as the 96-well triplicate replica plate. Open the foil on the triplicate replica plate. Take up a new pipet tip, pick up the sample and if the pipet program requires, discard first pipet action back into the pick up well. Dispense into the triplicate location of the 384-well plate working top to bottom and left to right matching the clean pipet tip used with the same location in the triplicate replica plate. Advance the LED display each sample. If you use the tip that matches the location on the 96-well plate it will decrease pipetting confu-

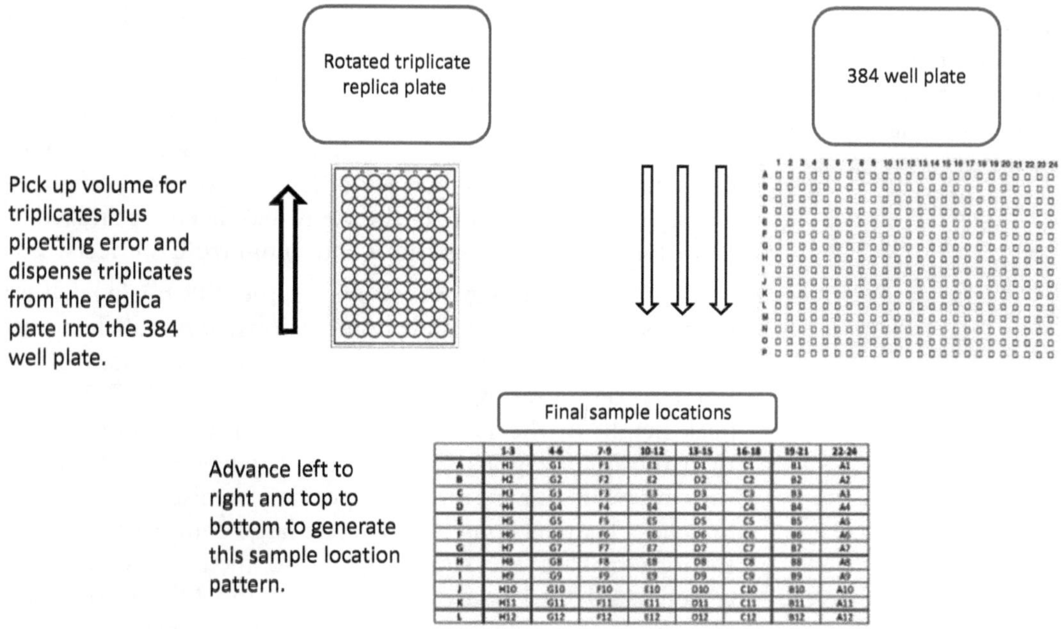

	1-3	4-6	7-9	10-12	13-15	16-18	19-21	22-24
A	H1	G1	F1	E1	D1	C1	B1	A1
B	H2	G2	F2	E2	D2	C2	B2	A2
C	H3	G3	F3	E3	D3	C3	B3	A3
D	H4	G4	F4	E4	D4	C4	B4	A4
E	H5	G5	F5	E5	D5	C5	B5	A5
F	H6	G6	F6	E6	D6	C6	B6	A6
G	H7	G7	F7	E7	D7	C7	B7	A7
H	H8	G8	F8	E8	D8	C8	B8	A8
I	H9	G9	F9	E9	D9	C9	B9	A9
J	H10	G10	F10	E10	D10	C10	B10	A10
K	H11	G11	F11	E11	D11	C11	B11	A11
L	H12	G12	F12	E12	D12	C12	B12	A12

Fig. 6 Work Flow to Create the 384-Well Assay Plate. The replica plate contains master mix and a single gDNA per well. Each well contains enough solution to be drawn up and repeat dispensed into triplicates in the 384-well assay plate. The replica plate is turned 90° clockwise to make the dimensions of the 96-well plate and 384-well plate identical when the samples are dispensed as triplicates

sion and errors. Multiple LED guides can be used to keep progress through the plates obvious. Some LED guides also have locations for two plates.

7. Continue until all samples have been pipetted. Add a sample of each of the homozygous controls for the SNP (*see* **Note 13**).
8. Seal the 384-well plate by separating the foil from its release liner and placing the foil on the top of the wells. Place the release liner on the top of the foil to protect the foil. Gently smooth air bubbles out of the foil using a straight edge object (*see* **Note 15**).
9. Being careful not to damage or get contamination on the foil or bottom of the plate, centrifuge the plate for 5 min to remove any air bubbles in the wells. Scratches in the foil, dirt particle, fingerprints, or air bubbles will disrupt light transfer through the plate and sample and reduce accuracy of the assay.
10. A usual assay is primer annealed by touchdown from 62 to 55 °C at 0.5° increments for a total of 55 cycles of anneal and 94 °C melt.
11. Data is acquired for 25 data points per degree melt after final complete melt at 94 °C, rapid cooling and complete melting from 70 to 90 °C.

3.3 Peak Tm and Peak Width Interpretation and Data Recording

1. Each SNP will have its own distinctive pattern, especially for the heterozygote. The strand swap of a G/C location creates a large conformational distortion to the mismatched amplicon pairs and a very wide profile results as shown in Fig. 3 where melting occurs over a 5 °C range. The two homozygous samples demonstrate that efficiency differences do not complicate genotype determination if the assay has been optimized to allow for intersample variations and minimize CA effects.
2. In the 96 triplicate samples in Fig. 2, the 288 tracings clearly demonstrate the major allele homozygous, minor allele homozygous, and HTZ genotypes. The PTm differences of the homozygous states are obvious, as is the shape of the HTZ. The peak height of the HTZ sample is much lower and broader than the homozygous sample. The shape of HTZ PTm will vary by SNP due to the site-specific chemistry at the mismatches. Transversions will generate large conformational distortions making the strands easier to melt. This assay was spiked at 20 % to assure that the MJA and MIA were clearly separated. It is obvious that the MIA population PTm is slightly lowered and broadened by the spike but retains a homozygous profile due to the predominance of the CTS-CBS amplicon. The melt initiation portion of the homozygous profiles is well separated due to the spike. The relative temperature relationship of the homozygous state is based on amplicon melt chemistry, not gene prevalence. Presence or prevalence of the MJA and MIA in any sample set can't be assumed. The area under the curve represents the quantity of amplicon and is approximately equal in all three genotypes. It is also obvious that the inter-sample variation of efficiency results in minor differences in PTm height. Inter-sample variations in CAI products result in slight variation in melt temperature. These effects are not significant to make genotype assignment ambiguous. Primer pair self-amplification, so-called primer dimers are much shorter amplicons. Samples without targets, i.e., negative control samples, demonstrate low temperature and low quantity melt profiles seen in the green tracings. Some SNPs will be more affected by carry over salts in the gDNA sample and the melt temperature of the gDNA samples will vary slightly from the melt temperatures of the control samples. The Mg^{2+} provided in the HRM supplies kit can be added to the synthetic template to adjust the melt temperature of the control sample (*see* **Note 16**).
3. As shown in Fig. 2, all wells can be visualized at once. The researcher must refer to their specific machine options to visualize wells in groups or singly to determine the well identity and match it with outcome conformity. This software is not

capable of SNP classification based on melt temperature and peak shape [5]. The software automatically scales the Y-axis to the highest efficiency outcomes. Visual inspection of the melting curves reveals three obvious profiles.

4. Placing the mouse over the melt profile tracings allows the operator to determine which well correlates with the tracing. Using the mouse select individual samples, a complete row or column or multiples of these to visualize and interrogate. It is easy to remove and replace the tracing from the display by selecting or deselecting the well in the upper left array. It is often easier to classify and record the outcomes with less than the entire sample set displayed. Displaying fewer samples at a time will allow lower efficiency samples to be evaluated. Remember, the PTm and peak melt shape are not affected by efficiency of amplification.
5. Use the layout generated by rotating the triplicate replica plate to create a data recording master sheet to mark the outcomes of each assay. Complete the data sheet and retain copies. A repeat reading can be done by a second operator or switching up the order of selecting the profiles to record.
6. We used the following method to assign genotype based on profile: (a) From the displayed profiles select a single genotype profile, identify the members of that tracing group by mousing over the profile, deselect these tracings from the displayed wells (if a tracing is misidentified, it can be adjusted by reselecting or deselecting as necessary), using the displayed wells panel record on the data sheet, which wells conformed to the first profile; (b) Return to the displayed profiles and select one of the two remaining profiles, identify the members of tracing groups as before (this should result in a single profile remaining); (c) Record the remaining wells as the third profile; (d) The data sheet will be filled for two profiles, the remaining profile is composed of the empty cells on the data sheet. All wells can be deselected and the profile can be verified by reselecting the wells. This method can be used for the whole plate or a subset of the plate. Any well can be selected or deselected multiple times.
7. The synthetic controls can be selected or deselected for comparison to the samples. Low efficiency samples can be evaluated without "wash out" of a Y-axis that is inappropriate to the sample by displaying them separately instead of in the presence of high efficiency reactions (*see* **Note 17**). The synthetic target confirms a sample as a low frequency allele or indicates further investigation such as Sanger sequencing should be completed to determine a novel finding.

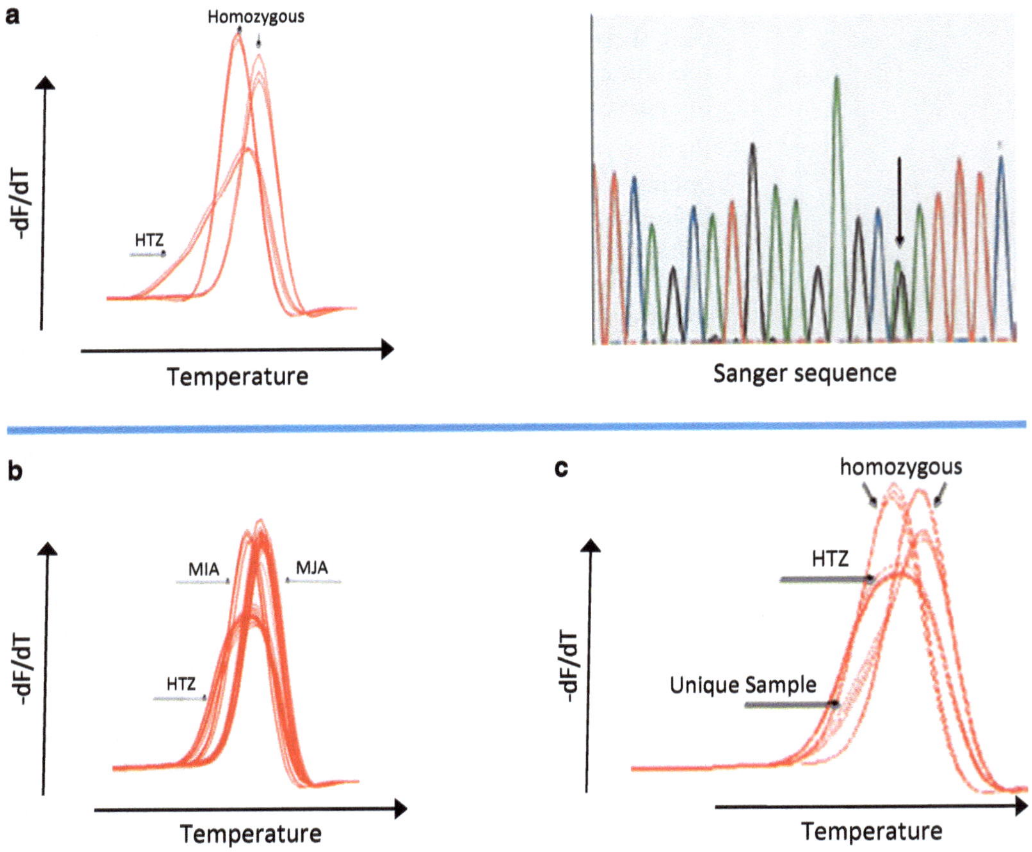

Fig. 7 Heterozygote Detection and Unique Outcome Identification. (**a**) The detection of heterozygotes is highly obvious with this assay. The distinctive wide peak of the heterozygote was verified by Sanger sequencing, the "gold standard" of sequence identity, shown in the upper right. The software generated sequence report for the Sanger reaction did not identify the heterozygous location. Technical interpretation of the HRM profile is faster, easier, and less ambiguous than reviewing Sanger data. (**b**) A low frequency MIA for this SNP is shown in triplicate tracings that coincide with the synthetic target control. Validation with a synthetic target and inclusion of the synthetic target on each assay plate is necessary to confirm assay function and genotype status. (**c**) The triplicate tracings of this single sample demonstrate a profile that does not match the three expected profiles for this SNP. This sample was subjected to amplification with the larger amplicon producing primer pair and the amplicon was sequenced revealing a unique genotype

8. Figure 7 illustrates the advantages and utility of this assay. The PTm of the homozygous cases and the profile of the HTZ cases are specific to each optimized SNP assay. Any sequence change within the amplicon will affect the profiles making this assay excellent at detecting very rare and unpredicted events. Unlike probe based methods that can only identify outcomes for which the investigator designs the query probes, this assay sorts the outcomes to the three predicted classes and identifies samples of further investigation saving resources and time. Figure 7, panel A demonstrates the simplicity of differentia-

tion of the three genotypes. While Sanger sequencing can be used to differentiate homozygous states it cannot determine HTZ status. The HTZ is marked with arrows in the melt profiles and the Sanger sequence reaction validation study. The Sanger data had to be interpreted to identify the HTZ site. Panel B demonstrates the need for the synthetic template as a validation of the MIA, especially when this is a rare event. The assay must demonstrate differentiation before samples are tested. Panel C is triplicate tracings of samples that conform to the expected genotypes and a single sample's triplicate tracings that does not conform. The primer pair for the large amplicon was used in standard PCR reaction (Expand HIFi Roche) and cleaned by PCR cleanup (Qiagen), quantified by spectrophotometry, and submitted for sequencing with each of the amplification primers following core facility instructions. Sanger sequencing confirmed a novel change within the amplicon target.

4 Notes

1. Purified gDNA will carry with it artifacts of the purification process and source material, contamination artifacts (CA). Contamination artifact interference (CAI) can affect either the amplification efficiency or the melt temperature. Amplification inhibition will result in a decreased quantity of amplicon. Since yield is not an outcome measure for this assay, decreased efficiency is not critical. However greatly reduced efficiency must be addressed. Salt concentrations affect amplicon melt temperatures and some targets are more sensitive to the presence of salts than others. The relationship of hotter and colder melt curve will not be affected but the PTm can be shifted by the presence of salts for some amplicons. Reducing the quantity of template used will also reduce the concentration of salt and CA in the reaction. The synthetic templates will have very low salt concentrations compared to purified gDNA samples. The synthetic template can also be evaluated with addition of Mg^{2+} commonly supplied in PCR kits. Synthetic template with added Mg^{2+} may have PTm that is a closer match to the gDNA. All control samples need to have equal quantities of Mg^{2+}.
2. SNPs which are triallellic [15] or SNPs where primers cannot be designed to place the in SNP site within an amplicon of ~100 bp can be evaluated with hydrolysis probes or by HRM through asymmetric PCR and the melting domain of an unlabeled extension blocked oligonucleotides [5]. Sequence spe-

cific probes with different fluorescent output wavelength can be synthesized and used with minor adaptions to this protocol. A probe is designed and labeled for each expected sequence. Switching to a probe-based assay is more expensive, more difficult, all probes must be used to accurately evaluate for HTZ samples and the assay is unable to detect any sequence for which the probes are not designed.

3. In our work with hundreds of samples we did identify a very small number of novel genotype sequences. These presented as unique melt patterns that did not match the three expected profiles. We amplified a longer segment of the same area of gDNA and a novel sequence was identified by Sanger sequencing. The profile that does not conform should be investigated further. Also, samples that do not create an amplicon for a single SNP but do create amplicons for other SNPs should be investigated for novel changes in the 3' primer locations. Amplify these templates with the longer amplicon primers and sequence to investigate primer site changes.
4. A study of the amplification of serial diluted gDNA and the synthetic control allows the user to select a starting concentration that generates a linear response, can relate the functional concentration of the gDNA to the synthetic template, and guards against the use of too much template. Amplification depends upon the physical accessibility of the gDNA to the primers and the polymerase. Inclusion of excess gDNA can blunt amplification as the reaction is saturated with the large molecules. Amplification efficiency and PTm can be affected by impurities that are carried along in the sample purification process. Additionally, the dye will not distinguish among double-stranded DNAs. Excess gDNA or synthetic template will take up dye, may produce confusing melt profiles, and generally decreases assay efficiency and data clarity.
5. LED back-lighted plate loading guide (LiteOne) was used to reduce confusion during pipetting. The guide can be programed to back light the next samples to load and advance through pushing a button or stepping on a pedal. The LED light travels easily through the plate plastic but the wavelength does not react with the assay dye. If such a device is unavailable it will be helpful to arrange a system to remind the user of their plate location. Tape, colored threads, markings on the plate, moving a temporary cover should be devised to reduce the human error potential at this step.
6. Testing the primers against the synthetic amplicons will suggest which pairs of primers can generate amplicons that have a length and SNP placement that allows melting profile differentiation. Commercial gDNA is used for testing the primer pair

for reproducibility and off site binding. Analysis of primer sequence with alignment tools will also predict off target binding issues and guide the user to increasing specificity through elongation of the primer or making minor placement adjustments. The best analysis is evaluation of primer function against gDNA. A touchdown protocol should be used to further guard against off site binding.

7. Control sample gDNA is necessary to validate the selected primer pair on DNA with the same purification and storage artifacts. This is a measurement of the effects of carry over components from the purification process. There is likely no way to obtain samples that will represent both homozygous states and the HTZ state when testing this. Samples that show homozygous characteristics can be mixed with the opposite homozygous synthetic template to preview heterozygous profile in an extracted gDNA environment.
8. SNP target sequence, especially for the MIA, may be very rare or not present in the sample set. Validation that the assay can differentiate the alleles needs to be made before samples are considered. Investigations designed to identify a rare event must be established with proof that discovery will be made if the rare event occurs. The synthetic template must always be shown to separate the MJA and the MIA before sample analysis starts.
9. SNP flanking sequence must be evaluated for primer placement. Accurate, robust primer binding requires that the area be free of repetitive sequence that would allow printer stutter and be unique in the genomic sample to avoid off site binding.
10. Primers must not have a SNP at the 3' location. Samples that do not generate amplicons for a single pair of primers should be investigated for a primer 3' MIA. MIA sequences within the primer generally do not affect the assay as the ends of the amplicon become primer or primer complement during amplification cycles. As in all situations of trying to find a rare event a single nucleotide change in short amplicons are more obvious than in a longer amplicon. For example, single events in a population of 100 are more profound than a single event in 500. Limiting the amplicon length to about 100 bp produces a double stranded DNA melt profile temperature range that is distinct from possible alternates. Primer dimers, usually about 50 bp, the synthetic template at 500 to 1000 bp or genomic DNA will have PTm that do not overlap the 100 bp amplicon. Highly damaged gDNA can contain 100 bp fragments and must not be analyzed.
11. A gradient PCR reaction can be performed using a standard PCR kit such as Expand HiFi (Roche) to establish the annealing

temperature. In general, a touchdown primer annealing protocol is a superior choice to limit off target priming and accommodate minor intersample binding temperature differences.

12. Product inserts and instruction sheets usually describe a 20 μl assay. In our system this volume makes the wells overfull and there was sample-to-sample contamination when applying the sealing foil to the overfull wells. Evaluation of performance with lesser volumes demonstrated the assay to be accurate at a much lower volume and we chose a 15 μl reaction to eliminate the contamination issue and reduce cost.

13. Make dilutions of the synthetic templates and use Cq to determine the functional concentration of the synthetic templates compared to their matched gDNA target. Make stock of each synthetic template at a concentration that matches the amplification efficiency of the control samples. Include the Cq match sample on each SNP assay plate. Dilute the hotter melt synthetic target to 20 % concentration and reserve for possible spike. Very small quantities of synthetic target will provide huge quantities of control and spike. Be sure to use caution not to contaminate the laboratory with this very high concentration source. If possible, prepare the synthetic template stock in a separate area from that of the assays such as a colleague's laboratory. Remove all PPE and dispose BSL1 waste away from the assay space following all relevant waste disposal rules.

14. Nearly equal homozygous melt temperatures can be separated by destabilizing the colder melting profile. This is accomplished by "spiking" the assay with a very small amount of the hotter melt synthetic template. A PTm presents the purity of amplicon produced as the shape of the curve and the quantity of amplicon produced as the area under the curve. Close inspection of the cold melt amplicon profile with a hot melt amplicon spike will show a slight broadening and shortening of the peak shape accompany the slight shift to colder PTm while it retains the normal overall appearance. The broadening reflects the earlier melting of the heterozygous amplicons. However, PCR efficiency is unaffected, the area under the curve remains unchanged, and the broader peak is shortened (*see* Fig. 2).

15. It is important to protect the plate and foil from scratches and dirt particles to get the maximum reproducible light transmission in every well. Do not rub the foil to the plate excessively as you can scratch it. The foil is often a static cling and not an adhesive. The foil will adhere by heat in the thermal cycler. Our protocol to protect the foil from scratches is to separate the release liner from the foil, place the foil on the assay plate, place the release liner on top of the foil on the plate, and smooth the foil gently with a wide blunt straight edge working from center to edge.

16. In SNP target assays that are sensitive to the salt concentration, the "salty" gDNA samples may show a different pair of PTms than the nearly "salt free" synthetic templates. A titration curve adding Mg^{2+} to the homozygous synthetic template reactions can be created to align the PTms.
17. No amplification may also be caused by polymorphisms, which occur in the location of one of the primers. In cases where there is no amplicon produced this should be considered and the longer amplicons should be processed and evaluated by sequencing.

References

1. Levy S, Sutton G, Ng PC, Feuk L, Halpern AL, Walenz BP, Axelrod N, Huang J, Kirkness EF, Denisov G, Lin Y, MacDonald JR, Pang AW, Shago M, Stockwell TB, Tsiamouri A, Bafna V, Bansal V, Kravitz SA, Busam DA, Beeson KY, McIntosh TC, Remington KA, Abril JF, Gill J, Borman J, Rogers YH, Frazier ME, Scherer SW, Strausberg RL, Venter JC (2007) The diploid genome sequence of an individual human. PLoS Biol 5:e254
2. Liew M, Pryor R, Palais R, Meadows C, Erali M, Lyon E, Wittwer C (2004) Genotyping of single nucleotide polymorphisms by high-resolution melting of small amplicons. Clin Chem 50:1156–1164
3. Er T-K, Chang JG (2012) Invited critical review: high resolution melting: applications in genetic disorders. Clin Chim Acta 414:197–220
4. Wittwer CT, Reed GH, Gundry CN, Vandersteen JG, Pryor RJ (2003) High-resolution genotyping by amplicon melting analysis using LCGreen. Clin Chem 49: 853–860
5. Lin CW, Er TK, Tsai FJ, Liu TC, Shin PY, Chang JG (2010) Development of a high resolution melting method for the screening of Wilson disease related ATP7B gene mutations. Clin Chim Acta 411:1223–1231
6. Wilkening S, Bader A (2004) Quantitative real-time polymerase chain reaction: methodical analysis and mathematical model. J Biomol Tech 15:107–111
7. Bruzzone CM, Tawadros PS, Boardman LS, Steer CJ (2013) Enhanced primer selection and synthetic amplicon templates optimize high-resolution melting analysis of single-nucleotide polymorphisms in a large population. Genet Test Mol Biomark 17:675–680
8. Bustin SA, Benes V, Garson JA, Hellemans J, Huggett J, Kubista M, Mueller R, Nolan T, Pfaffl MW, Shipley GL, Vandesompele J, Wittwer CT (2009) The MIQE guidelines: minimum information for publication of quantitative real-time PCR experiments. Clin Chem 55:611–622
9. Rosenfeld JA, Malhotra AK, Lencz T (2010) Novel multi-nucleotide polymorphisms in the human genome characterized by whole genome and exome sequencing. Nucleic Acids Res 38:6102–6111
10. Schmittgen TD, Zakrajsek BA, Mills AG, Gorn V, Singer MJ, Reed MW (2000) Quantitative reverse transcription-polymerase chain reaction to study mRNA decay: comparison of endpoint and real-time methods. Anal Biochem 285:194–204
11. Rajeevan MS, Vernon SD, Taysavang N, Unger ER (2001) Validation of array-based gene expression profiles by real-time (kinetic) RT-PCR. J Mol Diagn 3:26–31
12. Kontanis EJ, Reed FA (2006) Evaluation of real-time PCR amplification efficiencies to detect PCR inhibitors. J Forensic Sci 51: 795–804
13. de Juan I, Esteban E, Palanca S, Barragán E, Bolufer P (2009) High-resolution melting analysis of rapid screening of BRCA1 and BRCA2 Spanish mutations. Breast Cancer Res Treat 115:405–414
14. Evrard A, Rayna C, Boyer J-C, Le Gallic L, Lumbroso S (2007) Mutation scanning of the cytidine deaminase gene by high-resolution melting curve analysis using the Lightcycler® 480 System. Biochemica 3:13–14
15. Swen JJ, Baak-Pablo RF, Guchelaar HJ, van der Straaten T (2011) Alternative methods to a TaqMan assay to detect a tri-allelic single nucleotide polymorphism rs757210 in the HNF1β gene. Clin Chem Lab Med 50: 279–284

Chapter 3

High-Speed Droplet-Allele-Specific Polymerase Chain Reaction for Genotyping of Single Nucleotide Polymorphisms

Kazuyuki Matsuda and Takayuki Honda

Abstract

Single nucleotide alternations such as single nucleotide polymorphisms (SNPs) or single nucleotide mutations are useful genetic markers for molecular diagnosis, prognosis, drug response, and predisposition to diseases. Rapid identification of SNPs or mutations is clinically important, especially for determining drug responses and selection of molecular-targeted therapy. Here, we describe a rapid genotyping assay based on the allele-specific polymerase chain reaction (AS-PCR) by using our droplet-PCR machine (droplet-AS-PCR).

Key words Single nucleotide polymorphism, Single nucleotide mutation, Droplet-allele-specific PCR, Drug response, Molecular-targeted therapy

1 Introduction

Single nucleotide alternations (SNPs) are useful genetic markers for investigating interindividual differences in drug responses and predisposition to diseases [1–5]. Such genetic diagnoses should contribute to personalized therapy for selecting drugs and treatment regimens. In pharmacogenomics, SNPs such as CYP2C9 and VKORC1 greatly influence the effective warfarin maintenance dose [1, 2]. Warfarin therapy is typically commenced soon after the diagnosis of a disease is made, which exemplifies the need for rapid genotyping of SNPs relevant to pharmacogenomics. We have developed a droplet-PCR protocol for detection of influenza virus and a chimeric gene associated with leukemia by using a novel PCR machine (SEIKO EPSON, Nagano, Japan) with better thermal conductivity than conventional PCR machines, thus enabling rapid PCR amplification [6, 7]. Our droplet-PCR method is performed in a droplet of 1 μL in a reaction tube [6, 7]. The effect of partitioning the template DNA is limited, and only one droplet is used in the reaction. Therefore, the detection limit of our droplet

Peter Bugert (ed.), *Molecular Typing of Blood Cell Antigens*, Methods in Molecular Biology, vol. 1310,
DOI 10.1007/978-1-4939-2690-9_3, © Springer Science+Business Media New York 2015

PCR is lower than that of digital-droplet PCR. Our novel droplet-AS-PCR protocol also has a markedly reduced analysis time and is less labor-intensive. We subsequently applied our novel high-speed droplet-PCR machine technology for rapid SNP genotyping, in which genotypes were determined within 9 min while retaining specificity and sensitivity [8]. The total assay time of our droplet-PCR assay was further reduced when buccal cells (not subjected to DNA extraction) were used as specimens [8].

2 Materials

1. Droplet-PCR machine: The droplet-PCR machine (SEIKO EPSON, Nagano, Japan) has two connected heater blocks that regulate the temperature of each end of the reaction tube (Fig. 1) [6]. The reaction temperature of the two heater blocks is controlled consistently during denaturation and annealing/extension. To perform a rapid temperature transition, the reaction tube is filled with silicone oil, allowing the droplet of the PCR mixture to move easily in the tube during the mechanical rotation of the machine with the two connected heater blocks. Once the droplet is transferred from one end to another by gravity, the machine with the two heater blocks inverts to

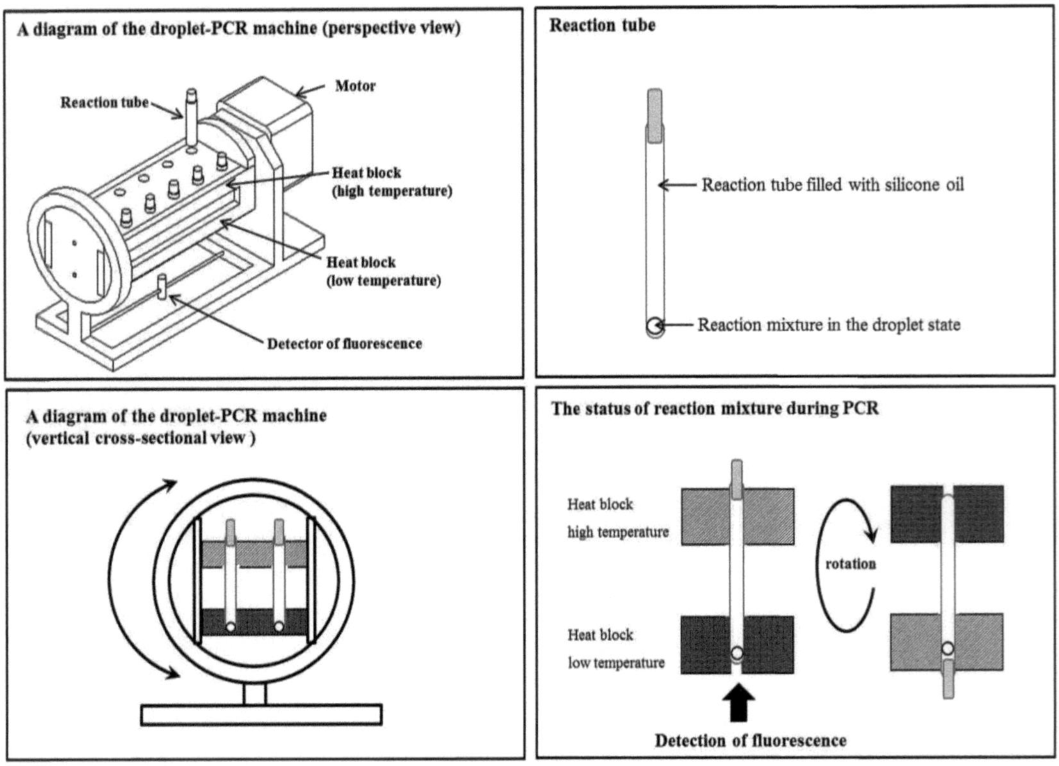

Fig. 1 Diagram of the droplet-PCR machine (*reproduced from* [8])

return the droplet. The PCR mixture in the droplet state is able to perform shuttle PCR in the reaction tube. The droplet-PCR machine includes a fluorescence detector that allows monitoring of the amount of PCR products after each extension step.

2. AS-PCR mixture components: The AS-PCR mixture included genomic DNA, Platinum Taq DNA polymerase (Life Technologies, Grand Island, NY), sense/antisense primers (*see* **Note 1**), TaqMan probe, and reaction buffer composed of Tris–HCl, KCl, and $MgCl_2$.

3 Methods

3.1 Preparation of AS-PCR Mixture

1. Add the following components to a sterile microcentrifuge tube on ice (final volume, 10 μL): 1 μL genomic DNA (up to 50 ng/μL) (*see* **Note 2**), 0.2 μL Platinum Taq DNA polymerase (5 U/μL), 0.8 μL sense primer (10 μM; final concentration: 0.8 μM), 0.8 μL antisense primer (10 μM; final concentration: 0.8 μM), 0.3 μL TaqMan probe (10 μM; final concentration: 0.3 μM), 1.25 μL dNTP (2 mM; final concentration: 250 μM), 2 μL 5× reaction buffer (*see* **Note 3**), 3.65 μL sterilized distilled water.
2. Mix gently and centrifuge briefly.

3.2 Droplet-AS-PCR

1. Add 1 μL of the AS-PCR mixture to a sterile PCR tube filled with silicone oil without introducing air bubbles (*see* **Note 4**). Confirm that the reaction mixture is in the droplet state (Fig. 1).
2. Insert the tube plug without introducing air bubbles (*see* **Note 4**).
3. Wipe the silicone oil off of the bottom wall surface of the reaction tube (*see* **Note 5**).
4. Place the reaction tube containing the AS-PCR mixture in the heating block of the droplet-PCR machine.
5. Perform droplet-AS-PCR with the following cycle profile: 95 °C for 10 s and 35 cycles at 95 °C for 4 s and 58–66 °C for 8 s (*see* **Note 6**).
6. Assess the amplification and identify the SNP type (Fig. 2) (*see* **Note 7**).

4 Notes

1. The design of the sense or antisense primers specific for the SNP genotype is important for AS-PCR amplification. Based on the amplification refractory mutation system (ARMS) [9], we found that insertion of nucleotides mismatched to the

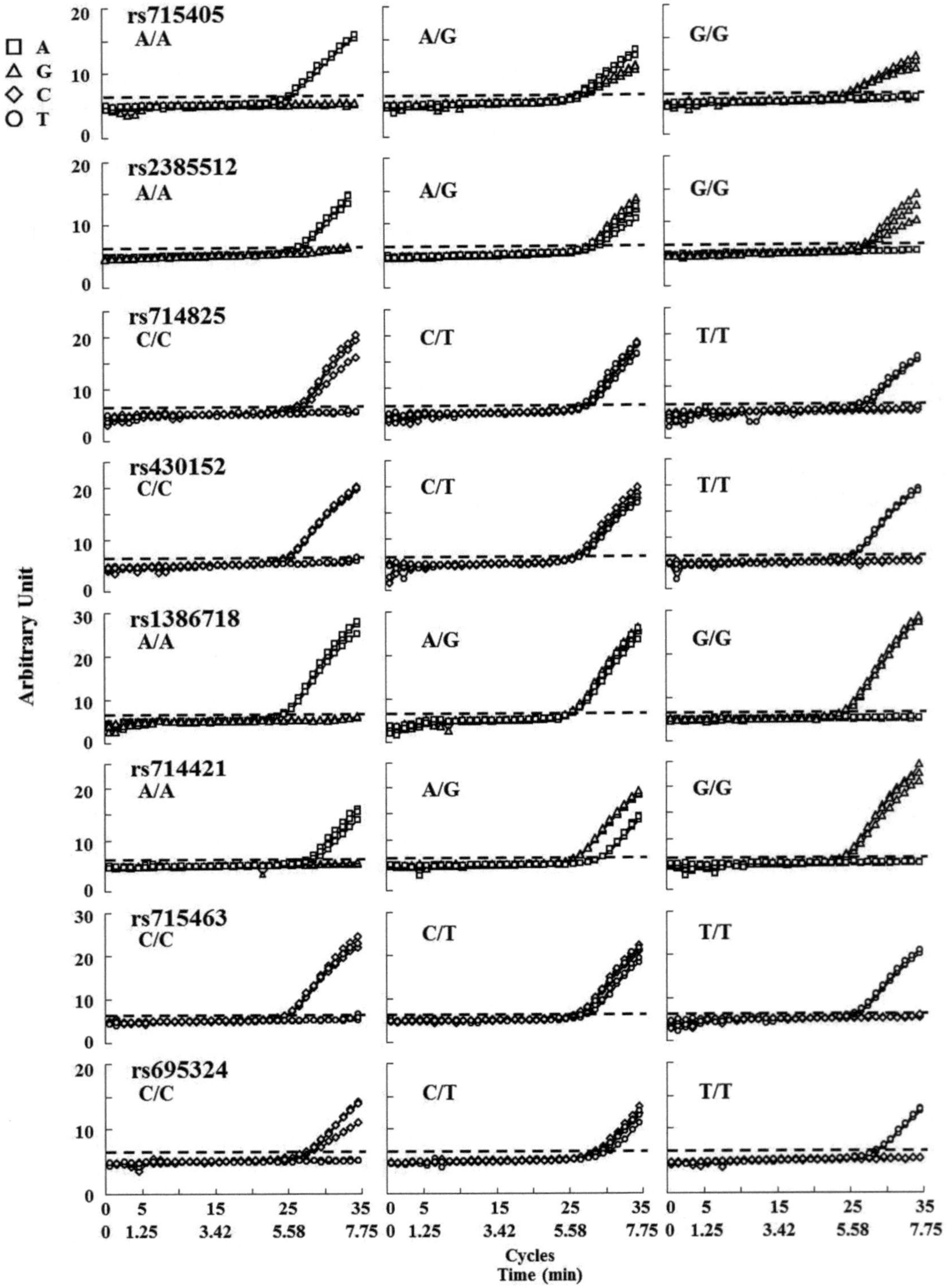

Fig. 2 Reactivity of the droplet-AS-PCR using genomic DNA extracted from PB. Amplification plots for eight SNP loci (rs715405, rs2385512, rs714825, rs430152, rs1386718, rs714421, rs715463, and rs695324) are shown. Genomic DNA homozygotic and heterozygotic at each of the eight SNP loci was used for evaluating amplification (AA/AG/GG for rs715405, rs2385512, rs1386718, and rs714421; CC/CT/TT for rs714825, rs430152, rs715463, and rs695324). *X*-axes indicate the cycles and time of PCR; *Y*-axes indicate the fluorescence level (arbitrary unit). We set the arbitrary standard for the fluorescence level at 6.7 (*dotted lines*) for evaluating amplification; amplification was considered positive when a fluorescence level over 6.7 was detected at two consecutive assay points (*reproduced from* [8])

template (base-pair mismatch) and modification with locked nucleic acids are effective for AS-PCR amplification [10–13]. However, we have not determined consistent types and positions for the base-pair mismatches and modified nucleotides, thus leaving room for experimentation. In our recent report on rapid identification of SNPs using droplet-AS-PCR, we designed AS primers that included an SNP-matched nucleotide at the 3′-end and a template-mismatched nucleotide at the -2 position from the 3′-end [8].

2. Genomic DNA extracted from peripheral blood using various extraction kits available from manufacturers can be used for SNP genotyping by using a droplet-PCR machine. For more rapid SNP genotyping, buccal cells can be used for analysis [8]. The buccal cells are treated with 20 mg/mL proteinase K in lysis buffer (50 mM Tris–HCl, pH 8.5, 100 mM NaCl, 1 mM EDTA, 0.5 % Tween-20, 0.5 % Nonidet-P40, and 20 mM dithiothreitol) at 50 °C for 1 min and then denatured at 95 °C for 1 min to inactivate proteinase K. The pretreated buccal samples without DNA extraction can be directly subjected to droplet-AS-PCR for SNP genotyping (Fig. 3).
3. The 5× reaction buffer is composed of Tris–HCl pH 9.0 (10–100 mM), KCl (0–80 mM), and $MgCl_2$ (1.5–10 mM). The concentration of Tris–HCl, KCl, and $MgCl_2$ has to be adjusted empirically.
4. The bubble introduced in the reaction tube prevents the droplet of the PCR mixture from moving smoothly between the high-temperature heat block and the low-temperature block. Care should be taken to avoid bubble formation when adding the PCR mixture to the reaction tube.
5. When inserting the tube plug, silicone oil escapes from the reaction tube. Silicone oil adhering to the bottom wall surface of the reaction tube prevents detection of fluorescence signals.
6. The temperature at the annealing and extension steps is target sequence- and primer-dependent. The cycle conditions have to be adjusted empirically.
7. The droplet-PCR machine includes a fluorescence detector that allows monitoring of the amount of PCR products after each extension step. Using samples for which the SNP types were predetermined by direct sequencing, we set an arbitrary standard for assessing positive amplification when the fluorescence level obtained from the positive samples was over three standard deviations above the mean value for negative samples with an alternative SNP type [8]. Setting a standard in this manner enables us to assess the amplification and identify the SNP genotype before all of the PCR cycles are completed.

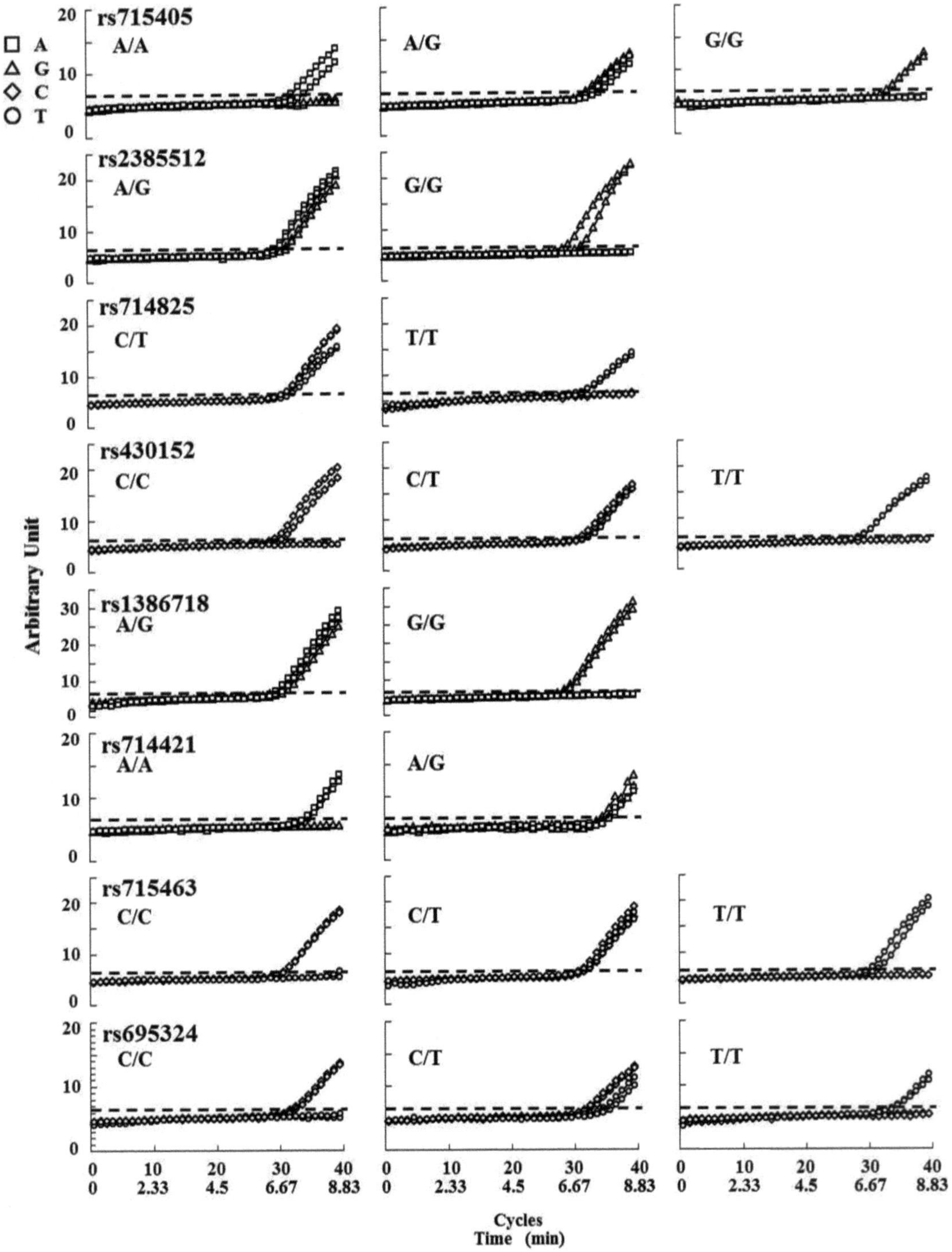

Fig. 3 Reactivity of droplet-AS-PCR using buccal cells without DNA extraction. Buccal cells were treated with proteinase K at 50 °C for 1 min, denatured at 95 °C for 1 min to inactivate the proteinase K, and then directly subjected to the droplet-AS-PCR assay without the DNA extraction step. Representative amplification plots for eight SNP loci (rs715405, rs2385512, rs714825, rs430152, rs1386718, rs714421, rs715463, and rs695324) are shown. The genotypes at the eight SNP loci were determined within 9 min when the fluorescence level of the amplification was over 6.7 at two consecutive assay points (*dotted lines*), as depicted in each figure (*reproduced from* [8])

References

1. Aomori T, Yamamoto K, Oguchi-Katayama A, Kawai Y, Ishidao T, Mitani Y, Kogo Y, Lezhava A, Fujita Y, Obayashi K, Nakamura K, Kohnke H, Wadelius M, Ekström L, Skogastierna C, Rane A, Kurabayashi M, Murakami M, Cizdziel PE, Hayashizaki Y, Horiuchi R (2009) Rapid single-nucleotide polymorphism detection of cytochrome P450 (CYP2C9) and vitamin K epoxide reductase (VKORC1) genes for the warfarin dose adjustment by the SMart-amplification process version 2. Clin Chem 55: 804–812
2. Yin T, Miyata T (2007) Warfarin dose and the pharmacogenomics of CYP2C9 and VKORC1: rationale and perspectives. Thromb Res 120:1–10
3. Oguro R, Kamide K, Katsuya T, Akasaka H, Sugimoto K, Congrains A, Arai Y, Hirose N, Saitoh S, Ohishi M, Miura T, Rakugi H (2012) A single nucleotide polymorphism of the adenosine deaminase, RNA-specific gene is associated with the serum triglyceride level, abdominal circumference, and serum adiponectin concentration. Exp Gerontol 47:183–187
4. Wagner KW, Ye Y, Lin J, Vaporciyan AA, Roth JA, Wu X (2012) Genetic variations in epigenetic genes are predictors of recurrence in stage I or II non-small cell lung cancer patients. Clin Cancer Res 18:585–592
5. Park C, Han S, Lee KM, Choi JY, Song N, Jeon S, Park SK, Ahn HS, Shin HY, Kang HJ, Koo HH, Seo JJ, Choi JE, Kang D (2012) Association between CASP7 and CASP14 genetic polymorphisms and the risk of childhood leukemia. Hum Immunol 73:736–739
6. Matsuda K, Yamaguchi A, Taira C, Sueki A, Koeda H, Takagi F, Sugano M, Honda T (2012) A novel high-speed droplet-polymerase chain reaction can detect human influenza virus in less than 30 min. Clin Chim Acta 413:1742–1745
7. Sueki A, Matsuda K, Taira C, Yamaguchi A, Koeda H, Takagi F, Kobayashi Y, Sugano M, Honda T (2013) Rapid detection of PML-RARA fusion gene by novel high-speed droplet-reverse transcriptase-polymerase chain reaction: possibility for molecular diagnosis without lagging behind the morphological analyses. Clin Chim Acta 415:276–278
8. Taira C, Matsuda K, Yamaguchi A, Sueki A, Koeda H, Takagi F, Kobayashi Y, Sugano M, Honda T (2013) Novel high-speed droplet-allele specific-polymerase chain reaction: application in the rapid genotyping of single nucleotide polymorphisms. Clin Chim Acta 424:39–46
9. Newton CR, Graham A, Heptinstall LE, Powell SJ, Summers C, Kalsheker N, Smith JC, Markham AF (1989) Analysis of any point mutation in DNA. The amplification refractory mutation system (ARMS). Nucleic Acids Res 17:2503–2516
10. Matsuda K, Sakashita K, Taira C, Tanaka-Yanagisawa M, Yanagisawa R, Shiohara M, Kanegane H, Hasegawa D, Kawasaki K, Endo M, Yajima S, Sasaki S, Kato K, Koike K, Kikuchi A, Ogawa A, Watanabe A, Sotomatsu M, Nonoyama S, Koike K (2010) Quantitative assessment of PTPN11 or RAS mutations at the neonatal period and during the clinical course in patients with juvenile myelomonocytic leukaemia. Br J Haematol 148:593–599
11. Taira C, Matsuda K, Kamijyo Y, Sakashita K, Ishida F, Kumagai T, Yamauchi K, Okumura N, Honda T (2011) Quantitative monitoring of single nucleotide mutations by allele-specific quantitative PCR can be used for the assessment of minimal residual disease in patients with hematological malignancies throughout their clinical course. Clin Chim Acta 412:53–58
12. Taira C, Matsuda K, Saito S, Sakashita K, Sugano M, Okumura N, Honda T (2012) Application of allele-specific quantitative PCR using genomic DNA to monitor minimal residual disease based on mutant gene levels following allogeneic hematopoietic stem cell transplantation in patients with hematological malignancies: comparison of mutant levels with autologous DNA percentage by short tandem repeat-PCR. Clin Chim Acta 413:516–519
13. Matsuda K, Sugano M, Honda T (2012) PCR for monitoring of minimal residual disease in hematologic malignancy. Clin Chim Acta 413:74–80

Chapter 4

Blood Grouping Based on PCR Methods and Agarose Gel Electrophoresis

Ana Maria Sell and Jeane Eliete Laguila Visentainer

Abstract

The study of erythrocyte antigens continues to be an intense field of research, particularly after the development of molecular testing methods. More than 300 specificities have been described by the International Society for Blood Transfusion as belonging to 33 blood group systems. The polymerase chain reaction (PCR) is a central tool for red blood cells (RBC) genotyping. PCR and agarose gel electrophoresis are low cost, easy, and versatile in vitro methods for amplifying defined target DNA (RBC polymorphic region). Multiplex-PCR, AS-PCR (Specific Allele Polymerase Chain Reaction), and RFLP-PCR (Restriction Fragment Length Polymorphism-Polymerase Chain Reaction) techniques are usually to identify RBC polymorphisms. Furthermore, it is an easy methodology to implement. This chapter describes the PCR methodology and agarose gel electrophoresis to identify the polymorphisms of the Kell, Duffy, Kidd, and MNS blood group systems.

Key words Blood group antigens, Genotyping, SNPs, PCR, Polymorphism

1 Introduction

The study of erythrocyte antigens continues to be an intense field of research, particularly after the development of molecular testing methods. More than 300 specificities have been described and have been classified by the International Society for Blood Transfusion (ISBT), as belonging to 33 blood group systems. Genes of all these systems have been cloned (http://www.isbt-web.org). Knowledge of the molecular bases of the blood group polymorphism enables the development of molecular biology typing methods and the identification of new mutations and provides a means to predict blood group phenotype from genomic DNA with a high degree of accuracy [1, 2]. Some of the variety of mechanisms that account for blood group polymorphism included single nucleotide polymorphism (SNP), gene deletion, single nucleotide deletion, sequence duplication, and intergenic recombination [2].

Peter Bugert (ed.), *Molecular Typing of Blood Cell Antigens*, Methods in Molecular Biology, vol. 1310, DOI 10.1007/978-1-4939-2690-9_4,

The red cell blood groups are composed of numerous antigens, of which the main ones are ABO, Rh, Kell, Duffy, Kidd, and MNS. The Rh system is a clinically important blood group because it induces Rh negative incompatible blood transfusion and hemolytic disease of the newborn [3]. The antigens of this system are encoded by two genes located on chromosome 1: *RHD* and *RHCE*. The most immunogenic and clinically important antigen is D (RH:1. *RHD*01* allele) because D antigens consist of at least 30 epitopes [1].

The Kell blood group system is complex and contains many antigens that are highly immunogenic. These antigens are the third most potent for triggering an immune reaction, after those of the ABO and Rh blood groups. These antigens are produced by alleles located on chromosome 7q33, including sets of antithetical antigens such as Kell (K, KEL:1,-2; *KEL*01.1* allele) and cellano (k, KEL:2; *KEL*02* allele), which differ in a single amino acid change (T193M) [4, 5].

The Duffy antigen is encoded by the *FY* gene, and Fy^a and Fy^b antigens are encoded by *FY*01* and *FY*02* alleles (125A > G). This first human gene recognized as being autosomal consists of two exons and its locus is on the chromosome 1q22-23 [6]. The common phenotypes of the Kidd blood group systems are encoded by two codominant alleles: *JK*01* and *JK*02*, located in the 18q12,3 region [7]. The MNS blood group system consists of 46 antigens carried on glycophorin A (GPA), glycophorin B (GPB), or on hybrids of these glycophorins, encoded by *GYPA* and *GYPB*, two closely linked loci located on chromosome 4 (4p28-q31). These proteins are single pass type I membrane glycoproteins that are heavily *O*-glycosylated. GPA carries an *N*-glycan [8].

The polymerase chain reaction (PCR) is a central tool for RBC genotyping. PCR and agarose gel electrophoresis are low cost, easy, and versatile in vitro method for amplifying defined target DNA (RBC polymorphic region). Usually, the method is designed to permit selective amplification of a specific target DNA sequence(s) within a heterogeneous collection of DNA sequences. To permit such selective amplification, some prior DNA sequence information from the target sequences is required. This information is used to design two oligonucleotide primers which are specific for the target sequence and which are often about 15–25 nucleotides long. After the primers are added to denatured template DNA, they bind specifically to complementary DNA sequences at the target site. In the presence of a suitably heat-stable DNA polymerase and DNA precursors (the four deoxynucleoside triphosphates, dATP, dCTP, dGTP, and dTTP), they initiate the synthesis of new DNA strands which are complementary to the individual DNA strands of the target DNA segment, and which will overlap each other. The PCR is a chain reaction because newly synthesized DNA strands will act as templates for further DNA synthesis in subsequent cycles. After about 25 cycles of DNA synthesis, the products of the PCR will include, in addition to the starting DNA, about 10^5 copies of the specific target sequence, an amount which is easily visualized as a discrete band of a specific size when submitted to agarose gel electrophoresis. A heat-stable DNA polymerase is used because the reaction involves sequential cycles composed of three steps: denaturation (typically at about 93–95 °C for human genomic DNA), reanneling (usually from about 50–70 °C depending on the T_m), and DNA synthesis (typically at about 70–75 °C) [9].

AS-PCR (Allele-Specific PCR) and RFLP-PCR (Restriction Fragment Length Polymorphism-PCR) techniques are frequently used to identify RBC polymorphisms. *RHCE*C/c* and *RHD* genotyping can be performed by a multiplex assay [10] and *RHD*pseudogene* (*RHD*ψ*, *RHD*04 N.01*) is detected using the AS-PCR [11]. The *RHCE*E/e*, *KEL*01.1/KEL*02*, *FY*01/FY*02*, *FY*01N.01* (GATA-1 mutation), and *JK*01/JK*02* (*SLC14A1* gene) genotyping can be performed by the RFLP-PCR technique [12, 13].

The aim of this chapter was to describe a PCR methodology to identify the polymorphisms of the Kell, Duffy, Kidd, and MNS blood group systems.

2 Materials

It is necessary to have separate rooms for pre-PCR and for post-PCR procedures. One should not exchange reagents and supplies between these rooms. Use ultrapure water (deionized water) to prepare all solutions and molecular grade reagents. The solutions and reagents must be in the ambient temperature. Before PCR reactions: clean the laminar flow or DNA workstation with 0.5 % hypochlorite solution and 70 % alcohol; irradiate by UV light for 30 min.

2.1 Reagents and Solutions

1. Taq polymerase: Perkin Elmer® or Invitrogen® or others products. The appropriate PCR buffer with 15 mM $MgCl_2$ is supplied with the enzyme.
2. 50 or 100 bp molecular weight marker (Gibco–BRL, Bethesda, MD, USA): prepare in the pre-PCR room: use 10 μL molecular weight marker (1 μg/μL), add 392 μL ultrapure water and mix by vortexing; add 98 μL 5× Ficoll and prepare aliquots; store at 4 °C.
3. dNTP solution (10 mM Gibco–BRL) 2.5 mM each: prepare in the pre-PCR room with micropipettes exclusively for this purpose: use 25 μL of each dNTP and add 900 μL ultrapure water; store 50 μL aliquots at −20 °C.

4. Agarose (molecular biology grade; Gibco–BRL).
5. Bromophenol blue gel loading buffer.
6. SYBR green (Invitrogen Life Technologies®, Grand Island, NY, USA) or ethidium bromide (10 mg/mL).
7. TBE (5×): dissolve 54 g Tris base and 27.5 g boric acid, add 20 mL EDTA 0.5 M pH 8 (20 mL), add ultrapure water to a final volume of 100 mL. 1× TBE is prepared by diluting 5× TBE with ultrapure water.
8. Genomic DNA isolated from 150 μL buffy coat or 500 μL EDTA blood using standard procedures such as phenol-chloroform extraction or commercial kits (e.g., QIAamp® DNA Blood Mini Kit; Qiagen, Valencia, CA) according to manufacturer's protocols (*see* **Note 1**). Estimate DNA concentration and quality by spectrophotometry (*see* **Note 2**).
9. Primer stock solutions (1 μg/μL): prepare in the pre-PCR room with micropipettes exclusively for this purpose: (1) Centrifuge tubes containing primers; (2) See the amount (μg) of the primer in the certificate of analysis and add the same volume (μL) of ultrapure water; (3) after 10 min, mix well by vortexing. Store at 4 °C for up to 48 h and after at −20 °C.
10. Primer working solutions (100 ng/μL): prepare a 1:10 dilution of the primer stock solution with ultrapure water (*see* **Note 3**). Verify the concentration (OD_{260}) and adjust the volume in the PCR reaction, if necessary.
11. Restriction enzymes (MBI Fermentas®, Canada) for RFLP-PCR: *Bsm*I for *KEL* 01/KEL* 02*; *Mnl*I for *JK* 01/JK* 02*; *Ban*I for *FY* 01/FY* 02*; *Sty*I for GATA-1 mutation *FY* 01N.01*.

2.2 Laboratory Equipment

1. Thermocycler with a 96-well block (*see* **Note 4**).
2. Electrophoresis horizontal apparatus and power supply: the size of the agarose gel should be 8 cm × 12 cm (9 wells comb) or preferably 10 cm × 10 cm (16 or 21 wells comb).
3. Gel documentation or gel imaging system.
4. UV–VIS Spectrophotometer.

3 Methods

3.1 RFLP-PCR for KEL, JK, and FY

RFLP-PCR is used for genotyping the antithetical Kell blood group antigens K (*KEL* 01.1*, KEL:1,-2) and k (*KEL* 02*, cellano, k, KEL:2), the antithetical Kidd blood group antigens Jk^a(*FY* 01*) and Jk^b(*FY* 02*), and the Duffy blood group system (Fy^a antigen, *FY* 01*; Fy^b antigen, *FY* 02*; GATA-1 mutation *FY* 01N.01*). Primers (Table 1) and amplification conditions were published previously [12–15].

Table 1
Primer sequences for RFLP-PCR of KEL, JK, and FY

	Primers	Sequence
*KEL*01/KEL*02*	KELS	5′-AAGCTTGGAGGCTGGCGCAT-3′
	KELR	5′-CCTCACCTGGATGACTGGTG-3′
*JK*02/JK*02*	JKABF	5′-CCCACCCTCAGTTTCCTTCC-3′
	JKABR	5′-GCGCCATGAACATTGCTCCC-3′
*FY*01/FY*02*	FYAB1	5′-TCCCCCTCAACTGAGAACTC-3′
	FYAB2	5′-AAGGCTGAGCCATACCAGAC-3′
GATA-mutation	FYN1	5′-CAAGGCCAGTGACCCCCATA-3′
	FYN2	5′-CATGGCACCGTTTGGTTCAG-3′

Table 2
PCR setup of one reaction for *KEL, JK, and FY*

17.25 μL	Ultrapure water
2.50 μL	10× PCR Buffer (with 15 mM $MgCl_2$)
1.00 μL	$MgCl_2$ 50 mM
0.50 μL	dNTP 10 mM
0.50 μL	Sense primer (100 ng/μL)
0.50 μL	Antisense primer (100 ng/μL)
0.25 μL	Taq Polymerase (5 U)
22.50 μL	*Mix volume*
2.50 μL	DNA (50–100 ng/μL)
25.00 μL	*Total volume*

3.1.1 PCR Amplification

1. Prepare a mix including reagents and primers according to Table 2.
2. Pipette 2.5 μL of the DNA in each sample strip; pipette 2.5 μL of water as the negative control; add 22.5 μL of the mix in each PCR tube and close the tubes (*see* **Notes 10** and **11**).
3. Use the following cycling program for amplification: 95 °C—15 min; 32 cycles with 94 °C—20 s, 62 °C—20 s, 72 °C—20 s; 72 °C—10 min; 4 °C (hold).

3.1.2 Agarose Gel Electrophoresis

1. Prepare a 2 % agarose gel: add 2 g of agarose in 100 mL of 1× TBE and heat in a microwave oven. Add 2 μL of staining reagent (SYBR green or ethidium bromide—10 mg/mL). Dispense the agarose in the gel stand of the horizontal electrophoresis apparatus and wait 15–20 min for complete solidification.

2. In each well, add 4 μL of the PCR product and 4 μL of bromophenol blue gel loading buffer.
3. Run the gel for 10 min and 150 V (5–7 V/cm).
4. Visualize and document the PCR products in the agarose gel on the documentation apparatus.

3.1.3 Enzyme Digestion

1. Prepare enzyme/buffer mixture according to manufacturer's recommendation: use 7.5 μL water and add 2 μL of the 10× enzyme buffer and 0.5 μL of the restriction enzyme.
2. Use 10 μL of PCR product and add 10 μL of the enzyme/buffer mixture.
3. Incubate overnight at 37 °C.
4. Prepare agarose gels (2 % for Kell and Duffy; 3 % for Kidd): add 2 or 3 g agarose in 100 mL of 1× TBE and heat in a microwave oven. Add 2 μL of staining reagent (SYBR green or ethidium bromide—10 mg/mL). Dispense the agarose in the gel stand of the horizontal electrophoresis apparatus and wait 15–20 min for complete solidification.
5. Mix 10 μL of the restriction digest with 4 μL bromophenol blue gel loading buffer and load 10 μL to the agarose gel.
6. For Kell and Duffy run the gel for 10 min at 70 V and 20 min at 90 V. For Kidd run the gel for 10 min at 70 V and 40 min at 80 V.
7. Visualize and document the results from restriction digest on the documentation apparatus.

3.1.4 Result Interpretation

1. For the Kell blood group alleles the PCR product is 156 bp in size and the *Bsm*I digestion results in 100 and 56 bp fragments (Fig. 1).

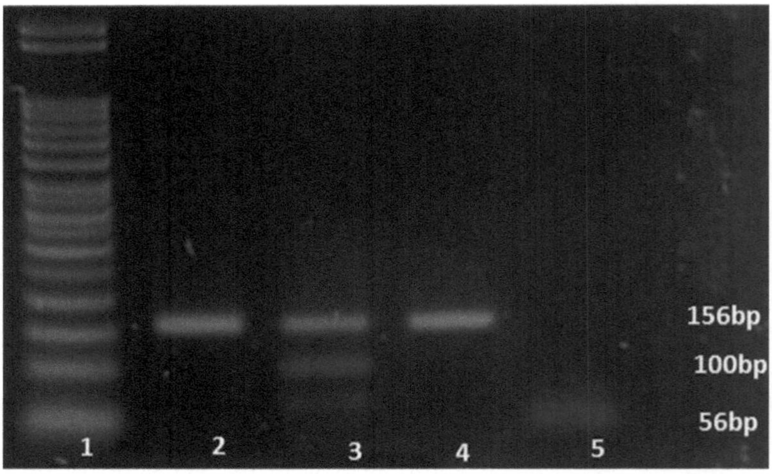

Fig. 1 Kell blood group genotyping. *Lane 1*: molecular weight marker; *lanes 2* and *4*: *KEL*02*; *lane 3*: *KEL*01.1/KEL*02*; *lane 5*: negative control (without DNA)

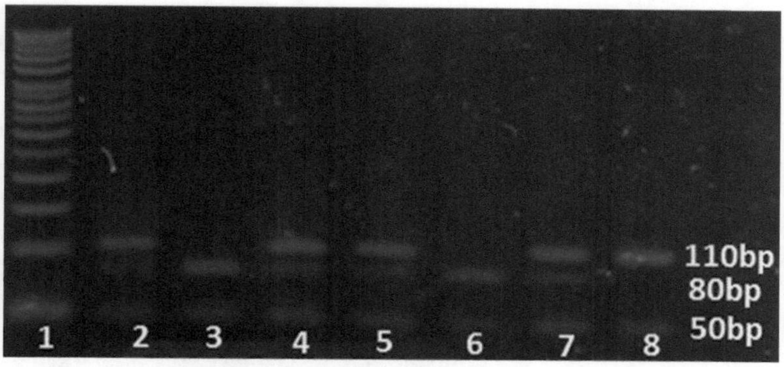

Fig. 2 Kidd blood group genotyping. *Lane 1*: molecular weight marker (50 bp); *lanes 2, 4, 5,* and *7*: *JK*01/JK*02*; lanes 3 and 6: *JK*01/JK*01*; *lane 8*: *JK*02/JK*02*

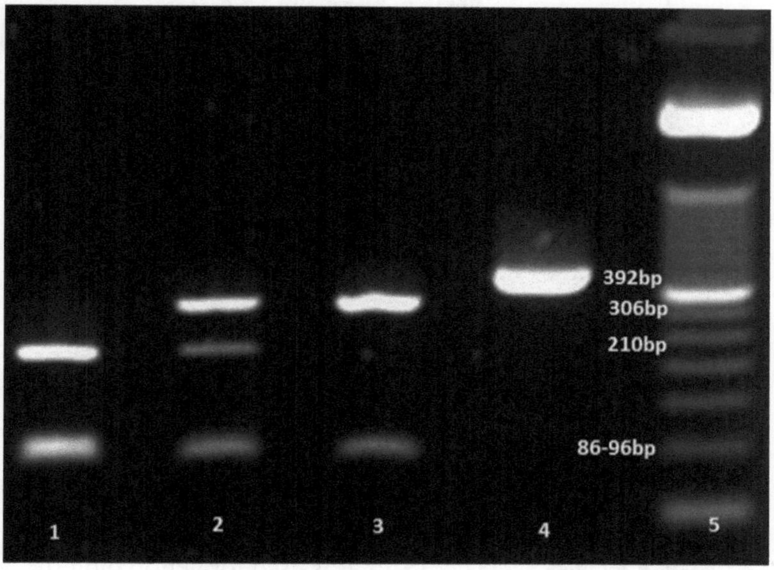

Fig. 3 *Duffy blood group* genotyping (*FY*A/FY*B*). *Lane 1*: *FY*01/FY*01* (*FY*A/FY*A*); *lane 2*: *FY*01/FY*02* (*FY*A/FY*B*); *lane 3*: *FY*02/FY*02* (*FY*B/FY*B*); *lane 4*: undigested PCR product; *lane 5*: molecular weight marker (50 bp)

2. For the Kidd blood group alleles the PCR product is 246 bp in size and the *Mnl*I digestion results in 110, 80, and 56 bp fragments (Fig. 2).
3. For the Duffy blood group alleles *FY* 01* and *FY* 02* the PCR product is 392 bp in size and the *Ban*I digestion results in 306 bp (*FY* 02*) or 210 bp and 86–96 bp fragments (Fig. 3). For the GATA-1 mutation the PCR product is 189 bp in size and the *Sty*I digestion results in 108 and 81 bp in samples without the GATA-1 mutation (GATA -67T). In samples with the mutation (GATA -67C) a 61 bp fragment is produced (Fig. 4) (*see* **Note 5**).

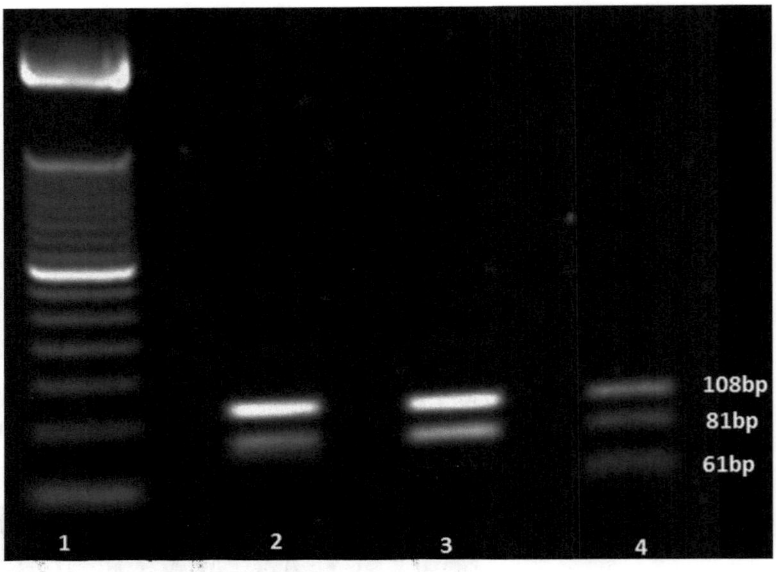

Fig. 4 Duffy blood group genotyping (GATA-1 -67T>C mutation). *Lane 1*: molecular weight marker (50 bp); *lanes 2* and *3*: no mutation (homozygous GATA -67T); *lane 4*: *FY*02/FY*01 N.01* (heterozygote GATA -67T>C)

Table 3
Primer sequences for AS-PCR of MN antigens

Primers	Sequences
GPA	5′-GTGAGGGAATTTGTCTTTTGCA-3′
GPA-N	5′-AAGAGGTTGAAGTGTGCATTGCCACCT-3′
GPA-M	5′-TGCCACACCAGTGGTACTTG-3′

3.2 AS-PCR for MNS

The AS-PCR is used for genotyping the MNS blood group system. Single nucleotide polymorphisms (SNPs) are responsible for the M/N and S/s allelic variants. The *GYPA* and *GYPB* genes encode for the GPA (M/N) and GPB (S/s) proteins, respectively. Primers and amplification conditions were previously published [16, 17].

3.2.1 AS-PCR for MN

1. Prepare a primer pool by mixing equal volumes of each of the three primers (Table 3).
2. Prepare a mix including reagents and primers according to Table 4 (*see* **Note 6**).
3. Pipette 2.5 μL of the DNA in each sample strip (*see* **Note 7**); pipette 2.5 μL of water as the negative control; add 22.5 μL of the mix in each PCR tube and close the tubes (*see* **Notes 10** and **11**).
4. Use the following cycling program for amplification: 94 °C—10 min; 32 cycles with 94 °C—30 s, 65 °C—30 s, 72 °C—30 s; 72 °C—5 min; 4 °C (hold).

Table 4
PCR setup of one reaction for MN genotyping

16.75 μL	Ultrapure water
2.50 μL	10× PCR Buffer (with 15 mM $MgCl_2$)
1.00 μL	$MgCl_2$ 50 mM
0.50 μL	dNTP 10 mM
1.50 μL	Pool primer (100 ng/μL)
0.25 μL	Taq Polymerase (5 U)
22.50 μL	*Mix volume*
2.50 μL	DNA (20–100 ng/μL)
25.00 μL	*Total volume*

Table 5
Primer sequences for AS-PCR of Ss antigens including *HGH* as internal control

Genes	Primers	Sequences
GYPB	GPYPB-S (Ss)	5′-GTATAAGAGAGCTTCATGACA-3′
GYPB 03*	GPYPB-S-as (S)	5′-CGATGGACAAGTTGTCCCA-3′
GYPB 04*	GPYPB-s-as (s)	5′-CGATGGACAAGTTGTCCCG-3′
HGH	HGH-S HGH-AS	5′-TGCCTTCCCAACCATTCCCTTA-3′ 5′-CCACTCACGGATTTCTGTTGTG TTTC-3′

3.2.2 AS-PCR for Ss

1. Prepare a primer mix for the S-specific PCR by mixing equal volumes of each of the four primers (Table 5): GPYPB-S, GPYPB-S-as, HGH-S, and HGH-AS.
2. Prepare a primer mix for the s-specific PCR by mixing equal volumes of each of the four primers (Table 5): GPYPB-S, GPYPB-s-as, HGH-S, and HGH-AS.
3. Prepare a mix including reagents and primers according to Table 6 (*see* **Note 8**).
4. Pipette 2.5 μL of the DNA in each sample strip (*see* **Note 7**); pipette 2.5 μL of water as the negative control; add 22.5 μL of the mix in each PCR tube and close the tubes (*see* **Notes 10** and **11**).
5. Use the following cycling program for amplification: 94 °C—9 min; 32 cycles with 94 °C—30 s, 62 °C—30 s, 72 °C—30 s; 72 °C—5 min; 4 °C (for ever).

Table 6
PCR setup of one reaction for S or s genotyping

16.25 μL	Ultrapure water
2.50 μL	10× PCR Buffer (with 15 mM $MgCl_2$)
1.00 μL	$MgCl_2$ 50 mM
0.50 μL	dNTP 10 mM
2.00 μL	Primer mix S or s (100 ng/μL)
0.25 μL	Taq Polymerase (5 U)
22.50 μL	*Mix volume*
2.50 μL	DNA (20–100 ng/μL)
25.00 μL	*Total volume*

3.2.3 Agarose Gel Electrophoresis

1. Prepare a 3 % agarose gel: add 3 g of agarose in 100 mL of 1× TBE and heat in a microwave oven. Add 2 μL of staining reagent (SYBR green or ethidium bromide—10 mg/mL). Dispense the agarose in the gel stand of the horizontal electrophoresis apparatus and wait 15–20 min for complete solidification.
2. In each well add 4 μL of the PCR product and 4 μL of bromophenol blue loading dye.
3. For MN genotyping run the gel for 30 min at 95 V (*see* **Note 9**). For Ss genotyping run the gel for 21 min at 95 V.
4. Visualize and document the PCR products in the agarose gel on the documentation apparatus.

3.2.4 Result Interpretation

1. In case of a positive genotype M, a fragment of 128 bp is amplified. A positive genotype N leads to a fragment of 147 bp in size. For MN both fragments will be present (Fig. 5).
2. An internal control fragment (*HGH*–432 bp) is amplified in all reactions. In case of a positive *GYPB* 03* (*GYPA* S*) or *GYPB* 04* (*GYPA* s*) genotype the 655 bp fragment is visible (Fig. 6).

4 Notes

1. The concentration and quality of DNA affects the PCR. The DNA concentration should be about 50–100 ng/μL and the $OD_{260/280}$ ratio should be 1.6–1.8.
2. The concentration of the DNA can be overestimated in spectrophotometric determination due to RNA contamination. Estimation of DNA concentration by agarose gel electrophoresis may be an alternative. Degraded DNA can leave a smear in the agarose gel.

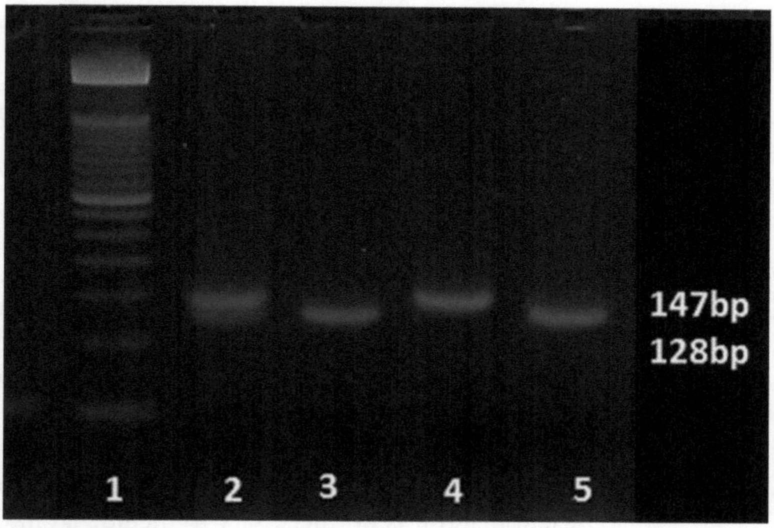

Fig. 5 MNS *blood group genotyping* (*GYPA*01* and *GYPA**02). *Lane 1*: molecular weight marker (50 bp); *lane 2*: *GYPA*01*/*GYPA*02* (MN); *lanes 3* and *5*: homozygotes *GYPA*01* (M); *lane 4*: homozygote *GYPA*02* (N)

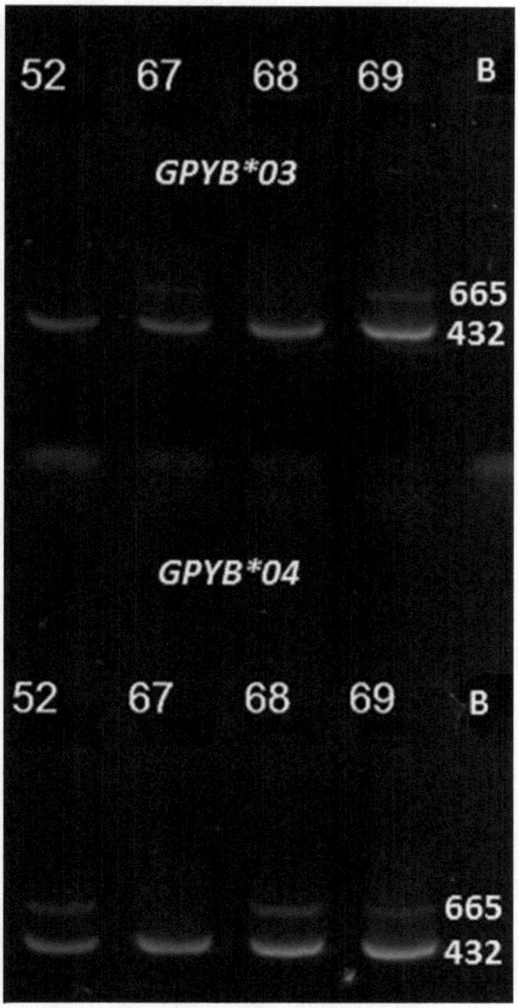

Fig. 6 MNS *blood group genotyping* (*GYPA*03* and *GYPA**04). Samples 52 and 68: homozygotes *GYPB*04* (s); sample 67: homozygote *GYPB*03* (S); sample 69: *GYPB*03*/*GYPB*04* (Ss)

3. The primers in working solutions can degrade due to the dilution and should be used not longer than 1 month.
4. Ensure calibration of the thermocycler.
5. Fy(a-b-) is rare among Caucasian and Asian populations, is common in African blacks, and is associated with a -67T>C substitution (*FY*01 N.01* allele): this mutation impairs the promoter activity in erythroid cells by disrupting a bind site for GATA-1 erythroid transcription factor, and it can protect the individuals from malaria infestation [18]. Individuals that had the allele *FY*01 N.01* can receive blood phenotyped as Fy^b because they had the expression of the Fy^b in other cells.
6. In case of MN genotyping both alleles are amplified in one reaction and it is not necessary to include an internal control. Due to codominant expression of the alleles, amplification will occur in any case.
7. Unspecific amplification may be due to high amounts of DNA. The DNA amount should be <200 ng per PCR (<100 ng for MN). If the volume of DNA needs to be changed (in order to adjust the concentration), also change the volume of water. The final reaction volume should be 25 μL.
8. The Ss genotyping by AS-PCR must be performed in two separate reactions because the PCR products for *GYPB*03* (*GYPA*S*) and *GYPB*04* (*GYPA*s*) have the same size (655 bp). Here, an internal control is used: HGH (human growth hormone—432 bp).
9. It is possible to separate bands with little difference in base pairs in the 3 % agarose gel. For this, it is necessary to adjust the running time and use a thicker agarose gel. If necessary cool down the gel in a cold chamber.
10. To ensure quality control of the PCR positive controls (reference DNA samples with known genotypes) and a negative control (without DNA) should be used.
11. Nonamplification: Hemoglobin or Heparin can inhibit the PCR amplification.

References

1. Daniels G (2002) Human blood groups. Blackwell Science, Oxford
2. Daniels G (2009) The molecular genetics of blood group polymorphism. Hum Genet 126:729–742
3. Colin Y, Chérif-Zahar B, Le Van Kim C et al (1991) Genetic basis of the RhD-positive and RhD-negative blood group polymorphism as determined by Southern analysis. Blood 78:2747–2752
4. Wagner T, Berer A, Lanzer G, Geissler K (2000) Kell is not restricted to the erythropoietic lineage but is also expressed on myeloid progenitor cells. Br J Haematol 110:409–411
5. Wagner T, Lanzer G, Geissler K (2002) Kell expression on myeloid progenitor cells. Leuk Lymphoma 43:479–485
6. Iwamoto S, Omi T, Kajii E, Ikemoto S (1995) Genomic organization of the glycoprotein D gene: Duffy blood group Fya/Fyb alloantigen

system is associated with a polymorphism at the 44-amino acid residue. Blood 85:622–626
7. You G, Smith CP, Kanai Y et al (1993) Cloning and characterization of the vasopressin-regulated urea transporter. Nature 365:844–847
8. Reid ME (2009) MNS blood group system: a review. Immunohematology 25:95–101
9. Strachan T, Read AP (1999) PCR, DNA sequencing and in vitro mutagenesis. Human molecular genetics. Wiley-Liss, New York, NY
10. Maaskant-Van Wijk PA, Faas BH, De Ruijter JA et al (1998) Genotyping of RHD by multiplex polymerase chain reaction analysis of six RHD-specific exons. Transfusion 38: 1015–1021
11. Singleton BK, Green CA, Avent ND et al (2000) The presence of on RHD pseudogene containing a 37 base pair duplication and a nonsense mutation in Africans with the Rh-negative blood group phenotype. Blood 95:12–18
12. Rios M, Cash K, Strupp A et al (1999) DNA from urine sediment or buccal cells can be used for blood group molecular genotyping. Immunohematology 15:61–65
13. Reid ME, Rios M, Yazdanbakhsh K (2000) Applications of molecular biology techniques to transfusion medicine. Semin Hematol 37: 166–176
14. Castilho L, Rios M, Bianco C et al (2002) DNA-based typing for the management of multiply-transfused sickle cell disease patients. Transfusion 42:232–238
15. Castilho L, Rios M, Pellegrino J Jr et al (2002) Blood group genotyping facilitates transfusion of beta-thalassemia patients. J Clin Lab Anal 16:216–220
16. Male DA, Phillips P, Turner DR (2002) Improved polymerase chain reaction-based glycophorin-A M/N blood group allelotyping. Vox Sang 83:170–171
17. Lavoiet J, Perreault J, St-Louis M (2008) Génotypage du systeme S et s par PCR en multiplex. Version 2. Département de Recherche et Développement, Québec
18. Tournamille C, Colin Y, Cartron JP et al (1995) Disruption of a GATA motif in the Duffy gene promoter abolishes erythroid gene expression in Duffy-negative individuals. Nat Genet 10: 224–228

Chapter 5

Parallel Donor Genotyping for 46 Selected Blood Group and 4 Human Platelet Antigens Using High-Throughput MALDI-TOF Mass Spectrometry

Stefan Meyer, Nadine Trost, Beat M. Frey, and Christoph Gassner

Abstract

Most blood group antigens are defined by single nucleotide polymorphisms (SNPs). Highly accurate MALDI-TOF MS has proven its potential in SNP genotyping and was therefore chosen for blood donor oriented genotyping with high-throughput capability, e.g., 380 samples per day. The Select Module covers a total of 36 SNPs in two single-tube reactions, representative of 46 blood group and 4 human platelet antigens. Using this tool, confirmatory blood group typing for RhD, RhCE, Kell, Kidd, Duffy, MN, Ss, and selected rare antigens is performed on a routine basis.

Key words Blood group gene, Blood group genotyping, High-throughput SNP typing, MALDI-TOF MS, Kell, Kidd, Duffy, MNSs, Rare blood group antigens, Blood donor

1 Introduction

1.1 Blood Groups and Single Nucleotide Polymorphisms

Today, over 300 blood group antigens have been characterized [1, 2]. Nearly all were observed in patient samples using serological techniques [3]. The analysis of the molecular basis for blood group expression has identified single nucleotide polymorphisms (SNPs) as the major causative DNA variation between these antigens. Almost all common SNPs have only two alleles, and the variation may encode for two different amino acids within the coding regions, typically leading to the two representatives of two antithetic blood group antigens as exemplified for Colton a and b, respectively [4].

Since it is relevant for all blood group systems and their respective genes, insertions and deletions of single or multiple nucleotides (nts) represent the second common mechanism for the molecular determination of blood group antigens. Positioned within coding regions, these "indel" variations lead to altered reading frames, usually preventing physical presence, or catalytic activity of the

Peter Bugert (ed.), *Molecular Typing of Blood Cell Antigens*, Methods in Molecular Biology, vol. 1310,
DOI 10.1007/978-1-4939-2690-9_5, © Springer Science+Business Media New York 2015

respective peptides as exemplified for by the famous deletion of G at coding nucleotide (cdnt) 261, inactivating the ABO glycosyltransferase, thereby encoding the ABO O phenotype [5]. In genotyping, short insertions and deletions may technically be addressed according to SNPs. Many of these SNPs, representing intra-genetic variation, are entered in specialized databases, comprehensively documented and selectively retrievable by their unique reference SNP (rs) ID number [6].

However, genetic single nt variations between paralogs, e.g., two genes as a result of gene duplication, usually coding for proteins with a similar function and/or structure, are not considered as SNPs. Typical examples are the genes *RHD/RHCE* and *GYPA/GYPB* of the RhD/RhCE and MNSs blood group systems, respectively [7, 8]. Genetic dissimilarity between such highly homologous genes may be limited to 3.6 % of all cdnt (45 dissimilarities of 1,254 cdnt), as exemplified for the two genes *RHD* and *RHCE*, encoding the peptides specific for RhD and Rhce, respectively [7]. Again, molecular diagnosis of such inter-genetic variation is technically similar to common SNP detection and widely used since decades [9]. Dependent on the existence of paralogous loci, hybrid-genes represent the third common molecular mechanism for blood group antigen determination. Representative examples for such results of gene conversion events may be encountered within the Rh and MNSs blood group systems, occasionally [8, 10, 11].

1.2 Errors in Predicting Blood Group Phenotypes from Genotypes

SNP based genotyping of blood groups, is surprisingly accurate, considering the fact that most techniques rely on the exclusive detection of one single SNP for the prediction of a whole peptide (antigen, phenotype), usually consisting of several 100 amino acids, encoded by three times as many cdnts. However, minimizing the pleiority of potential reasons for technical failures applying robust techniques, e.g., MALDI-TOF MS, still the genetic background itself represents some risks for the correct prediction of blood group phenotypes deduced from genotypes. Most, if not all such “genotyping errors” may be explained by rarely occurring genetic variants of commonly known alleles, and therefore rather be interpreted as highly specific “indicators” further adding to the genetic complexity, than as profane “errors”.

At least two different genetic backgrounds may cause such genetically reasoned “genotyping errors.” One is the whole world of unexpressed alleles, the other a growing number of very rare mutant alleles, interacting specifically with primer binding sites nearby the diagnosed SNP of interest [12]. Blood group null phenotypes, e.g., found as ABO O, K_0, Jr-, or Lan negative phenotypes, are well recognized to be encoded by many more alleles, than only by a single one, solely responsible for the respective null phenotype [13–17].

1.3 Different Requirements in Donor Versus Recipient Genotyping

In recipient typing, typically, only individual samples are analyzed at varying time-points, due to the urgency and impact of the results on transfusion decisions. In contrast, genotyping of repetitive donors is time insensitive and aims to type as many blood group systems and donors' samples as possible. Also requirement for analytic accuracy represents a striking difference between donor- and recipient-specific genotyping: For instance, unconsidered null-alleles remain unidentified, and donor typing would accept these, because such heterozygous "pretender-results" would phenotypically behave as homozygous. So, there is no harm to the patient, if being transfused according to its heterozygous phenotype. In recipients on the other hand, such untrue heterozygous "pretender-results" could potentially lead to fatal transfusion reactions and would genetically best be addressed by a technique currently unavailable, e.g., the affordable whole blood group genome within 2 h. However, recipients' whole blood group genomes within a timely manner will probably stay illusive for the foreseeable future, whereas donors' SNP based blood group genotypes are readily available.

1.4 "High-Throughput" Genotyping

Although a variety of different blood group genotyping methods [1, 3, 18] have been claimed to possess capability for "high-throughput," there are no commonly accepted numerical characteristics for this figure. Impressive sample throughput may also be generated using pooling strategies, in order to identify certain analytes of relatively low frequencies, e.g., such as viruses, or rare blood group alleles [19]. However, efficiency of such strategies is directly dependent on the frequency and number of analytes investigated in parallel, and needs to be optimized based on mathematical models. Currently and on the other hand, Next-Generation Sequencing, may well be used for the generation of an excessive number of SNP genotypes from a single, or a small number of samples and as such be qualified of being capable for high throughput. Still, this type of information may not fulfil present-day requirements for transfusion services.

Consequently, capability for high-throughput may be expressed considering (1) the type and (2) wanted number of samples, (3) the number of SNPs of interest and still, though of minor impact (*see* **Note 1**) (4) the time interval needed for their analysis. Using matrix-assisted laser desorption/ionization, time-of-flight mass spectrometry (MALDI-TOF MS) blood group genotyping, a single multiplex reaction, e.g., covering 16 SNPs allows for genotyping of approximately 3,840 blood donor DNAs per day (10 times 384 different DNAs), or roughly 60,000 SNP genotypes within 1 day. In its 384-well microtiter plate version, throughput limitations may rather result from a lack of donor numbers (*see* **Note 2**), insufficient DNA sample number extraction, underscaled PCR cycling production line, or limited manpower, then from the analytical capacity of the mass spectrometer itself. In fact, in our institute, the average throughput need for the described "Select Module" is far below the described maximal throughput capacity and lies at some 10,000 samples per year. A typical daily typing batch size consists of 384 DNA samples, simultaneously analyzed by two single multiplexes, covering the described 36 SNPs of interest (Table 1). As a result, approximately 14,000 SNPs are genotyped per day, which to our opinion, may still be considered as "high-throughput".

1.5 Core Analytical Procedures of MALDI-TOF MS

The core analytical procedures of MALDI-TOF MS based SNP genotyping are shown in Fig. 1. As claimed by the provider, multiplexing levels, e.g., simultaneous amplifications of polymerase chain reaction (PCR) fragments of up to 40 genomic target DNA sequences seems to be feasible. However, the presented Select Module consists of two multiplexes, with amplifications allowing the simultaneous genotyping of 23 and 13 SNPs, representative of gender determination plus 30 blood group in 1, and 16 blood group and 4 human platelet antigens in the other, respectively (Table 1). Amplification is followed by the degradation of dNTPs and an allele-specific single base extension of a primer that anneals directly adjacent to the SNP of interest. Resulting single-stranded, nucleic acid oligomer analytes of 15–30 base-pairs (bp) in length (4,300–9,000 Da range) are then desalted applying anion-exchange resin material and transferred to a silicon chip with pre-spotted matrix crystal (e.g., 3-hydroxy picolinic acid) containing patches.

Laser-irradiation induces the desorption and ionization of the analytes causing the +1 positively charged molecules to accelerate into a vacuum flight tube towards a detector. Separation occurs by the time of flight (TOF), which is proportional to the mass of the individual molecules. Low mass molecules arrive in a shorter time than those of higher masses, and molecules of different masses are thereby separated. After data processing, a spectrum is produced with relative intensity on the y-axis and mass/charge on the x-axis (Fig. 2). The method directly measures the mass of the molecules of interest, without using any surrogate, such as fluorescence.

1.6 General Applications of MALDI-TOF MS Based Genotyping

MALDI-TOF MS was initially introduced in proteomics applications, while the full potential for DNA analysis was demonstrated in 1995 [20]. The special and advantageous features of mass spectrometry qualify the technology adapted for genotyping as an advanced system for automated high-throughput analysis of SNPs [21]. MALDI-TOF MS also proved its ability in the reliable quantification of certain alleles and genetic variants in non-Mendelian mixtures of DNAs, e.g., fetal DNA in maternal plasma, or somatically mutated DNA in cancerous tissue [22–24]. Reproducibly, the respective sensitivity limits were shown to be as low as 5 % [23, 25]. The advantage of short amplicon lengths and minimal

Table 1
Detected blood group antigens included in the two multiplexes of the MALDI-TOF MS based Select Module

ISBT#	Blood group	Gene (HGNC)	On	Allele name 1	Allele name 2	nt position	nt 1	nt 2	Amino a.	Antigens	Allele ct.	SNP ct.	plex	rs #
001	ABO A, B, O2/O1	*ABO*	9q	*[ABO*G261]*	*[ABO* delG261]*	261	G	delG	fsThr88Pro	1	2	1	2	no rs
002	M/N	*GYPA*	4q	*GYPA*01*	*GYPA*02*	59	C	T	Ser20Leu	2	2	1	2	rs7682260
002	S/s	*GYPB*	4q	*GYPB*03*	*GYPB*04 (wt)*	143	C	T	Thr48Met	2	2	1	1	rs7683365
002	S, s/U–	*GYPA/GYPB*	4q	*GYPA*	*GYPB*	i1 + 15914	G	C	–	1	1	1	2	no rs
002	M, N/ Henshaw	*GYPA/GYPB*	4q	*GYPA*01, 02*	*GYPB*06.01*	59	Y	G	Leu20Trp	1	1	–	2	no rs
004	RhD+/RhD–	*RHD/RHCE*	1p	*RHD*01 (wt)*	*RHD*01N.01*	455	A	[C]	Asn152[Thr]	2	2	1	1	no rs
004	RhD+/RhD–	*RHD/RHCE*	1p	*RHD*01 (wt)*	*RHD*01N.01*	787	G	[A]	Gly263[Arg]	–	–	1	1	no rs
004	RhD+/RhD–	*RHD/RHCE*	1p	*RHD*01 (wt)*	*RHD*01N.01*	1362	A	[T]	–	–	–	1	1	no rs
004	RhD+/RhD–	*RHD/RHCE*	1p	*RHD*01 (wt)*	*RHD*04N.01*	504–541	–	ins 37bp	–	–	1	1	1	no rs
004	RhD+/RhD–	*RHD/RHCE*	1p	*RHD*01 (wt)*	*RHD*01N.06*	1006	G	C	Gly336Gly	–	1	1	1	no rs
004	RhD+/RhD–	*RHD/RHCE*	1p	*RHD*01*	*RHCE*all (wt)*	1362	[A]	T	–	–	–	–	1	no rs
004	Rhc/RhC	*RHCE*	1p	*RHCE*01 (03) (wt)*	*RHCE*02 (04)*	i2 + 3095	–	ins 109bp	–	2	2	1	2	no rs
004	Rhc/RhC	*RHCE*	1p	*RHCE*01 (03) (wt)*	*RHCE*02 (04)*	307	C	T	Ser103Pro	–	–	1	2	rs676785
004	RhC, Rhc/ RhC^w	*RHCE*	1p	*RHCE*all*	*RHCE*02.08*	122	A	G	Gln41Arg	1	1	1	1	rs138268848
004	Rhe/RhE	*RHCE*	1p	*RHCE*01 (02)*	*RHCE*03 (04)*	676	G	C	Pro226Ala	2	2	1	2	rs609320
005	Lu^a/Lu^b	*BCAM*	19q	*LU*01*	*LU*02 (wt)*	230	A	G	His77Arg	2	2	1	1	rs28399653

(continued)

Table 1
(continued)

ISBT#	Blood group	Gene (HGNC)	On	Allele name 1	Allele name 2	nt position	nt 1	nt 2	Amino a.	Antigens	Allele ct.	SNP ct.	plex	rs #
006	K/k	*KEL*	7q	*KEL*01.1*	*KEL*02 (wt)*	578	T	C	Met193Thr	2	2	1	2	rs8176058
006	K,k/K_{mod}	*KEL*	7q	*KEL*01M.01*	*KEL*02 (wt)*	578	G	C	Arg193Thr	–	1	–	2	rs8176058
006	Kp^a/Kp^b	*KEL*	7q	*KEL*02.03*	*KEL*02 (wt)*	841	T	C	Trp281Arg	2	1	1	2	rs8176059
006	Js^a/Js^b	*KEL*	7q	*KEL*02.06*	*KEL*02 (wt)*	1790	C	T	Pro597Leu	2	1	1	1	rs8176038
006	K, k/K_0	*KEL*	7q	*KEL*02 (wt)*	*KEL*02N.06, 02N.01*	i3+1g>m	G	M	–	1	2	1	1	no rs
008	Fy^a/Fy^b	*DARC*	1q	*FY*01, or FY*A*	*FY*02, or FY*B*	125	G	A	Gly42Asp	2	2	1	2	rs12075
008	Fy^b/Fy^x	*DARC*	1q	*FY*wt*	*FY*02M*	265	C	T	Arg89Cyt	–	1	1	2	no rs
008	$Fy^{a,b}$/Fy null	*DARC*	1q	*FY*wt*	*FY*02N.01*	P-67t>c	T	C	–	1	1	1	1	no rs
009	Jk^a/Jk^b	*SLC14A1*	18q	*JK*01, or JK*A*	*JK*02, or JK*B*	838	G	A	Asp280Asn	2	2	1	1	rs1058396
009	$Jk^{a,b}$/Jk null	*SLC14A1*	18q	*JK*wt*	*JK*02N.01, 01N.06, 02N.02*	i5-1g>m	G	M	–	1	3	1	1	rs78937798
009	$Jk^{a,b}$/Jk null	*SLC14A1*	18q	*JK*wt*	*JK*01N.03*	582	C	G	Tyr194Stop	–	1	1	1	rs34756616
010	Di^a/Di^b	*SLC4A1*	17q	*DI*01*	*DI*02 (wt)*	2561	T	C	Leu854Pro	2	2	1	1	no rs
010	Wr^a/Wr^b	*SLC4A1*	17q	*DI*02.03*	*DI*02 (wt)*	1972	A	G	Glu658Lys	2	2	1	1	rs75731670
011	Yt^a/Yt^b	*ACHE*	7q	*YT*01 (wt)*	*YT*02*	1057	C	A	His353Asn	2	2	1	1	rs1799805
013	SC:1, SC:2	*ERMAP*	1p	*SC*01 (wt)*	*SC*02*	169	G	A	Gly57Arg	2	2	1	1	rs56025238
014	Do^a/Do^b	*ART4*	12p	*DO*01*	*DO*02 (wt)*	793	A	G	Asn265Asp	2	2	1	1	no rs

015	Co^a/Co^b	*AQP1*	7p	*CO*01.01 (wt)*	*CO*02*	134	C	T	Ala45Val	2	2	1	1	rs28362692
016	LW^a/LW^b	*ICAM-4*	19p	*LW*05 (wt)*	*LW*07*	299	A	G	Gln100Arg	2	2	1	1	rs77493670
023	In^a/In^b	*CD44*	11p	*IN*01*	*IN*02 (wt)*	137	G	C	Arg46Pro	2	2	1	1	rs121909545
n.a.	Vel+/Vel–	*SMIM1*	1p	*[SMIM1*Vel+]*	*[SMIM1*Vel-]*	64–80	–	del 17bp	–	1	2	1	2	no rs
n.a.	[HPA-1a/b]	*ITGB3*	17q	*[ITGB3*001] (HPA-1a) (wt)*	*[ITGB3*002] (HPA-1b)*	176	T	C	Leu59Pro	2	2	1	2	rs5918
n.a.	[HPA-5a/b]	*ITGA2*	5q	*[ITGA2*001] (HPA-5a) (wt)*	*[ITGA2*002] (HPA-5b)*	1600	G	A	Glu534Lys	2	2	1	2	rs10471371
n.a.	[Female]/[male]	*GYG2/paralog*	Xp/Yp	*[GYG2*Xfemale] (wt)*	*[GYGpar*Ymale]*	i2 + 3291	C	[A]	–	–	2	1	1	no rs

Blood groups are ordered according to their official International Society of Blood Transfusion (ISBT) numbers. For the human platelet antigens (HPA), and gender genotyping, no ISBT numbers are available. Every line is representative of one antithetic antigen pair. Values in square brackets are no blood groups (column "blood group"), or do not represent official ISBT allele terminology (columns "allele name"), or are single nucleotide (nt) variations between two paralog genes (column "nt" and amino a.). Gene names are given according to the HUGO Gene Nomenclature Committee (HGNC). Nt values are given in International Union of Pure and Applied Chemistry (IUPAC) notation. Amino a. for amino acid, "ct." for count, and "rs" for reference SNP. (wt) indicates the more frequent allele, occurring among Caucasians. "i" stands for intron, "ins" for an insertion, "del" for a deletion, and "bp" for base pairs. Beside citations given, additional important information regarding blood group polymorphisms was retrieved from NCBI dbSNP and OMIM [6, 40]

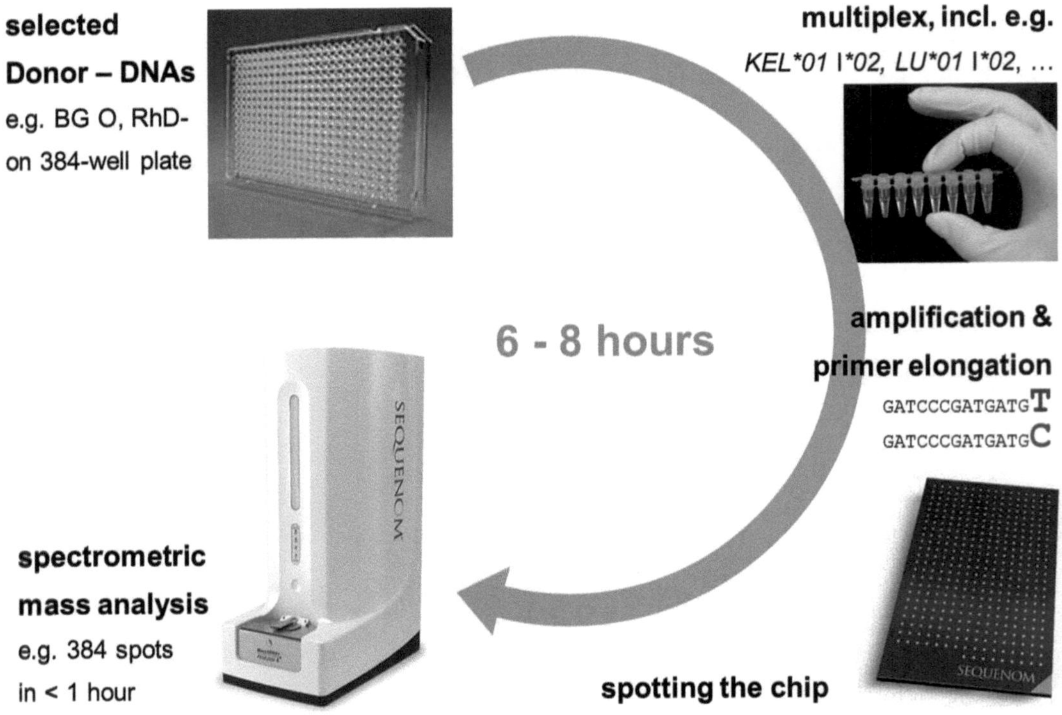

Fig. 1 Schematic representation of the MALDI-TOF MS based high-throughput blood group genotyping procedure applying the Select Module

requirement for template DNA amounts further expand the range of application to forensics, pathology (formalin-fixed and paraffin-embedded tissue) and the analysis of DNA methylation patterns [26–29].

1.7 MALDI-TOF MS Based Blood Group Genotyping of Donors

To date, MALDI-TOF MS based genotyping has been successfully applied in "non-invasive" determination of fetal blood group *RHD* and *KEL*01* status [30, 31]. Apart from those reports and starting in 2006, at least four different groups reported on their results using MALDI-TOF MS for donor genotyping of blood groups, or human platelet antigens (HPA), so far [24, 32–36]. MALDI-TOF MS analysis in comparison to PCR using Sequence Specific Priming (PCR-SSP) and a novel real-time PCR high-resolution melt curve (HRM) analysis, delivered 100 % concordance rates for all investigated HPA and blood group Indian genotypes, respectively [33, 35]. A third group of researchers reported about polymorphisms linked to 22 different blood groups, that both the error rate of the MALDI-TOF MS assay, as measured by the strand concordance rate, and the no-call rate were very low (0.1 %) [32]. With respect to donor genotyping, all authors positively commented on the ability of MALDI-TOF MS based methodology for automation, high throughput, and cost efficiency.

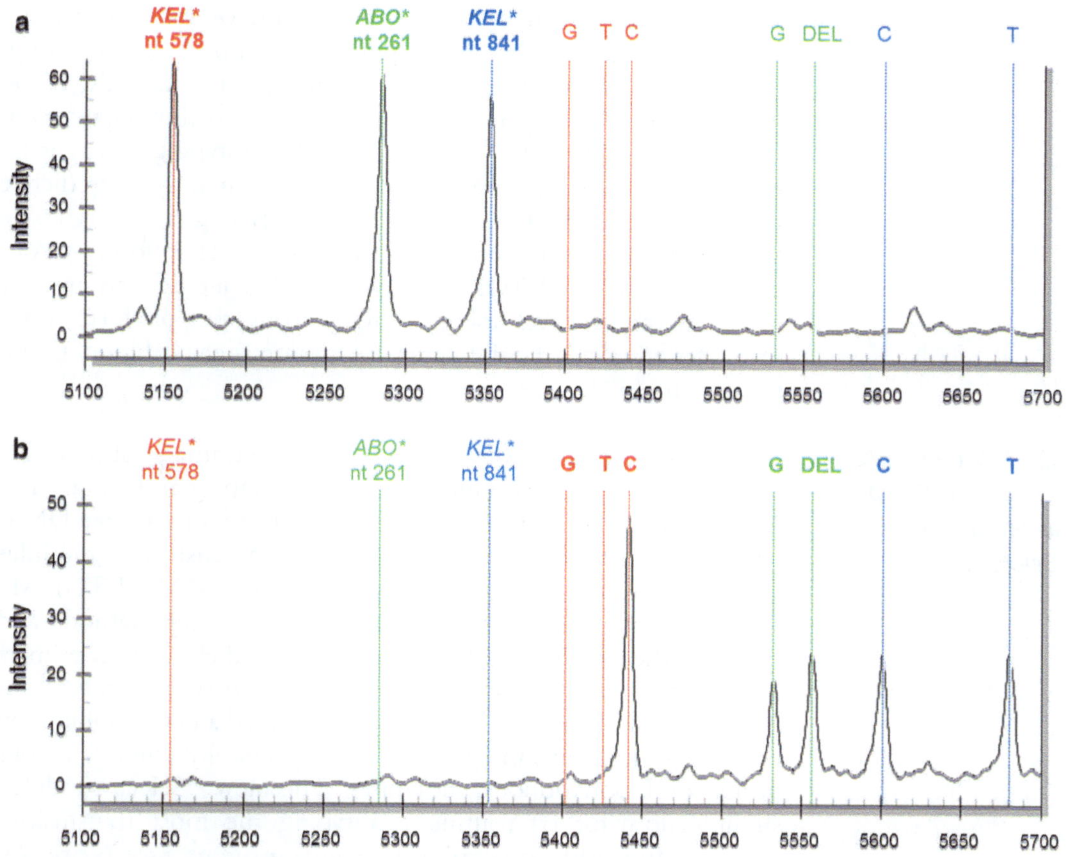

Fig. 2 MALDI–TOF mass spectrum of three SNPs (out of 13), specific for *KEL*01* vs. *02* (e.g., K vs. k, plus *KEL*01M.01*), [*ABO*G261*] vs. [*ABO*delG261*], and *KEL*02* vs. *KEL*02.03* (e.g., Kp^a vs. Kp^b) in multiplex 2 of the Select Module from a negative control sample (no-template control, H_2O) (**a**), and an exemplary DNA sample (**b**). For every SNP the calculated mass of the unextended primer (UEP) before base extension reaction (**a**) and the masses of the corresponding extended primers (**b**) are marked by *dashed lines* (*colour-coded* per SNP assay). As expected in the no template control sample (**a**) only peaks of UEPs were detectable. The mass spectrum of all SNPs showed either one or two extension products in homozygous (*KEL** coding nt 578 CC), or in an approximate 1:1 ratio in heterozygous (*ABO** coding nt 261 G/del, *KEL** coding nt 841 CT) genotypes of the respective SNP (**b**). For SNP details, also refer to Table 1

Above mentioned key statements were confirmed by our own experience using MALDI-TOF MS in genotyping of 170 alleles predictive of 101 blood group and platelet antigens [34]. The method also allowed for reliable differentiation of *RHD* hetero- and homozygous individuals, at multiple genetic positions in individual samples by calculating the *RHD/RHCE* MALDI-TOF MS peak area quotient [34]. A more detailed analysis of 4,000 Swiss blood donor samples delivered genotype/phenotype concordance rates between 99.93 and 100 % for the blood groups Kell, Kidd, and Duffy, respectively. Genotyping proved its practicability in the daily routine setting and qualitatively outperformed serology. Technology was ideal for time-insensitive donor genotyping and allowed for a broad range of throughput needs. We therefore suggested that, from a technological point of view, serotyping should be replaced by genotyping for donors' blood groups encoded by *KEL*, *SLC14A1*, and *DARC* [36]. Currently, 6,000 blood group MN and Ss phenotypes from Swiss donors are compared to their MALDI-TOF MS derived genotyping data. Again, robustness, accuracy, reproducibility, and phenotype-predictive value of MALDI-TOF MS based genotyping are impressive (unpublished data, manuscript in preparation). Therefore, we concluded, that MALDI-TOF MS based blood group genotyping may represent the one technological high-throughput platform, optimally covering all requirements for donor specific blood group genotyping [34].

1.8 MALDI-TOF MS Based Blood Group Genotyping Using "Select Module"

Obviously, there are several reasons to take advantage of MALDI-TOF MS in high-throughput blood group genotyping. The MALDI-TOF MS platform does not need fixed formats like DNA-chips, and users are therefore free to select and customize modules of their interest. Of note, this flexibility of the MALDI-TOF MS technology is unique among all other genotyping methods and based on the simple fact, that amplification and elongation primers are the only variable determinant of all (!) sorts of applications based on SNP detection. Therefore, we defined a new combination of certain blood group specific SNPs, specifically tailored to our needs for blood donor genotyping. This new "Select Module" should allow for (i) routine genotyping the most transfusion-relevant and additional blood group antigens (*see* **Note 2**), e.g., such as K/k, $Jk^{a/b}$, or MN and Ss, the (ii) simultaneous genetic prediction of rare blood group phenotypes, e.g., such as Kp^b and Vel negativity, (iii) minimizing costs for this purpose and (iv) consider additional advantages arising from genetic typing.

The presented Select Module finally consists of two multiplexes, allowing the parallel genotyping of 23 and 13 SNPs in two single tubes per DNA sample, respectively (Table 1). Beside given specificities addressing (i) and (ii) given above, the Select Module includes a low resolution *RHD* genotyping capability, rather thought as a tool for aspects of confirmation, than considered for comprehensive *RHD* gene analysis. With respect to (iv) given above, specificities for HPA-1 and HPA-5 were included in order to identify potential platelet donors with rare platelet antigen constellations. And, serving as a security measure, assays specific for the cdnt deletion G261 of the *ABO* gene and an inter-genetic single nt variation between *GYG2* on chromosome X and a highly homologous sequence on chromosome Y, allowed for the prediction of blood group O and gender, respectively [5, 37]. Both genotypes were then routinely compared to the respective existing phenotypic pre-values of every donor in order to exclude erroneous qualitative serial sample mix-up, e.g., bottom to top, or left to right flips of the 96-, or 384-well microtiter plates handled in the course of the analytical procedure.

Validation of the Select Module was done on 1,520 previously genotyped individual donor DNA samples and showed full concordance, e.g., identical results for all 54,720 SNP genotypes tested when comparing the results of the previously published methods to the new Select Module [34, 36]. Costs consist of material costs of € 1.20 (US$ 1.65, August 2014) and 2.1 min of labour per DNA extraction (using Chemagen technology, PerkinElmer, Baesweiler, Germany) and material costs of € 8.75 (US$ 12.00, August 2014) and 2.4 min of labour per two multiplexes (complete typing), not including overhead, amortization costs for hardware and yearly maintenance fees. Since published guidelines of the national blood transfusion service of the Swiss Red Cross prescribe duplicate testing of donors' blood groups on an independent second sample [38], the Select Module is considered as highly attractive alternative in comparison to a second typing done by serology. Further validation is underway in order to fulfil Swiss national requirements for an approval of the Select Module as an officially accepted method for second testing of confirmatory character, in the course of the routinely performed blood group typing in duplicate.

2 Materials

2.1 Genomic DNA

1. Beside manual DNA preparation using Nucleon BACC 3 reagents (Gen-Probe Life Sciences Ltd, Manchester, UK), automated DNA preparation has been implemented, applying the Chemagen magnetic bead technology (PerkinElmer, Baesweiler, Germany) in its automated 96-well microtiter plate format.
2. Preparation was done from 0.2 mL and 6 mL EDTA anticoagulated blood (*see* **Note 3**), for the automated and manual protocol, resulting in approximately 8 μg (in 100 μl eluate) and 400 μg total genomic DNA, respectively (*see* **Note 4**).
3. For the automated method, all individual donor samples, e.g., 3 mL EDTA anticoagulated blood were barcoded. The "chemagen 96-deep well microtiter input plate" and respective data files were generated using standard operation procedures and pipetting robots by Tecan (Tecan Group AG, Maennedorf, Switzerland), or Hamilton (Hamilton AG, Bonaduz, Switzerland) linked to our in-house blood management software.

2.2 Thermal Cyclers

Four Veriti DX 384-well thermal cyclers (0.02 mL, Applied Biosystems by Life Technologies, Zug, Switzerland) (*see* **Note 5**).

2.3 Hardware and Software for Mass Spectrometry

1. All hardware and software for mass spectrometry were provided by Sequenom GmbH, Hamburg, Germany a division of Sequenom Inc., San Diego, USA. Mass spectrometry package included:

2. MassARRAY® Analyzer 4, with capacity for the analysis of up to two times 384 SpectroCHIP®s per load.
3. MassARRAY® Nanodispenser RS-1000.
4. Server for data management and software MassARRAY® Genotyper 4.v.
5. Delivery of the 384-well microtiter plate format system additionally includes a complete lay out for a 96-well microtiter plate format procession.
6. Alternatively, a pure 96-well microtiter plate format for reduced costs may be considered and will also abrogate the need for two Liquid Handler Stations.
7. Additional equipment was two MassARRAY® Liquid Handler Stations (Matrix).
8. Additional software needed was MassARRAY Quantitate Gene Expression 3.v* also including the software tool MassArray Assay Design mentioned later in this article (*see* **Note 6**).

2.4 Consumables for Mass Spectrometry

1. Complete MassARRAY iPLEX Pro Genotyping Reagent Set including all reagents for the genotyping 10 x 384 DNA samples with 1 multiplex (Sequenom GmbH, Hamburg, Germany).
2. Amplification and elongation primers of adequate quality (*see* **Note 7**) were provided by Metabion (Metabion International AG, Planegg, Germany).

2.5 Water, Purity Requirements

Usage of ultrapure water is highly recommended for all washing and flushing steps performed by the Liquid Handler Stations and the Nanodispenser during the whole typing procedure. Volumes needed range between 2 and 5 l per 2 × 384 well plate run. Water should have a resistivity of 18.2 MΩ × cm and was purified in-house using a Milli-Q Direct system (Merck Millipore, Zug, Switzerland).

3 Methods

This section can hardly describe all the details needed to be considered and conducted in performing a high-throughput MALDI-TOF MS Select Module genotyping on multiples of 384 DNA samples per run. However, the following paragraphs provide a good overview of the work-flow (Fig. 1) and procedures performed and add further details. Readers with increased thirst for knowledge regarding this may wish to contact the manufacturer and further consult detailed standard operation procedure manuals for this purpose. All SNPs were genotyped following the standard Sequenom MassARRAY iPLEX Pro genotyping procedure.

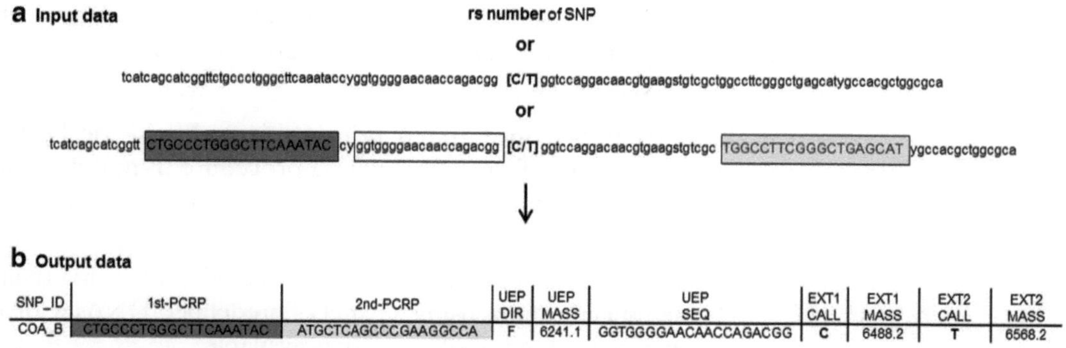

Fig. 3 Data in- and output using Assay Designer software exemplified for blood group Colton a/b polymorphism specific SNP of the Select Module multiplex reaction 1. (**a**) Data entry either requires only a list of rs numbers (*upper option* represented as "rs"), or DNA sequence given in IUPAC notation, spanning approximately 50–300 base-pairs (bp) flanking sequence of SNP given with the variation and in *square brackets* (*middle and lower options*). Sequence given in *lowercase letters* allows for an unrestricted calculation of amplification primer binding sites (*middle option*), *uppercase letter* (*shaded in dark and light grey*) constrict calculation of primer binding sites to a preferred region, or even a genetically required exact position (*lower option*). Binding site of the unextended primer (*unshaded box, lower option*) will be determined by the software, but the user is free to demand forward or reverse orientation if required (not shown in figure). (**b**) The output file delivers the DNA sequence of the amplification (first-primer, second-primer) and unextended primers (UEP), the orientation of UEP (forward or reverse) and the mass of the unextended and each version of the extended primers, respectively

3.1 Assay Design

1. Use the assay design software (TYPER 4.0, Sequenom) and online assay design tools (MySequenom, Sequenom) to select PCR amplification primer pairs, which uniquely amplified only the genomic region of interest, considering all database retrievable allelic variants.
2. The software continue to group the pairs into multiplexes and to validate all pairs within one multiplex for undesired cross-reactions among each other, with paralog genes and other homologous regions of the genome.
3. Finally, the software choose orientation and sequence of the extension primers, and the expected molecular weights of all expected elongated products, representing the 2–4 alleles potentially present at each SNP position and calculated mass distribution for compatibility with the mass analysis window.
4. In- and output files are comparably prosaic with respect to their generation, content, and handling as shown in Fig. 3. The output file of the Assay Designer is formatted for direct use further downstream in the genotyping process under the Assay Editor function of the TYPER 4.0 software.

3.2 Primer Mixes for Multiplex Amplification and Elongation

Of note, flexibility of the MALDI-TOF MS technology is unique among all other genotyping methods and based on the simple fact, that amplification and elongation primers are the only variable determinant of all sorts of applications based on SNP detection.

Downstream genotyping is widely facilitated using specific primer mix concentrates for (1) the amplification and (2) elongation reactions, respectively.

1. Both types of concentrated primer mixes should ideally be prepared ahead of the actual typing procedure in multiples of amounts needed for single typing runs and kept frozen at –20 °C for up to at least 6 months.
2. These batches of primer mixes should be controlled for their claimed specifications using a panel of predefined DNAs with a maximal reproduction of genotypes available.
3. For amplification, concentration of all primers in the final reaction volume of a 4.8 µL multiplex reaction is 100 nM.
4. Concentration of the elongation primers is much higher and varies, depending on the expected mass of the elongated product. The larger the product, or the respective unextended primer, the higher is its concentration in the final reaction volume of 8.6 µL elongation reaction and typically lies between 590 and 1,180 nM.
5. Primer orders need to account for the high quality requirements of the elongation primers (*see* **Note** 7), and appropriate synthesis scales. The micromolar amounts of elongation primers needed for MALDI-TOF MS genotyping are a relevant cost factor, whereas costs for amplification primers are insignificant.

3.3 Prearrangements of DNAs, Amplification, and SAP Treatment

1. Use four Chemagen 96-well microtiter output plates as matrices and pre-PCR Liquid Handler Stations as automated 96-well pipettors to generate working plates for the appropriate dilution of 384 different DNAs, and the final transfer to two 384-well microtiter amplification plates (2 h). Air-dry the DNAs overnight.
2. All enzymes, reagents and consumables needed for genotyping are provided within the complete MassARRAY iPLEX Pro Genotyping Reagent Set. Prepare the two amplification cocktails for the two multiplexes each with a calculated excess of 30 % in two separate tubes.
3. Aliquot the amount of three times 150 µL to each well of rows 1, and 7, and from there dispense five times 25 µL to each remaining empty well of a 96-well V-bottom plate using an automated 8-channel pipettor.
4. Transfer the final 4.8 µL to each 384-well of the amplification plate using the pre-PCR Liquid Handler Station (1 h).
5. Perform amplification of each DNA for both Select Module multiplexes on the two different 384-well amplification plates, also taking advantage of a “hot start” thermocycling procedure. Use two pre-PCR Veriti DX 384-well thermocyclers to facilitate parallel work-flow of the two 384-well plates (cycling:

2 h 45 min). From here on, carry out all steps in the post-PCR area.

6. Transfer the shrimp alkaline phosphatase (SAP) reaction mixture to all wells, again using automated pipettors and the post-PCR Liquid Handler Station. Non-incorporated dNTPs are enzymatically dephosphorylated by SAP, which ensures exclusive single nt extension in the next step. SAP reactions are carried out in the two post-PCR Veriti DX 384-well thermal cyclers (45 min).

3.4 Elongation of Unextended Primers, Spotting of Chip

1. The extension reactions calculated with an excess of 54 % contain buffer, termination mix, *Thermus aquaticus* Polymerase (TAQ) enzyme, and extension primers. The use of ddNTPs instead of dNTPs ensures exclusive single nt extension of the unextended primers (UEP 2 h 30 min).
2. Resulting single-stranded, nucleic acid oligomer analytes of 15–30 bp in length (4,300–9,000 Da range) are then desalted applying anion-exchange resin material (45 min) and transferred by the MassARRAY® Nanodispenser RS-1000 to a silicon chip with pre-spotted matrix crystal (e.g., 3-hydroxy picolinic acid) containing patches.
3. The Nanodispenser simultaneously aspirates 24 samples by 24 grooved needles just by capillary force. It delivers the impressively low volume of only 10 nL per sample with high accuracy. The dispensed volume is regulated, only by adjusting the speed of the needles the chip is hit with (30 min).
4. After spotting, chip is transferred into the vacuum chamber of the mass spectrometer.

3.5 Mass Spectrometry and Data Generation

1. Complete data flow is documented. In brief, data arrangement of the original four "chemagen 96-well microtiter output plates" is done using the Plate Editor function of the TYPER 4.0 software and results in the final 384-well plate file. The Assay Editor function of the TYPER 4.0 software holds all relevant "output files" of the Assay Designer (*see* Subheading 3.1), thereby providing specific information for each multiplex to be linked to each plate file. Finally, the 384-well plate file is linked to the chip using the software tool Chip Linker.
2. The mass spectrometry system is equipped with an N2 laser with 337-nm wavelength (pulse max energy of 100 microJ and 0.5 ns pulse width) for use with matrix components absorbing light of this wavelength. Every single spot of the chip, e.g., all analytes of one multiplex and one individuals' DNA (1 spot), are analyzed by 15 laser pulses (3 positions, 5 pulses each) and mathematically processed further downstream.
3. Spotting and laser operation are controlled by additional control spots. Ahead of sample analysis, calibration is performed using a 3-oligo mass/amount calibrant and water.

4. Data analysis is performed using Assay Analyser function of the TYPER 4.0 software, allowing for a comprehensive analysis of every single SNP, every single sample, e.g., peak area for all allele-specific analytes in any given assay, and systemic performance of every single run, e.g., call and extension rate.
5. A comprehensive mass-spectrum, visualizing all detected peaks of every SNP of every single DNA sample is provided (Fig. 2). TYPER 4.0 output files have a standardized format and may therefore easily be converted into other files, or used for selective data retrieval.
6. In order to translate TYPER 4.0 derived SNP genotyping data into predicted blood group phenotypes, a computer spreadsheet program (Microsoft Excel, Microsoft, Redmond, WA) fulfilled all our needs satisfactorily. This way, data were "humanized" and could be used for comparisons to their serological pre-values, statistical analysis, served as documents and offered a way for the transfer to our in-house blood management system (*see* **Note 8**).

4 Notes

1. Alternatively, individual steps of the lab process can also be run over night, or the process can be interrupted at any time (e.g., after amplification, SAP treatment, elongation, and resin purification), and resumed at any later time point. Products are stable for up to 6 months if stored in sealed microtiter plates at −20 °C.
2. In Switzerland, the minimal mandatory immune-hematological blood group antigen determination for every erythrocyte concentrate includes duplicate serotyping for ABO and RhD on two independent samples before their blood is transfused for the first time. Started in 2012, additionally all RhD negative donors are molecularly tested once for the presence of the *RHD* gene before the first usage of their blood, mandatorily [19, 39]. Expanded phenotyping for RhC/c, RhCw, RhE/e, Kell, Kidd, Duffy, MN, and Ss phenotypes is only done depending on the regional requirements, influenced by the local presence of "high-end" medicine, and usually covers between 20 and 80 % of all donors. Only donors selected for expanded phenotyping are also considered as candidates for genotyping by the MALDI-TOF MS based Select Module.
3. Dependent on the number of DNAs per time interval expected, EDTA blood may also be stored at 4 °C for up to 2 weeks before extraction. Alternatively, collection might take place externally and last for longer than 2 weeks. In this case, EDTA blood may simply be frozen at −20 °C, before shipped collectively using

cool-packs, or frozen ice. However, care should be taken, that collection tubes withstand the freezing/thawing procedure without being ruptured. In both cases, EDTA blood needs thorough stirring before transfer to the "chemagen 96-deep well microtiter input plate", best achieved using commercially available "head-over-head" mixers. Still, samples having been stored at −20 °C might need time-consuming labor for the manual removal of coagulated material with wooden sticks.

4. For MALDI-TOF MS analysis, approximately 20–30 ng of genomic DNA per each of the two multiplex reactions were used. Due to the high concentration conformity of the automatically extracted DNAs, laborious single DNA UV quantification was abandoned and replaced by the simplified usage of a fixed volume of 0.4 μL of the "chemagen eluate" per multiplex [34].

5. Four Veriti DX 384-well thermal cyclers used in our laboratory are labelled for in vitro diagnostic use, with a list price of € 13,800 each (US$ 19,400, September 2011). In order to maintain validity of the in vitro diagnostic use label, hardware requires inspection by the manufacturer on a yearly basis. In our department for Molecular Diagnostics and Research (MOC), barrier between pre- and post-amplification area is represented by a 10 m^2 room, serving as a gate. Air conditioning in this room and the post-amplification area has a separate circle and accounts for (1) appropriate cooling, in order to discharge thermal heat produced by the thermal cyclers located the gate, and (2) a slight atmospheric underpressure. The two doors for entering the room, or leaving it towards the post-amplification area, may only be opened alternatively and never simultaneously. This way, potential PCR product contaminations will always be directed towards the "uncritical" post-amplification area.

6. The mass spectrometry package was provided by Sequenom GmbH, Hamburg, Germany a division of Sequenom Inc., San Diego, USA. In 2014, parts of Sequenom Inc. have been acquired and are now firming as Agena Bioscience, San Diego, USA. The hardware and software package included a MassARRAY® Analyzer 4, with capacity for the analysis of up to 2 × 384 SpectroCHIP®s per load, a MassARRAY® Nanodispenser RS-1000, a server for data management and software MassARRAY® Genotyper 4.v* with a total list price of € 349,000.00 (US$ 502,200.00, June 2011). Additional equipment was 2 × MassARRAY® Liquid Handler Stations (Matrix) with a list price of € 53,500 each (US$ 77,000, June 2011). Additional software was the MassARRAY Quantitate Gene Expression 3.v* including the MassARRAY Assay Design tool with a list price of € 39,500 (US$ 56,800, June 2011).

According to the manufacturer, yearly maintenance of all hardware components is mandatory.

7. Self-evidently, manufacturing process of single elongation primers needs to account for oligonucleotides of unique length. Mass detection of elongated primers with contaminant adducts of +1 or −1 nts in length would seriously worsen single peak-quality of the spectrum.
8. Currently, our IT department is on its way to establish a direct transfer from TYPER 4.0 (raw) data to our in-house blood management system.

Acknowledgements

Financial support for the development of the Select Module was granted by the Humanitarian Foundation of the Swiss Red Cross (SRC); the Blood Transfusion Service Zurich, SRC, Switzerland and the Swiss blood transfusion umbrella organization Blutspende SRK Schweiz, Bern, Switzerland. SM, NT, and BMF are employees of the Blood Transfusion Service Zurich, SRC, Switzerland, and have not disclosed any conflicts of interest. CG is employee of the Blood Transfusion Service Zurich, SRC, Switzerland, and acts as a consultant for Inno-Train GmbH, Kronberg im Taunus, Germany.

References

1. Daniels G (2013) Human blood groups, 3rd edn. Blackwell Science, Oxford
2. Committee on Terminology for RBC Surface Antigens [database on the Internet] (2012) http://www.isbtweb.org/working-parties/red-cell-immunogenetics-and-blood-group-terminology/blood-group-terminology/blood-group-allele-terminology/
3. Denomme GA, Johnson ST, Pietz BC (2011) Mass-scale red cell genotyping of blood donors. Transfus Apher Sci 44:93–99
4. Halverson GR, Peyrard T (2010) A review of the Colton blood group system. Immunohematology 26:22–26
5. Yamamoto F, Clausen H, White T, Marken J, Hakomori S (1990) Molecular genetic basis of the histo-blood group ABO system. Nature 345:229–233
6. dbSNP, NCBI Build 138, Phase I [database on the Internet] (2013) http://www.ncbi.nlm.nih.gov/projects/SNP/
7. Mouro I, Colin Y, Cherif-Zahar B, Cartron JP, Le Van Kim C (1993) Molecular genetic basis of the human Rhesus blood group system. Nat Genet 5:62–65
8. Reid ME (2009) MNS blood group system: a review. Immunohematology 25:95–101
9. Gassner C, Schmarda A, Kilga-Nogler S, Jenny-Feldkircher B, Rainer E, Muller TH et al (1997) RHD/CE typing by polymerase chain reaction using sequence-specific primers. Transfusion 37:1020–1026
10. Wagner FF, Gassner C, Muller TH, Schonitzer D, Schunter F, Flegel WA (1998) Three molecular structures cause rhesus D category VI phenotypes with distinct immunohematologic features. Blood 91:2157–2168
11. Wagner FF, Frohmajer A, Flegel WA (2001) RHD positive haplotypes in D negative Europeans. BMC Genet 2:10
12. Gassner C, Utz I, Schennach H, Ramoni A, Steiner H, Scholz S et al (2013) Novel RHD alleles with weak hemagglutination and genetic Exon 9 diversity: weak D Types 45.1, 75, and 76. Transfusion 53(Suppl 2): 2954–2959
13. Amado M, Bennett EP, Carneiro F, Clausen H (2000) Characterization of the histo-blood group O(2) gene and its protein product. Vox Sang 79:219–226

14. Kormoczi GF, Wagner T, Jungbauer C, Vadon M, Ahrens N, Moll W et al (2007) Genetic diversity of KELnull and KELel: a nationwide Austrian survey. Transfusion 47:703–714
15. Saison C, Helias V, Ballif BA, Peyrard T, Puy H, Miyazaki T et al (2012) Null alleles of ABCG2 encoding the breast cancer resistance protein define the new blood group system Junior. Nat Genet 44:174–177
16. Zelinski T, Coghlan G, Liu XQ, Reid ME (2012) ABCG2 null alleles define the Jr(a-) blood group phenotype. Nat Genet 44: 131–132
17. Helias V, Saison C, Ballif BA, Peyrard T, Takahashi J, Takahashi H et al (2012) ABCB6 is dispensable for erythropoiesis and specifies the new blood group system Langereis. Nat Genet 44:170–173
18. Haer-Wigman L, Ji Y, Loden M, de Haas M, van der Schoot CE, Veldhuisen B (2013) Comprehensive genotyping for 18 blood group systems using a multiplex ligation-dependent probe amplification assay shows a high degree of accuracy. Transfusion 53(Suppl 2):2899–2909
19. Gowland P, Gassner C, Hustinx H, Stolz M, Gottschalk J, Tissot JD et al (2014) Molecular RHD screening of RhD negative donors can replace standard serological testing for RhD negative donors. Transfus Apher Sci 50:163–168
20. Tang K, Fu D, Kotter S, Cotter RJ, Cantor CR, Koster H (1995) Matrix-assisted laser desorption/ionization mass spectrometry of immobilized duplex DNA probes. Nucleic Acids Res 23:3126–3131
21. Jurinke C, van den Boom D, Cantor CR, Koster H (2002) The use of MassARRAY technology for high throughput genotyping. Adv Biochem Eng Biotechnol 77:57–74
22. Li Y, Wenzel F, Holzgreve W, Hahn S (2006) Genotyping fetal paternally inherited SNPs by MALDI-TOF MS using cell-free fetal DNA in maternal plasma: influence of size fractionation. Electrophoresis 27:3889–3896
23. Fumagalli D, Gavin PG, Taniyama Y, Kim SI, Choi HJ, Paik S et al (2010) A rapid, sensitive, reproducible and cost-effective method for mutation profiling of colon cancer and metastatic lymph nodes. BMC Cancer 10:101
24. Garritsen HS, Xiu-Cheng Fan A, Lenz D, Hannig H, Yan Zhong X, Geffers R et al (2009) Molecular diagnostics in transfusion medicine: in capillary, on a chip, in silico, or in flight? Transfus Med Hemother 36:181–187
25. Vivante A, Amariglio N, Koren-Michowitz M, Ashur-Fabian O, Nagler A, Rechavi G et al (2007) High-throughput, sensitive and quantitative assay for the detection of BCR-ABL kinase domain mutations. Leukemia 21: 1318–1321
26. Cerezo M, Cerny V, Carracedo A, Salas A (2009) Applications of MALDI-TOF MS to large-scale human mtDNA population-based studies. Electrophoresis 30:3665–3673
27. Xiu-Cheng Fan A, Garritsen HS, Tarhouny SE, Morris M, Hahn S, Holzgreve W et al (2008) A rapid and accurate approach to identify single nucleotide polymorphisms of mitochondrial DNA using MALDI-TOF mass spectrometry. Clin Chem Lab Med 46:299–305
28. Jaremko M, Justenhoven C, Abraham BK, Schroth W, Fritz P, Brod S et al (2005) MALDI-TOF MS and TaqMan assisted SNP genotyping of DNA isolated from formalin-fixed and paraffin-embedded tissues (FFPET). Hum Mutat 25:232–238
29. Docherty SJ, Davis OS, Haworth CM, Plomin R, Mill J (2010) DNA methylation profiling using bisulfite-based epityping of pooled genomic DNA. Methods 52:255–258
30. Li Y, Finning K, Daniels G, Hahn S, Zhong X, Holzgreve W (2008) Noninvasive genotyping fetal Kell blood group (KEL1) using cell-free fetal DNA in maternal plasma by MALDI-TOF mass spectrometry. Prenatal Diagn 28: 203–208
31. Bombard AT, Akolekar R, Farkas DH, Van Agtmael AL, Aquino F, Oeth P et al (2011) Fetal RHD genotype detection from circulating cell-free fetal DNA in maternal plasma in non-sensitized RhD negative women. Prenatal Diagn 31:802–808
32. Montpetit A, Phillips MS, Mongrain I, Lemieux R, St-Louis M (2006) High-throughput molecular profiling of blood donors for minor red blood cell and platelet antigens. Transfusion 46:841–848
33. Garritsen HS, Fan AX, Bosse N, Hannig H, Kelsch R, Kroll H et al (2009) Matrix-assisted laser desorption/ionization time-of-flight mass spectrometry for genotyping of human platelet-specific antigens. Transfusion 49:252–258
34. Gassner C, Meyer S, Frey BM, Vollmert C (2013) Matrix-assisted laser desorption/ionisation, time-of-flight mass spectrometry-based blood group genotyping–the alternative approach. Transfus Med Rev 27:2–9
35. Lopez GH, McBean RS, Wilson B, Irwin DL, Liew YW, Hyland CA et al (2014) Molecular typing for the Indian blood group associated 252G>C single nucleotide polymorphism in a selected cohort of Australian blood donors. Blood Transfus 18:1–8
36. Meyer S, Vollmert C, Trost N, Bronnimann C, Gottschalk J, Buser A et al (2014) High-throughput Kell, Kidd, and Duffy matrix-

assisted laser desorption/ionization, time-of-flight mass spectrometry-based blood group genotyping of 4,000 donors shows close to full concordance with serotyping and detects new alleles. Transfusion 54(12):3198–3207

37. Santos FR, Pandya A, Tyler-Smith C (1998) Reliability of DNA-based sex tests. Nat Genet 18:103

38. Blood Donation Service Switzerland SRC. Guidelines of the Swiss Red Cross Blood Donation Service (2013) Chapter 11 B, immuno-haematological donor typing. https://sbsc-bsd.ch/dokuman/DokumenteBSD/Allgemeines/tabid/107/language/de/Default.aspx

39. Crottet SL, Henny C, Meyer S, Still F, Stolz M, Gottschalk J et al (2014) Implementation of a mandatory donor RHD screening in Switzerland. Transfus Apher Sci 50:169–174

40. Online Mendelian Inheritance of Men [database on the Internet] (2014) http://www.ncbi.nlm.nih.gov/omim/

Chapter 6

PCR with Sequence-Specific Primers for Typing of Diallelic Blood Groups

Gabriele Rink, Erwin A. Scharberg, and Peter Bugert

Abstract

PCR with sequence-specific primers (PCR-SSP) is a cost-effective and robust method for the analysis of single nucleotide polymorphisms (SNPs). Many blood group antigens and the antithetic antigens are based on a diallelic SNP in the coding region of the corresponding blood group gene. Here, we describe PCR-SSP protocols for genotyping 24 blood group antigens based on 12 diallelic SNPs. We also provide protocols for molecular determination of the rare blood group phenotypes Yk^{a-} and Vel−.

Key words Single nucleotide polymorphism (SNP) genotyping, Blood group antigen, PCR-SSP, Molecular blood typing

1 Introduction

Since 1900 more than 300 red cell antigens have been discovered. They are defined serologically by the use of a specific antibody. Antigens receiving ISBT numbers (assigned by the ISBT Working Party on Red Cell Immunogenetics and Blood Group Nomenclature) must have been shown to be inherited characters [1]. A blood group system consists of one or more antigens controlled at a single gene locus, or by two or more very closely linked homologous genes with little or no observable recombination between them. Currently recognized antigens within blood group systems are shown in Table 1.

The knowledge of the genetic background of a blood group antigen is the prerequisite for the development and use of genotyping methods. Nowadays almost every blood group antigen can be typed by analysis of a corresponding DNA marker. Most blood group antigens differ from their antithetic partner by the alteration of a single nucleotide in the DNA sequence of the blood group gene (Table 2). By genotyping of these single nucleotide polymorphisms (SNPs) the blood group phenotype can reliably be derived.

Peter Bugert (ed.), *Molecular Typing of Blood Cell Antigens*, Methods in Molecular Biology, vol. 1310, DOI 10.1007/978-1-4939-2690-9_6, © Springer Science+Business Media New York 2015

Table 1
Blood group systems

System	Number of antigens	Antigens
001 ABO	4	A, B, AB, A1
002 MNS	46	M, N, S, s, U, He, Mi^a, M^c, Vw, Mur, M^g, Vr, M^e, Mt^a, St^a, Ri^a, Cla, Ny^a, Hil, M^v, Far, S^D, Mit, Dantu, Hop, Nob, En^a, En^{a}KT, 'N', Or, DANE, TSEN, MINY, MUT, SAT, ERIK, Os^a, ENEP, ENEH, HAG, ENAV, MARS, ENDA, ENEV, MNTD
003 P1Pk	3	P1, P^k, NOR
004 RH	54	D, C, E, c, e, f, Ce, C^w, C^x, V, E^w, G, Hr$_0$, Hr, hr^s, VS, C^G, CE, D^w, c-like, cE, hr^H, Rh29, Go^a, hr^B, Rh32, Rh33, Hr^B, Rh35, Be^a, Evans, Rh39, Tar, Rh41, Rh42, Crawford, Nou, Riv, Sec, Dav, JAL, STEM, FPTT, MAR, BARC, JAHK, DAK, LORC, CENR, CEST, CELO, CEAG, PARG, CEVF
005 LU	20	Lu^a, Lu^b, Lu3, Lu4, Lu5, Lu6, Lu7, Lu8, Lu9, Lu11, Lu12, Lu13, Lu14, Lu16, Lu17, Au^a, Au^b, Lu20, Lu21, LURC
006 KEL	35	K, k, Kp^a, Kp^b, Ku, Js^a, Js^b, Ul^a, K11, K12, K13, K14, K16, K17, K18, K19, Km, Kp^c, K22, K23, K24, VLAN, TOU, RAZ, VONG, KALT, KTIM, KYO, KUCI, KASH, KELP, KETI, KHUL, KYOR
007 LE	6	Le^a, Le^b, Le^{ab}, Le^{bH}, ALe^b, BLe^b
008 FY	5	Fy^a, Fy^b, Fy3, Fy5, Fy6
009 JK	3	Jk^a, Jk^b, Jk3
010 DI	22	Di^a, Di^b, Wr^a, Wr^b, Wd^a, Rb^a, WARR, ELO, Wu, Bp^a, Mo^a, Hg^a, Vg^a, Sw^a, BOW, NFLD, Jn^a, KREP, Tr^a, Fr^a, SW1, DISK
011 YT	2	Yt^a, Yt^b
012 XG	2	Xg^a, CD99
013 SC	7	Sc1, Sc2, Sc3, Rd, STAR, SCER, SCAN
014 DO	8	Do^a, Do^b, Gy^a, Hy, Jo^a, DOYA, DOMR, DOLG
015 CO	4	Co^a, Co^b, Co3, Co4
016 LW	3	LW^a, LW^b, LW^{ab}
017 CH/RG	9	Ch1, Ch2, Ch3, Ch4, Ch5, Ch6, WH, Rg1, Rg2
018 H	1	H
019 XK	1	Kx
020 GE	11	Ge2, Ge3, Ge4, Wb, Ls^a, An^a, Dh^a, GEIS, GELP, GEAT, GETI
021 CROM	18	Cr^a, Tc^a, Tc^b, Tc^c, Dr^a, Es^a, IFC, WES^a, WES^b, UMC, GUTI, SERF, ZENA, CROV, CRAM, CROZ, CRUE, CRAG
022 KN	9	Kn^a, Kn^b, McC^a, Sl1, Yk^a, McC^b, Sl2, Sl3, KCAM
023 IN	4	In^a, In^b, INFI, INJA
024 OK	3	Ok^a, OKGV, OKVM

(continued)

Table 1
(continued)

System	Number of antigens	Antigens
025 RAPH	1	MER2
026 JMH	6	JMH, JMHK, JMHL, JMHG, JMHM, JMHQ
027 I	1	I
028 GLOB	1	P
029 GIL	1	GIL
030 RHAG	4	Duclos, Ol^a, DSLK, RHAG4
031 FORS	1	FORS1
032 JR	1	Jr^a
033 LAN	1	Lan
034 VEL	1	Vel

Table 2
Examples of blood group antigens based on diallelic SNPs

System (ISBT No.)	Gene	Antigen/ antithetic	SNP*	Number in dbSNP
MNS (002)	*GYPA*	M (MNS1)	175C, 187G (20Ser, 24Gly)	rs7682260
		N (MNS2)	175T, 187A (20Leu, 24Glu)	rs7687256
	GYPB	S (MNS3)	199T (48Met)	rs7683365
		s (MNS4)	199C (48Thr)	
Lutheran (005)	*BCAM*	Lu^a (LU1)	274A (77His)	rs28399653
		Lu^b (LU2)	274G (77Arg)	
		LU8	655T (204Met)	rs28399656
		LU14	655A (204Lys)	
Kell (006)	*KEL*	K (KEL1)	698T (193Met)	rs8176058
		k (KEL2)	698C (193Thr)	
		Kp^a (KEL3)	1051T (281Trp)	rs8176059
		Kp^b (KEL4)	1051C (281Arg)	
		Js^a (KEL6)	2000C (597Pro)	rs8176038
		Js^b (KEL7)	2000T (597Leu)	
Duffy (008)	*DARC*	Fy^a (FY1)	365G (42Gly)	rs12075
		Fy^b (FY2)	365A (42Asp)	
Kidd (009)	*SLC14A1*	Jk^a (JK1)	1070G (280Asp)	rs1058396
		Jk^b (JK2)	1070A (280Asn)	
Diego (010)	*SLC4A1*	Di^a (DI1)	2710T (854Leu)	rs2285644
		Di^b (DI2)	2710C (854Pro)	
		Wr^a (DI3)	2121A (658Lys)	rs75731670
		Wr^b (DI4)	2121G (658Glu)	

(continued)

Table 2 (continued)

System (ISBT No.)	Gene	Antigen/ antithetic	SNP*	Number in dbSNP
Cartwright (011)	*ACHE*	Yt^a (YT1) Yt^b (YT2)	1196C (353His) 1196A (353Asn)	rs1799805
Scianna (013)	*ERMAP*	SC1 SC2	335G (57Gly) 335A (57Arg)	rs56025238
Dombrock (014)	*ART4*	Do^a (DO1) Do^b (DO2)	1159A (265Asn) 1159G (265Asp)	rs11276
Colton (015)	*AQP1*	Co^a (CO1) Co^b (CO2)	244C (45Ala) 244T (45Val)	rs28362692
Landsteiner-Wiener (016)	*ICAM4*	LW^a (LW5) LW^b (LW7)	338A (100Gln) 338G (100Arg)	rs77493670
Knops (022)	*CR1*	Kn^a (KN1) Kn^b (KN2) McC^a (KN3) McC^b (KN6) Sl^a (KN4) Vil (KN7) Yk^a (KN5)	4708G (1561Val) 4708A (1561Met) 4795A (1590Lys) 4795G (1590Glu) 4828A (1601Arg) 4828G (1601Gly) 4223T (1408Met)	rs41274768 rs17047660 rs17047661 rs3737002
Indian (023)	*CD44*	In^a (IN1) In^b (IN2)	252C (46Pro) 252G (46Arg)	–

*Nucleotide position in the coding sequence of the gene

A large variety of techniques for SNP genotyping has been developed during the last two decades [2]. Among the first methods that were developed the PCR with allele (or sequence) -specific primers (PCR-SSP) is the most common. PCR-SSP is a very cost-effective and robust method for the analysis of a limited number of SNPs in single or a low number of samples. This made PCR-SSP to an attractive method for routine labs and, therefore, genotyping kits for various blood groups were the first that became commercially available [3, 4].

Here, we describe PCR-SSP methods for typing of several blood group antigens from different systems. Most antigens and the antithetic antigens are based on diallelic SNPs in the corresponding blood group gene leading to a single amino acid change in the protein.

2 Materials

Prepare all solutions using ultrapure water and analytical grade chemicals. All pipetting steps should be performed using sterile filtered tips.

2.1 Buffer Stocks

1. 1 M Tris–HCl, pH 8.3: Add about 800 mL water to a 1-L glass beaker with a magnetic stir bar. Put in on the magnetic stirrer and adjust the stirrer speed. Weigh 121 g Tris and transfer to the beaker. Dissolve the Tris and add concentrated HCl while continuously measuring pH. After a pH of 8.3 is reached add water to a final volume of 1 L. Store at room temperature.
2. 3 M KCl: Weigh 223.7 g KCl and transfer to a 1-L glass beaker. Add water to a final volume of 1 L and dissolve the KCl using a magnetic stirrer. Store at room temperature.
3. 1 M $MgCl_2$: Weigh 203.3 g $MgCl_2$ hexahydrate (*6 H_2O) and transfer to a 1-L glass beaker. Add water to a final volume of 1 L and dissolve the $MgCl_2$ using a magnetic stirrer. Store at room temperature.
4. 0.5 M EDTA: Weigh 186.1 g EDTA and transfer to a 1-L glass beaker with a magnetic stir bar. Add about 800 mL water and put it on the magnetic stirrer. Add sodium hydroxide pellets to reach approximately pH 8 (*see* **Note 1**). Completely dissolve the EDTA and add water to a final volume of 1 L. Store at room temperature.
5. 1 % bovine serum albumin (BSA): Weigh 10 g BSA fraction V (A3733; Sigma-Aldrich GmbH, Taufkirchen, Germany) and transfer to a 100-mL glass beaker. Add water to a final volume of 100 mL and dissolve the BSA. Store aliquots of 10 mL at –20 °C.

2.2 PCR Reagents

1. PCR reaction buffer (10×): Mix 10 mL 1 M Tris–HCl (pH 8.3), 16.7 mL 3 M KCl, 1.5 mL 1 M $MgCl_2$, 10 mL 1 % BSA, and 61.8 mL water. Use 0.22 μM syringe filters for sterile filtration of the PCR buffer. Store aliquots of 10 mL at –20 °C.
2. Nucleotide (dNTP) mix (2 mM each): Add 9.2 mL water to a 15-mL Falcon tube and add 200 μL of each dNTP stock solution (dATP, dCTP, dGTP, dTTP; 100 mM; Bioron GmbH, Ludwigshafen, Germany) (*see* **Note 2**). Mix well by vortexing and store aliquots of 1 mL at –20 °C.
3. Gel loading buffer (10×): Weigh 100 mg Cresol Red (Sigma Aldrich) and dissolve in 10 ml water. In a 15-mL Falcon tube mix 5 mL glycerol, 4 mL water and 1 mL Cresol Red solution.
4. Red buffer mix (RBX): Mix equal volumes (e.g., 1 mL) each of the 10× PCR buffer, the 2 mM dNTP mix and the 10× gel loading buffer. Mix well by vortexing and store aliquots of 500 μL at –20 °C.
5. Taq DNA polymerase: 5 U/μl DFS-Taq DNA polymerase (Bioron) (*see* **Note 3**).

6. Primer mixtures (2×): Primer stock solutions of 100 μM in water or 10 mM Tris–HCl pH 8.3 should be stored at −20 °C. For each blood group antigen a 2× primer mixture is prepared in a 1.5 mL-tube by adding 5 μL of the specific primer, 5 μL of the corresponding generic primer (Table 3), and 1 μL each of the internal control primer F and R (*see* **Note 4**). Adjust to a final volume of 250 μl by adding 238 μl water (*see* **Note 5**).

Table 3
Primers for blood group antigen typing by PCR-SSP

Primer mix	Antigen specificity	Primer nucleotide sequence (5′–3′)	PCR product size (bp)
1	LU8	ctctcccagagggctacat	218
2	LU14	ctctcccagagggctacaa	218
1 & 2	(generic)	gaggtcaaaggccagcacag	
3	Js^a (KEL6)	tgcctgggggctgccc	187
4	Js^b (KEL7)	tgcctgggggctgcct	187
3 & 4	(generic)	ggcccttgacacttgcatac	
5	Di^a (DI1)	gggtggtgaagtccacgct	190
6	Di^b (DI2)	ggtggtgaagtccacgcc	189
5 & 6	(generic)	tcctgcctgccctagttctg	
7	Yt^a (YT1)	catcaacgcgggagacttcc	145
8	Yt^b (YT2)	catcaacgcgggagacttca	145
7 & 8	(generic)	gggaggacttctgggacttc	
9	SC1	ctctctccctctggcccg	136
10	SC2	ctctctccctctggccca	136
9 & 10	(generic)	cccttatattccggcatcagatc	
11	Do^a (DO1)	gttgacctcaactgcaaccagtt	192
12	Do^b (DO2)	gttgacctcaactgcaaccagtc	192
11 & 12	(generic)	ctccacatccctcctgaaag	
13	LW^a (LW5)	cgggttgggtgtcttacca	196
14	LW^b (LW7)	cgggttgggtgtcttaccg	196
13 & 14	(generic)	agagcgactgtcaactaccc	
15	Kn^a (KN1)	ggagaacagctgtttgagcttg	258

(continued)

Table 3 (continued)

Primer mix	Antigen specificity	Primer nucleotide sequence (5′–3′)	PCR product size (bp)
16	Kn^b (KN2)	ggagaacagctgtttgagctta	258
17	McC^a (KN3)	ccccctcggtgtatttctactaata	174
18	McC^b (KN6)	cccctcggtgtatttctactaatg	173
19	Sl^a (KN4)	gctccagaagttgaaaatgcaatta	141
20	Vil (KN7)	gctccagaagttgaaaatgcaattg	141
15 & 20	(generic)	ccatctgccattggtctggcactgc	
21	Yk^a (KN5)	ctcaaagtcattaattgggatcg	230
22	Yk^{a-}	ctcaaagtcattaattgggatca	230
21 & 22	(generic)	gagcttcatcccaaggtaac	
23	In^a (IN1)	ggtcgctacagcatctctcc	212
24	In^b (IN2)	ggtcgctacagcatctctcg	212
23 & 24	(generic)	ccattcagctgtgggaaagg	
25	Vel(+)	gcagcagggacggagtca	216
26	Vel(−)	gcagcagggacggagtcc	199
25 & 26	(generic)	ccaaaggctgcggtttgctg	

2.3 Agarose Gel Electrophoresis Reagents

1. 50× TAE electrophoresis buffer: Add about 700 mL water to a 1-L glass beaker with a magnetic stir bar. Weigh 242 g Tris and transfer to the beaker. Add 57 mL acetic acid and 100 mL 0.5 M EDTA. Dissolve the Tris and measure the pH (should be approximately 8). Add water to a final volume of 1 L. Store at room temperature.
2. TAE electrophoresis buffer (1×): To prepare 10 L electrophoresis buffer use 9.8 L water and add 200 mL 50× TAE buffer. Mix extensively and store at room temperature.
3. Agarose gel (2 %): Weigh 2 g agarose and transfer to a 250-mL Erlenmeyer flask. Add 100 mL TAE buffer (1×) and heat in a microwave oven until the agarose is completely dissolved. Cool down to approximately 60 °C and add 5 μl GelRed™ (10,000× in DMSO; Biotium Inc., Hayward, CA, USA) (*see* **Note 6**). Mix well and pour the agarose gel.
4. DNA size marker: A ready-to-use DNA size marker with fragments in the range of 50–2,000 bp such as MWM2 (Biovendis Ltd., Mannheim, Germany) is preferred.

3 Methods

The PCR-SSP methods were tested on different standard PCR cyclers including GeneAmp 9700 (Applied Biosystems), PTC200 (Bio-Rad), or Mastercycler (Eppendorf) each equipped with a 96-well sample block and a heated lid. Genomic DNA used for PCR-SSP should be prepared by commercial DNA isolation kits according to manufacturers' specifications.

3.1 PCR-SSP Setup

1. Primer and format selection: Select the 2× primer mixtures for the antigens that need to be typed in the DNA sample and decide about the PCR format: 8-tube strip for up to 4 SNPs (8 reactions) or 96 well plate for larger numbers of SNPs or DNA samples (*see* **Note 7**).
2. Mastermix: Calculate the number of reactions for each DNA and prepare one mastermix per DNA in a 1.5-mL tube. E.g., typing of 4 SNPs (8 antigens = 8 reactions): mix 27 μL RBX, 18 μL DNA (5–20 ng/μL), and 0.8 μL Taq polymerase (5 U/μL).
3. PCR setup: Load 5 μL of each desired primer mix to the PCR tubes and add 5 μL master mix to each PCR tube. Close the PCR tubes, mix well, and spin down.
4. PCR cycling: Use the same cycling program for all PCR-SSP (Table 4).

3.2 Agarose Gel Electrophoresis

1. Sample loading: Load 8 μL of each PCR on the agarose gel. Load the specified volume of DNA size marker to one lane.
2. Electrophoresis: Perform electrophoresis with approximately 10 V/cm distance between the electrodes in the electrophoresis chamber. Electrophoresis is completed when the cresol red has moved in the gel approximately 1.5–2 cm from the loading position.

Table 4
Standard cycling program for PCR-SSP

Step	Temperature [°C]	Time [s]	Number of cycles
1	95	120	
2	94 65	20 60	10
3	94 61 72	20 60 30	20
4	10	Hold	

3.3 Result Evaluation

1. Documentation: By placing the gel on a UV transilluminator the DNA fragments in the gel are visualized. Documentation can be performed by using a camera device.
2. Read-out of genotypes: For read-out of the genotype of a diallelic SNP the results of the two corresponding PCR-SSPs (one PCR-SSP per allele) have to be evaluated. The larger PCR product (upper band) corresponds to the internal control and the smaller PCR product (lower band)—if present—represents the allele-specific PCR-SSP product (Fig. 1). If only the internal control band is present this PCR-SSP is negative, i.e., the SNP allele (blood group antigen) is absent. In case of presence of the PCR-SSP product the internal control fragment may be weak or even absent. In either case the PCR-SSP is positive, i.e., the SNP allele (blood group antigen) is present (*see* **Note 8**).

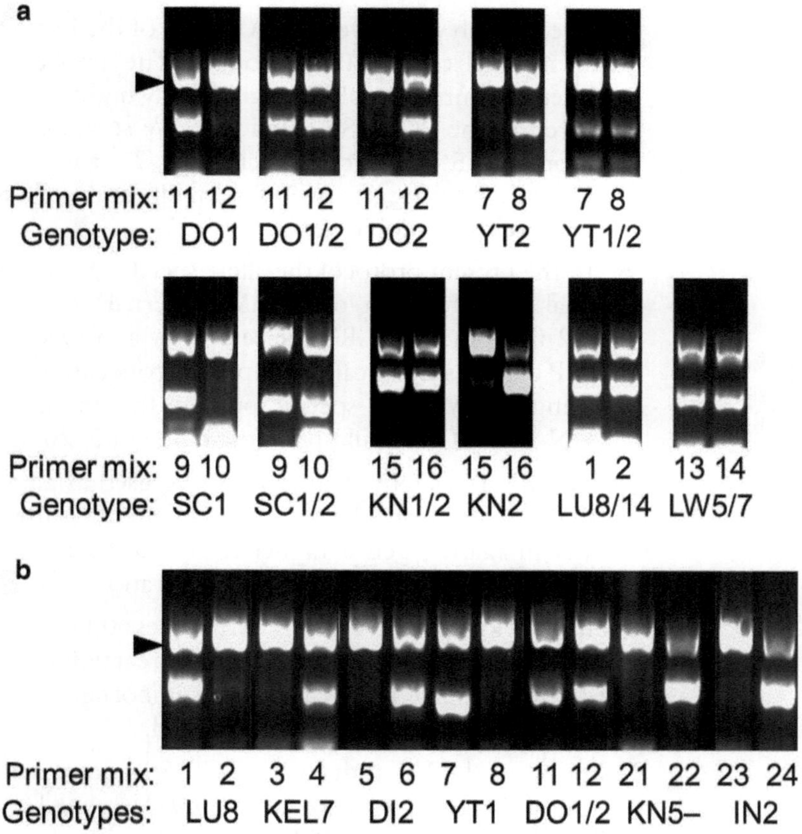

Fig. 1 Representative results from PCR-SSP typing of blood group antigens. (**a**) DNA samples from donors with known blood group phenotypes were used for validation of the PCR-SSP protocols. All samples revealed the expected genotypes for the different blood groups. (**b**) In this example a patient with unknown blood group antigens was investigated for LU8/14, Js^a/Js^b, Di^a/Di^b, Yt^a/Yt^b, Do^a/Do^b, Yk^a and In^a/In^b. From the genotypes it can be deduced that the patient is positive for the antigens LU8, Js^b, Di^b, Yt^a, Do^a, Do^b, In^b and negative for LU14, Js^a, Di^a, Yt^b, Do^a, Do^b, In^a and Yk^a

4 Notes

1. EDTA in water has a low pH and starts to dissolve at pH 8. Therefore, to get a 0.5 M EDTA solution it is important to increase the pH by adding NaOH either by using NaOH pellets or a 10 N solution.
2. Instead of using separate stocks of the four dNTPs many suppliers offer ready-to-use dNTP mixtures with a standard concentration of 2 mM of each dNTP. These mixtures can be used as well; however, costs are usually higher compared to single dNTP stocks at 100 mM concentration.
3. Any thermostable DNA polymerase can be used. The amount of units per reaction may be adapted due to differences between enzymes regarding stability and activity. Do not use enzymes with 3′–5′ proof reading activity. This will lead to positive results in PCR-SSP even when the DNA allele is not present.
4. Use a highly conserved DNA region of the human genome as an internal control PCR product. The amplicon size of the internal control should be significantly higher (>500 bp) compared to the PCR-SSP amplicons. We suppose the use of the F-primer 5′-ggttggccaatctactcccagg-3′ and the R-primer 5′-gctcactcagtgtggcaaag-3′ for amplification of a 540 bp fragment of the β-globin gene.
5. In the present protocol the allele-specific primers are used at a final concentration of 1 mM (internal control primers at 0.2 mM) in the PCR. The sensitivity and specificity of PCR-SSP depends significantly on primer concentrations [5]. When using 1 mM allele-specific primers the amount of genomic DNA per PCR should be in the range of 5–20 ng.
6. GelRed™ is a DNA stain that can be used as an alternative to ethidium bromide. The toxicity of GelRed™ is lower and sensitivity in agarose gels is higher compared to ethidium bromide due to a better signal-to-background ratio.
7. High or low profile 0.2 mL PCR tubes, tube strips or 96 well plates can be used. Because of the low reaction volume of 10 μL a tight sealing of the PCR tubes is important. Domed caps or specialized adhesive films are preferred.
8. In case of the Vel antigen the PCR-SSP determines the genotype of the 17 bp deletion in the *SMIM1* gene [6]. Individuals that show a negative PCR-SSP result with the Vel(+) allele-specific primer and a positive result with the Vel(−) primer are expected to have the Vel− blood group phenotype. The same is true for the Yk^a antigen, i.e., individuals that are negative in PCR-SSP with the Yk^a primer and positive with the Yk^{a-} primer are expected to be negative for the high prevalence antigen Yk^a.

References

1. Storry JR, Castilho L, Daniels G, Flegel WA, Garratty G, Francis CL, Moulds JM, Moulds JJ, Olsson ML, Poole J, Reid ME, Rouger P, van der Schoot E, Scott M, Smart E, Tani Y, Yu LC, Wendel S, Westhoff C, Yahalom V, Zelinski T (2011) International Society of Blood Transfusion Working Party on red cell immunogenetics and blood group terminology: Berlin report. Vox Sang 101:77–82
2. St-Louis M (2014) Molecular blood grouping of donors. Transfus Apher Sci 50:175–182
3. Inno-Train Diagnostik GmbH. http://www.inno-train.de
4. BAG Health Care GmbH. http://www.bag-healthcare.com/
5. Bugert P, Lese A, Meckies J, Zieger W, Eichler H, Klüter H (2003) Optimized sensitivity of allele-specific PCR for prenatal typing of human platelet alloantigen single nucleotide polymorphisms. Biotechniques 35:170–174
6. Ballif BA, Helias V, Peyrard T, Menanteau C, Saison C, Lucien N, Bourgouin S, Le Gall M, Cartron JP, Arnaud L (2013) Disruption of SMIM1 causes the Vel– blood type. EMBO Mol Med 5:751–761

Chapter 7

High-Resolution Melting Analysis for Genotyping Duffy Blood Group Antigens

Ewa Łukasik, Kazimiera Waśniowska, Magdalena Grodecka, Edyta Majorczyk, and Marcin Czerwiński

Abstract

Antigens of the Duffy (Fy) blood group are significant in medical transfusions since they may cause serious post-transfusion reactions and hemolytic disease of the fetus and newborn. Results of serotyping performed on donors with reduced or abolished erythrocyte Duffy expression may be misleading, since the Duffy antigen is also present on non-erythroid cells. In such cases only DNA-based genotyping may reveal the actual Duffy antigen status. Here we describe the high-resolution melting (HRM) method for Duffy genotyping, which is a new post-PCR analysis method used for identifying genetic variations in nucleic acid sequences. It is based on the PCR melting curve technique where single nucleotide polymorphism (SNP) in DNA determines a characteristic shape of the melting curve and melting temperature (Tm) of a sample. HRM analysis for *FY* genotyping can discriminate SNPs in the *FY* gene through detection of small differences in melting profiles of variants when compared to controls. Recently, we have shown the usefulness of HRM analysis in elucidation of the molecular basis of Duffy-negative phenotype in a Polish family and in large-scale Duffy genotyping.

Key words High-resolution melting (HRM) analysis, Blood group genotyping, Duffy antigen, Single nucleotide polymorphism (SNP), *FY* gene

1 Introduction

Duffy (Fy) blood group antigens are located on seven-transmembrane *N*-glycoprotein, expressed on erythrocytes and endothelial cells, which act as chemokine and malarial receptors [1, 2]. The Duffy blood group system consists of two major antigens, Fy^a and Fy^b, encoded by two codominant alleles designated *FY*A* and *FY*B*. *FY*A* and *FY*B* alleles differ by a single

Peter Bugert (ed.), *Molecular Typing of Blood Cell Antigens*, Methods in Molecular Biology, vol. 1310, DOI 10.1007/978-1-4939-2690-9_7, © Springer Science+Business Media New York 2015

nucleotide polymorphism (SNP) at position 125G>A of the *FY* gene that results in Gly42Asp amino acid change in the Fy^a and Fy^b antigens, respectively. The expression of the Duffy protein may be altered by the *FY*X* or *FY*B-33* alleles. The *FY*X* allele, found almost exclusively in Caucasians, is correlated with weak expression of Fy^b antigen. Fy^x antigen differs from the native Fy^b by the Arg89Cys and Ala100Thr amino acid substitutions due to SNPs: 265C>T and 298G>A in *FY*B* allele. The *FY*B-33* allele, frequent in Africans but very rare in Caucasians and Asians, is associated with SNP −33T>C in the promoter region of the *FY* gene, which suppresses erythroid expression of this gene [2]. The presence of antigen Fy^a and/or Fy^b on the erythrocytes determine three Duffy-positive phenotypes: Fy(a+b−), Fy(a−b+), and Fy(a+b+), while the Duffy-negative phenotype Fy(a−b−) is the result of the homozygous state of the *FY*B-33* alleles or the heterozygous state of the *FY*B-33* and *FY*X* alleles in Duffy genotype [3]. In order to identify all the *FY* alleles, we performed high-resolution melting (HRM) genotyping [3, 4].

High-resolution melting (HRM) is a novel technique for high-throughput post-PCR analysis of DNA variants [5]. It enables one to rapidly detect and categorize genetic mutations, especially single nucleotide polymorphisms (SNPs) or identify new variants in an analyzed fragment of a gene in multiple DNA samples without the need of nucleotide sequencing [6, 7]. HRM analysis is based on the melting temperature (Tm) evaluation at which 50 % of the DNA-double helix dissociates into single strands. In HRM genotyping, the region of interest is amplified by PCR, in the presence of double-stranded DNA-binding fluorescent dye. After the PCR step, the product is gradually melted by increasing the temperature, which results in a decrease of the fluorescence signal. The fluorescent dye is released during denaturation of double-stranded DNA and this effect is measured continuously on a specialized instrument to generate a characteristic melting curve. The resulting melting profile reflects the mix of amplicons present, and depends on the number of hydrogen bonds (GC pairs content), length of DNA double helix, sequence and its heterozygosity. The variations in the nucleic acid sequences, expressed by the different melting profiles, are distinguishable from each other by differences in melting temperatures (Tm) and curve shapes. The HRM method depends on melting curve analysis by fluorescent data, which has been made possible by both the improvement of instruments measuring sensitivity (high-resolution) and the discovery of saturating DNA dyes. Instruments for HRM, based on either capillary or the microtiter plate system (96 or 384 samples are analyzed simultaneously) are capable of detecting temperature alterations with high resolution (about 200 points per 1 °C) [8, 9]. HRM genotyping can be used to predict blood groups, resolve blood group incompatibilities and identify variant alleles and mutations [3, 10–12].

HRM analysis of several fragments of the *FY* gene can be used to detect any nucleotide polymorphism in a gene encoding Duffy blood group antigens. Duffy genotyping is particularly useful in determining Duffy antigens when antibodies are not available or are weakly reactive with Fy antigen, e.g., to confirm the presence of Fy^x antigen on erythrocytes. Recently, we have shown that HRM analysis, to genotype the Duffy blood group antigens, can be used to resolve all discrepancies between Duffy phenotype and genotype. Our data showed that the Duffy-negative phenotype in three Polish family members results from a rare combination of the *FY*B-33/FY*X* alleles. These individuals phenotyped as Duffy-negative can be exposed to Fyb + blood units with no risk of alloimmunization because their genotypes indicate Fy^x phenotype [3]. Here we present the protocols of HRM analysis to scan three fragments of the *FY* gene (Fy-33, FyAB, and FyX) to determine SNPs characterizing Duffy alleles, which allows for fast, precise, high-throughput analysis of multiple DNA samples without the need of nucleotide sequencing.

2 Materials

Reagents for HRM analysis and reaction conditions should be previously optimized to increase the performance of the HRM analysis (including instrument calibration for background and HRM dye). It is of utmost importance that variation is strictly avoided by improper assay design and optimization decisions. All reagents and solutions should be prepared using ultrapure water, and stored at room temperature (unless indicated otherwise) or according to the instructions of the manufacturer. A number of chemicals used in molecular biology can be hazardous. It is important that anyone working in a laboratory is aware of the information supplied in the form of MSDS (Material Safety Data Sheets).

2.1 Blood Sample and Leukocytes Preparation

1. Whole blood samples collected in closed-tubes with EDTA anticoagulant.
2. Erythrocyte lysis buffer, final concentration: 10 mM Tris–HCl pH 7.6, 5 mM $MgCl_2$, and 10 mM NaCl (*see* **Note 1**): Add 5 ml of 2 M Tris–HCl pH 7.6, 2.5 ml of 2 M $MgCl_2$, and 5 ml of 2 M NaCl to a 1-l graduated cylinder. Add water to a volume of 1-l and mix well.
3. Water for molecular biology, DEPC (Sigma-Aldrich, St. Louis, MO, USA).
4. 1.5 and 50 ml polypropylene reaction tubes.

5. Centrifuge for 50 ml reaction tubes (3K15; Sigma-Aldrich).
6. Microcentrifuge for 1.5 ml reaction tubes (5424 R; Eppendorf, Germany)

2.2 DNA Extraction from the Nucleus of the Leukocytes

1. Invisorb Spin Blood Midi Kit (STRATEC Molecular GmbH, Berlin, Germany), which contains all the necessary components: Proteinase K, Lysis and Binding and Wash Buffers, Tubes and Spin Filters (*see* **Note 2**).
2. 98 % ethanol.
3. Thermomixer for 70 °C (Thermomixer comfort; Eppendorf).

2.3 Equipment and Reagents for PCR Amplification and Sequencing (See Note 3)

1. MJ Mini gradient PCR apparatus (Bio-Rad, Hercules, CA, USA).
2. 0.2 ml PCR reaction tubes.
3. AmpliTaq Gold® DNA Polymerase (Applied Biosystems, Life Technologies, Carlsbad, CA, USA).
4. GeneAmp® 10× PCR Gold Buffer (Applied Biosystems).
5. 25 mM $MgCl_2$ (Applied Biosystems).
6. 10 mM dNTP (Fermentas, Thermo Scientific, Waltham, MA, USA).
7. Primers (5 μM; Table 1): Prepare each primer at a concentration of 5 μM in water. Store at −20 °C.
8. Genomic DNA (100 ng/μl): Prepare DNA solution at ~100 ng/μl in water. Store at −20 °C.
9. Bioinformatics software to analyze the results of sequencing (e.g., Finch TV).

2.4 Equipment and Reagents for PCR-HRM Analysis

1. 7500 Fast Real-Time PCR System (Applied Biosystems) (*see* **Note 4**).
2. HRM v2.0.1 Software (Applied Biosystems).
3. MicroAmp™ Optical 96-Well Reaction Plate with Barcode (Applied Biosystems).
4. MicroAmp™ Optical Adhesive Film (Applied Biosystems).
5. MeltDoctor™ HRM Master Mix (Applied Biosystems), which contains appropriate and optimized concentrations of: AmpliTaq Gold® 360 DNA Polymerase, dNTPs, $MgCl_2$, and double-stranded DNA-binding dye (*see* **Note 5**).
6. Primers (5 μM; Table 1): Prepare each primer at a concentration of 5 μM in water. Store at −20 °C (*see* **Note 6**).
7. Genomic DNA (~20 ng/μl): Prepare DNA solution at ~20 ng/μl in water. Store at −20 °C (*see* **Note 7**).

Table 1
Primer sequences used in this study

Primer/direction[a]	Location nt	Sequence (5′–3′)
DuffyAmpPromF[b]	nt -313 to -295	CTCAATCTCCCTTTCCAC
DuffyAmpPromR[b]	nt 219–235	AGGCACCAAGAGACCAG
DuffyAmpCodF[b]	nt 49–66	TCAAGTCAGCTGGACTTC
DuffyAmpCodR[b]	nt 807–824	GTTGACAACAGCAACAGC
DuffySeqPromR[b]	nt 57–72	ACTGAGGGGCAAACAG
DuffySeqCodF[b]	nt 87–104	CTATGGTGTGAATGATTC
DuffySeqCodR[b]	nt 344–328	ACGGGCACCACAATGCT
Fy-33F[a]	nt -106 to -87	CGTGGGGTAAGGCTTCCTGA
Fy-33R[a]	nt 1–20	CTGTGCAGACAGTTCCCCAT
FyABF[a]	nt 41–60	CTGAGAACTCAAGTCAGCTG
FyABR[a]	nt 181–200	AGGATGAAGAAGGGCAGTGC
FyXF	nt 228–247	CAGCACTGTCCTCTTCATGC
FyXR	nt 360–379	CAGAGCTGCGAGTGCTACCT

F and R—forward and reverse primer, respectively

Amp for Amplification, *Seq* for sequencing, *Prom* for promoter region, *Cod* for coding region (modified reproduction from ref. 3 with permission from Elsevier)

[a]Primer sequences suggested by Tanaka et al. [10]

[b]Primer sequences that we use for amplifying and sequencing promoter and coding regions of the *FY* gene

3 Methods

3.1 Blood Sample and Leukocytes Preparation

1. Collect the blood into tubes containing EDTA as an anticoagulant (*see* **Note 8**).
2. Transfer the blood (e.g., ~5 ml) into 50 ml tubes. Add erythrocyte lysis buffer to a volume of 40 ml and mix well (*see* **Note 9**).
3. Centrifuge at 1,500 × *g* for 10 min, at 18 °C.
4. Discard half of the volume of the supernatant and mix carefully to resuspend the cell pellet with the rest of the supernatant.
5. Refill the tube with the erythrocyte lysis buffer.
6. Mix well and centrifuge at 1,500 × *g* for 10 min, at 18 °C.
7. Discard the whole supernatant (*see* **Note 10**).
8. Repeat **steps 5**–**7**.

9. Add 2 ml of erythrocyte lysis buffer and resuspend the cell pellet.
10. Transfer the suspension into two 1.5 ml Eppendorf tubes.
11. Centrifuge at 587 × *g* for 5 min, at 18 °C.
12. Carefully remove the supernatant with a pipette (*see* **Note 11**).
13. Proceed with genomic DNA isolation or store the pellet at −20 °C.

3.2 DNA Extraction from the Nucleus of the Leukocytes

Isolate human genomic DNAs from the obtained leukocyte pellet using Invisorb Spin Blood Midi Kit (STRATEC, Germany) according to the manufacturer's recommendations with the following modifications:

1. For lysis of erythrocytes, use freshly made erythrocyte lysis buffer (10 mM Tris–HCl pH 7.6, 5 mM $MgCl_2$ and 10 mM NaCl) instead of the reagent from the kit (Buffer EL).
2. Elute DNA from the Spin Filters by adding water, instead of the reagent from the kit (Elution Buffer D) (*see* **Note 12**).
3. Determine DNA concentration and purity by A_{260}/A_{280} ratio using NanoDrop 2000 or Picodrop Microliter spectrophotometer (*see* **Note 13**).
4. Adjust the concentration of DNA to 20 ng/μl. Store at −20 °C.

3.3 PCR and Sequencing of the Promoter and Coding Regions of the FY Gene (see Note 14)

1. Carry out the PCR reaction in 20 μl reaction mix that contains (final concentrations): 1 U AmpliTaq Gold® DNA Polymerase, 1× buffer for Polymerase, 1.5 mM $MgCl_2$, 0.2 mM each dNTP, 0.2 μM of each primer (Table 1), 100 ng genomic DNA.
2. Run the PCR using the recommended conditions for the appropriate fragment (Table 2).

Table 2
PCR conditions for amplification of the promoter and the coding region

PCR stage	Fragment of the promoter region (°C)	Fragment of the coding region (°C)	Time
Initial denaturation	94	94	7 min
Amplification 30 cycles	94	94	30 s
	55	56	30 s
	72	72	2 min
Final extension	72	72	10 min

HRM – DNA samples screening for determine the Duffy polymorphism in FyX fragment

Materials:

1. one 96-well plate;
2. DNA samples from 25 donors (20 ng/μl)
3. DNA samples of controls appropriate for FyX fragment: known variant types: [1]wild type: 265C/C + 298G/G; [2]265C>T + 298G>A; [3]265C/C + 298G>A; [4]265C/C + 298A/A; [5]265T/T + 298A/A; [6]265C>T + 298A/A
4. Primer FyXF (5 μM)
5. Primer FyXR (5 μM)
6. MeltDoctor™ HRM Master Mix
7. H_2O for molecular biology

Method:

1. Add 1 μl of DNA sample (20 ng/μl) to each of three wells (do it in triplicates). *Remember: the last three wells are the negative control, do not add DNA into them! (wells H10, H11, H12).*
2. Prepare Premix consists of:
   - MeltDoctor™ HRM Master Mix : 100 x 10 μl = 1000 μl
   - Primer FyXF (5 μM) : 100 x 2 μl = 200 μl
   - Primer FyXR (5 μM) : 100 x 2 μl = 200 μl
   - H_2O : 100 x 5 μl = 500 μl
3. Add 19 μl of Premix to each well.
4. Place the plate into PCR-HRM instrument.
5. Program and run real-time PCR-HRM in the following conditions:

HRM condition:

1. Holding
   - 95°C 10'
2. Cycling 40x
   - 95°C 30"
   - 68°C 30"
   - 72°C 30"
3. Melting
   - 95°C 10"
   - 60°C 1'
   - 95°C 30"
   - 60°C 15"

Schematic diagram of a 96-well plate

	1	2	3	4	5	6	7	8	9	10	11	12
A	← control 1 →			← control 2 →			← control 3 →			← control 4 →		
B	← control 5 →			← control 6 →			← sample 1 →			← sample 2 →		
C	← sample 3 →			← sample 4 →			← sample 5 →			← sample 6 →		
D	← sample 7 →			← sample 8 →			← sample 9 →			← sample 10 →		
E	← sample 11 →			← sample 12 →			← sample 13 →			← sample 14 →		
F	← sample 15 →			← sample 16 →			← sample 17 →			← sample 18 →		
G	← sample 19 →			← sample 20 →			← sample 21 →			← sample 22 →		
H	← sample 23 →			← sample 24 →			← sample 25 →			← (-) control →		

Fig. 1 Sample protocol for PCR-HRM analysis for the FyX fragment

3. Samples prepared for sequencing are sent to a specialized company (Genomed, Warsaw, Poland). The results of nucleotide sequencing are analyzed with bioinformatics software (Finch TV 1.4.0).

3.4 PCR-HRM Analysis

Before starting HRM analysis, optimize the PCR conditions and reactions (*see* **Note 15**). To determine Duffy polymorphism, scan three fragments of the *FY* gene using primers listed in Table 1: Fy-33 fragment for the promoter region of 160 bp including SNP −33T > C; FyAB fragment for the coding region of 160 bp including SNP 125G > A; FyX fragment for the coding region for 152 bp including SNPs 265C > T and 298G > A. A sample protocol for PCR-HRM analysis for the FyX fragment is shown in Fig. 1.

Table 3
Components of the HRM-PCR

Components	Volume (μl)	Final concentration
MeltDoctor™ HRM Master Mix	10	1×
Primer Forward (5 μM)	2	0.5 μM
Primer Reverse (5 μM)	2	0.5 μM
Genomic DNA (20 ng/μl)	1	1.0 ng/μl
Water	5	–
Total volume	20	

Table 4
Conditions for the HRM-PCR

PCR stage	Fy-33 fragment		FyAB fragment		FyX fragment	
Initial denaturation	95 °C	10 min	95 °C	10 min	95 °C	10 min
Amplification 40 cycles	95 °C 67 °C 72 °C	20 s 20 s 20 s	95 °C 65 °C 72 °C	15 s 20 s 20 s	95 °C 68 °C 72 °C	30 s 30 s 30 s
Melting/dissociation	95 °C 50 °C 95 °C 60 °C	10 s 60 s 30 s 15 s	95 °C 60 °C 95 °C 60 °C	15 s 60 s 30 s 15 s	95 °C 60 °C 95 °C 60 °C	10 s 60 s 30 s 15 s

1. Add the required volumes of each component (Table 3) to the appropriate well of a PCR plate (*see* **Note 16**).
2. Prepare each sample in triplicate (*see* **Note 17**).
3. Seal the reaction plate with optical adhesive film.
4. Confirm that the liquid is at the bottom of the wells in the reaction plate (*see* **Note 18**).
5. Program a new experiment to amplify and melt the DNA, according to the guidelines for your instrument.
6. Put the plate into the instrument and run the HRM-PCR using the recommended conditions (Table 4) for an appropriate fragment (*see* **Note 19**).

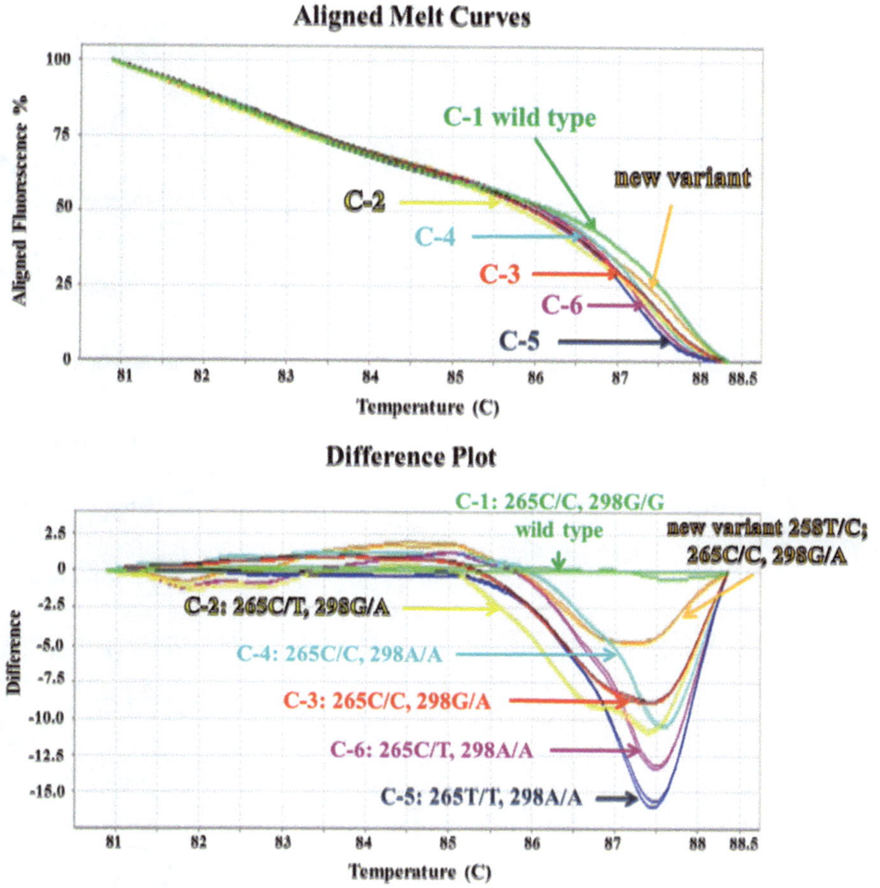

Fig. 2 PCR-HRM analysis of the FyX fragment of the *FY* gene, according to the protocol for the FyX fragment. The results are shown as Aligned Melt Curves plot (*above*) and Difference Plot (*below*). HRM curves, representing different SNPs of donors and control samples, are indicated by *arrowheads* in the Difference Plot. Wild type control was selected as the reference

7. Analyze the results using HRM software: The high-resolution melting data are presented in four graphs: Derivative Melt Curves plot and Raw Melt Curves plot, which scale the data in the Aligned Melt Curves and Difference Plot. The last two plots, present better the differences between variants. The Aligned Melt Curves plot displays the melt curves as percent melt over temperature and presents real differences in melt curve behavior of sequence variants. The Difference Plot displays the results of subtracting sample curves from the single reference run in the same experiment (Figs. 2 and 3).

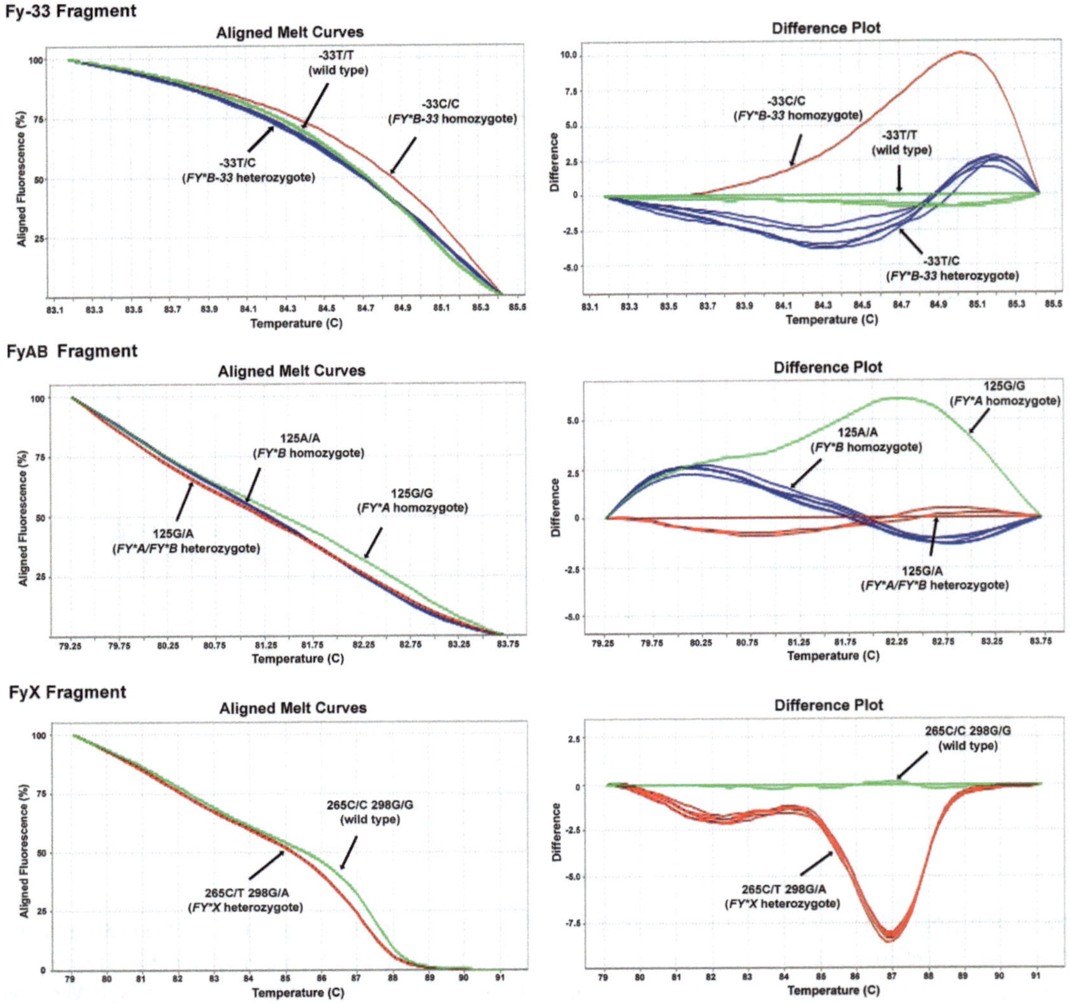

Fig. 3 PCR-HRM analysis of two coding fragments: FyAB and FyX and promoter fragment: Fy-33 of the *FY* gene. The results for all fragments are shown as normalized-shifted melting curves (*left*) and difference plots (*right*). HRM curves representing different SNPs of the Polish family members and control samples indicated by *arrowheads* were obtained for each analyzed fragment. Wild-type controls for the Fy-33 and FyX fragments and heterozygote control of the FyAB fragment were selected as the reference, reproduced from ref. 3 with permission from Elsevier

4 Notes

1. Erythrocyte lysis buffer should be fresh, made just before use. It is recommended to have ready-to-use components (e.g., 100 ml of each), stored at room temperature: 2 M Tris–HCl pH 7.6 (dissolve 24.2 g Tris in 80 ml H_2O, adjust pH to 7.6 with concentrated HCl at room temperature and add water to a final volume of 100 ml; pH of Tris buffer changes significantly with temperature); 2 M $MgCl_2$ (dissolve 4.06 g $MgCl_2 \times 6H_2O$ in 100 ml water); 2 M NaCl (dissolve 11.68 g NaCl in 100 ml water).

2. For HRM analysis, DNA should be isolated under non-salt conditions. Salt carryover may subtly change the thermodynamics of DNA melting transition, which can complicate the interpretation of the DNA melt curves, leading to lower reproducibility and higher error rates in HRM variant calls. Buffers with too high or too low pH can also carry over and impact HRM analysis. Dilution of the sample (in water) can help. We recommend using buffers and protocols of isolation that provide high yield and purity of the isolated genomic DNA.

3. HRM analysis may be preceded by the usual PCR reaction and sequencing of the promoter and the coding regions of the *FY* gene, of a few samples, to determine the controls for HRM genotyping. It is always recommended in HRM analysis to compare the melting profiles of the unknown and examined samples to the known and sequenced controls. Moreover, if there are any new melting profiles in HRM analysis, usual PCR and sequencing of the appropriate region of the *FY* gene are needed. The protocol of PCR reaction for amplifying fragments of the promoter and coding regions of *FY* gene is described in Subheading 3.3. The sequencing of these fragments is outsourced to a specialized company.

4. HRM analysis requires a PCR thermal cycler and an instrument with optics capable of collecting the numerous fluorescent data points. Alternatively, PCR can be performed on a thermal cycler followed by transfer to a real-time instrument for sample melt and data analysis. HRM analysis software needs to be capable of handling the large amount of data generated during HRM experiments.

5. We use Master Mix which has appropriate amounts of all necessary reagents for real-time PCR reaction: AmpliTaq Gold® 360 DNA Polymerase, dNTPs, $MgCl_2$ and high-resolution melting dye. If other reagents are used, HRM analysis has to be validated and optimized. Hot-start enzymes are recommended, since they increase the primer specificity. In addition, whichever dye is chosen, all the reactions should be optimized for that specific dye. Each dye interacts uniquely with the reaction components and amplicons, impacting the final results of the analysis. HRM-dye should have high fluorescence when bound to dsDNA, low fluorescence in the unbound state and should not inhibit PCR reaction.

6. Primer selection is a crucial step in HRM method setting. The primers need to be designed for maximum performance and must be specific to the region of interest. It is advisable to design three sets of primers and choose at least one that is highly active. The primer pair should be specific to the target and produce a minimum of nonspecific products and primer-dimers. Amplicons, with a length of ~200 bp, containing single nucleotide polymorphism (SNPs), are recommended

for HRM analysis. General guidelines for designing the primers include: a length of approximately 25 bp, an annealing temperature between 58 and 60 °C, and GC content between 30 and 80 % in each primer. Therefore, the specificity of primers must be checked, both in silico and under experimental conditions. The best annealing temperatures for each primer pair as well as numbers of cycles in a typical PCR reaction should also be determined. The appropriate length of the amplicons and their homogeneity should be confirmed by agarose electrophoresis.

7. Low-quality DNA may produce nonspecific PCR products. The amount of DNA template used in PCR should be consistent between samples, because large differences in starting templates can impact the resulting Tm.
8. If the blood samples are collected in advance, they should be stored at 4 °C.
9. The instructions for the Invisorb Spin Blood Midi Kit include DNA extraction from whole blood. We modified the protocol; first we isolated the leukocytes from the blood using fresh erythrocyte lysis buffer and then we extracted the DNA from leukocytes using reagents from the kit.
10. Do not remove the cell pellet!
11. If the pellet is red, wash again with erythrocyte lysis buffer.
12. We use H_2O for molecular biology for DNA elution from the Spin Filter. We elute two times, with 100 μl of H_2O and with 50 μl of H_2O. The DNA is collected and stored in two 1.5 ml Eppendorf tubes, each time.
13. The DNA-purity: A_{260}/A_{280} should be between 1.6 and 2.0. Concentration of DNA in the sample can be determined using A_{260}. An A_{260} of 1 indicates 50 μg/ml of double-stranded DNA.
14. Fragments of the promoter and coding regions of the *FY* gene may be amplified by PCR and sequenced using primers listed in Table 1. For determining the SNP-33T>C, the promoter region is amplified using DuffyPromAmpF and DuffyPromAmpR primers that flank a segment of 603 bp. The coding region, which includes the SNPs 125G>A, 265C>T and 298G>A, is amplified using DuffyCodAmpF and DuffyCodAmpR primers, that flank a segment of 776 bp. PCR products may be sequenced using the following primers: DuffySeqPromR for promoter regions, and DuffySeqCodF and DuffySeqCodR (Table 1) for coding regions.
15. Before commencing the determination of the Duffy polymorphism, the experimental conditions should be first checked. It is critical that the HRM instrument, all the reagents and conditions for each analyzed fragment work well in the laboratory environment.

16. If many samples are to be analyzed, first add DNA to each well. A premix can be prepared in an Eppendorf tube, which consists of an appropriate and calculated amount of HRM Master Mix, primer pair specific for each fragment and water. Remember to include excess volume in your calculations.
17. We recommend including replicates for significance, e.g., triplicates. Running multiple replicates makes it possible to more accurately define the variation within replicates of the same genotype or within different samples of the same sequence. If it is possible, include controls for each target sequence: samples with a known variant type (e.g., wild type control, homozygote control, heterozygote control) and a negative control—a sample without DNA.
18. If there is a need to wait before running the HRM experiment, protect the plate from light and store it at 4 °C. The plate should be allowed to warm up to room temperature before the run.
19. The instrument that we use allows to verify in real-time that the samples were amplified and melted. Typically, the fluorescence levels exceed the threshold between 20 and 30 cycles. During the Melt stage, Tm peak of each well is also seen. If there are any outliers (except the negative control), it is necessary to note in which well they are found. They may produce erroneous HRM results. Repeat the analysis of the sample, if necessary.

References

1. Grodecka M, Bertrand O, Karolak E et al (2012) One-step immunopurification and lectinochemical characterization of the Duffy atypical chemokine receptor from human erythrocytes. Glycoconj J 29:93–105
2. Daniels G (2013) Duffy blood group system. In: Daniels G (ed) Human blood groups, 3rd edn. Wiley-Blackwell, West Sussex, pp 324–341
3. Karolak E, Grodecka M, Suchanowska A et al (2013) Molecular characterization of the Fy(a-b-) phenotype in a Polish family. Transfus Apher Sci 49:313–317
4. Karolak E, Wasniowska K, Grodecka M et al (2013) Frequency of Duffy gene polymorphism in Polish population studied by High Resolution Melting (HRM) analysis. Vox Sang 105(Suppl 1):198–199
5. Wittwer CT, Reed GH, Gundry CN et al (2003) High-resolution genotyping by amplicon melting analysis using LCGreen. Clin Chem 49:853–860
6. Liew M, Pryor R, Palais R et al (2004) Genotyping of single-nucleotide polymorphisms by high-resolution melting of small amplicons. Clin Chem 50:1156–1164
7. Reed GH, Kent JO, Wittwer CT (2007) High-resolution DNA melting analysis for simple and efficient molecular diagnostics. Pharmacogenomics 8:597–608
8. Gundry CN, Vandersteen JG, Reed GH et al (2003) Amplicon melting analysis with labeled primers: a closed-tube method for differentiating homozygotes and heterozygotes. Clin Chem 49:396–406
9. Vossen RH, Aten E, Roos A et al (2009) High-resolution melting analysis (HRMA): more than just sequence variant screening. Hum Mutat 30:860–866
10. Tanaka M, Takahahi J, Hirayama F et al (2011) High-resolution melting analysis for genotyping Duffy, Kidd and Diego blood group antigens. Leg Med (Tokyo) 13:1–6
11. Soejima M, Fujimoto R, Agusa T et al (2012) Genetic variation of FUT2 in a Vietnamese population: identification of two novel Se enzyme-inactivating mutations. Transfusion 52:1268–1275
12. Hsu K, Lin YC, Chang YC et al (2013) A direct blood polymerase chain reaction approach for the determination of GP.Mur (Mi.III) and other Hil+Miltenberger glycophorin variants. Transfusion 53:962–971

Chapter 8

Molecular *RHD-RHCE* Analysis by Multiplex PCR of Short Fluorescent Fragments

Yann Fichou and Claude Férec

Abstract

Several hundred variant alleles have been reported within the homologous *RHD* and *RHCE* genes that encode the antigens involved in the human Rh blood group system, which is of the main interest in the field of both transfusion and obstetrical medicine. Although these variants can be mostly characterized at the molecular level by sequence-specific primer polymerase chain reaction (SSP-PCR) and/or direct sequencing, some allelic combinations remain unresolved by conventional methods. Typically exon deletion or hybrid genes may be difficult to assess in a heterozygous context. Here we describe a qualitative and quantitative method to resolve copy number variations in the *RH* gene exons by quantitative multiplex polymerase chain reaction (PCR) of short fluorescent fragments (QMPSF).

Key words Blood group, Hybrid gene, Polymerase chain reaction, QMPSF, *RHCE*, *RHD*

1 Introduction

The Rh blood group system is the most complex and polymorphic erythrocyte blood group including 54 antigens reported to date [1], among which the D, C, c, E, and e antigens are the most clinically relevant in the field of both transfusion and obstetrical medicine [2]. Since the discovery and the characterization of the two homologous *RHD* and *RHCE* genes, which encode, respectively, the antigens carried by the RhD and RhCE proteins [3–9], several hundred variants have been identified at the genetic level with typical ethnic/geographic associated patterns. *RH* gene variations have appeared through several mutational mechanisms within both the coding and noncoding sequences (RhesusBase version 2.0: www.uni-ulm.de/~fwagner/RH/RB2/) ranging from single-nucleotide variants (SNVs) (substitutions, insertions, and deletions), short indels, exon deletions and rearrangements, a combination of those latter mechanisms defining complex haplotypes, up to the whole deletion of the *RHD* gene, resulting

Peter Bugert (ed.), *Molecular Typing of Blood Cell Antigens*, Methods in Molecular Biology, vol. 1310,
DOI 10.1007/978-1-4939-2690-9_8, © Springer Science+Business Media New York 2015

in differential phenotypic expressions that may be characterized by panels of monoclonal antibodies [10].

While SNVs and short indels may be easily identified by direct sequencing and/or sequence-specific primer PCR (SSP-PCR) with different detection systems in a low- to high-throughput format engineered by academic laboratories or industrials [11–16], gene rearrangement and deletion can be visualized by the qualitative, PCR-based approach described by Maaskant-van Wijk et al. [17] at the end of the last century. Although very convenient and reliable this method is only applicable to hemizygous *RHD* samples, whereas *D-CE* hybrid genes in a heterozygous context cannot be resolved. We and others then thought to develop a quantitative method to assess hybrid genes in such a context [18, 19]. In a recent paper we reported the setup of a novel, convenient qualitative and quantitative PCR-based assay to investigate exon copy number variations and polymorphisms within both the *RHD* and *RHCE* genes [18]. This strategy displays many advantages, including the fact that the reaction is carried out in a closed-tube format, thereby reducing the chemical exposure of the technicians to potential harmful compounds; the whole procedure to treat 16 samples takes 4–5 h from DNA extraction to the final result, which is a rapid process for such a molecular analysis; and the method takes advantage of the universal fluorescent labeling [20, 21], which uses a single fluorescent dye-conjugated primer to label all PCR products, thus contributing to reduce the cost of reagents. Beyond these interesting features, the approach has proven its potency to characterize the most common hybrid gene structures found in diverse ethnic populations, to identify the common deletion of *RHD* exon 10 found in individuals originated from Western France [22], and most importantly to resolve some allelic combinations of compound *RHD* heterozygous samples.

Here we describe the technical procedure to carry out molecular QMPSF analyses of both the *RHD* and *RHCE* genes.

2 Materials

2.1 Primer Design and Mix

Two sets of ten gene-specific primer pairs, amplifying DNA markers that correspond to the 10 exons to be targeted, are designed for the *RHD* (NM_016124.3) and the *RHCE* (NM_020485.4) genes, respectively. Two additional sets of primers are designed to target the *HFE* (NM_000410.3) gene on chromosome 6, and the *F9* (NM_000133.3) gene on chromosome X. These products are positive amplification markers for all DNAs, while the *HFE* amplification product also serves as a normalization calibrator for quantifying exon copy numbers.

1. Export *RHD*, *RHCE*, *HFE*, and *F9* genomic sequences from UCSC Genome Browser hg19 (http://genome.ucsc.edu/).

2. Align the reference sequences of *RHD* and *RHCE* by ClustalOmega (www.ebi.ac.uk/Tools/msa/clustalo/) with default parameters.
3. Manually design primer pairs to target *RHD* and *RHCE* exons with at least one primer within an exonic sequence when possible (*see* **Note 1**).
4. Design primers for PCR amplification of *F9* and *HFE* markers with PrimerQuest[SM] (Integrated DNA Technologies, Coralville, IA, USA) (*see* **Note 2**).
5. Check all primer pairs by UCSC In-Silico PCR (http://genome.ucsc.edu/cgi-bin/hgPcr?command=start) (*see* **Note 3**).
6. Add a 16-bp nonhuman, universal sequence with a 4-bp spacer and a heptamer sequence to the 5′-end of forward and reverse primers [22, 23], respectively (*see* **Note 4**) (Table 1).
7. Prepare one mix per marker including the respective forward (F) and reverse (R) primers at a final concentration ratio (F:R) of 50 nM/5 μM in DNase-free water. Store at 4 °C.

Table 1
PCR primers for *RHD* and *RHCE* QMPSFs by universal fluorescent labeling

Gene	Exon	Size (bp)	Orientation[a]	Primer sequence[b] (5′ → 3′)	Concentration (nM)
HFE	2	254	F	U-AGCAGGACCTTGGTCTTTCCTT	2.0[c]; 1.5[d]
			R	H-ACCCTTGCTGTGGTTGTGAT	200[c]; 150[d]
F9	7	238	F	U-ACCATGACATTGCCCTTCTGGA	1.0[c]; 0.5[d]
			R	H-AGACATGTGGCTCGGTCAACAA	100[c]; 50[d]
RHD	1	247	F	U-CTCCATAGA**G**AGGCCAGCACA**A**	1.0
			R	H-CTGCTTCCAGTGTTAGGGC**C**	100
	2	172	F	U-CTTGGGCTTCCTCACCTC**G**A**G**	1.0
			R	H-TGTGATGACCACCTTCCCAG**A**	100
	3	122	F	U-CAGTC**G**TCCTGGCTCTCC**C**	0.5
			R	H-CTTCCCCAAGACAGCA**T**CC**A**	50
	4	221	F	U-ACTACCACATGAAC**A**TGA**T**GCAC**A**	3.0
			R	H-CCATTCTGCTCAGCCCAAGTA**G**	300
	5	159	F	U-GCTCTGCTGAGAAGTCCAATC**G**	1.0
			R	H-GCTCACC**T**TGCTGATCTTCC**C**	100
	6	191	F	U-TGGCTGGGCTGATCTCC**G**	0.5
			R	H-GCCAATAAGAGAATGC**G**CC**G**	50

(continued)

Table 1
(continued)

Gene	Exon	Size (bp)	Orientation[a]	Primer sequence[b] (5′ → 3′)	Concentration (nM)
	7	301	F	U-ACA**G**CTCC**A**TCATG**GG**CT**A**CA**A**	1.5
			R	H-CCAAGGTAGGGGCTGGACA**G**	150
	8	308	F	U-CTGGAGGCTCTGAGAGGTT**G**A**G**	1.0
			R	H-ACTGTCGGTGTCAGTAGTGCCATT	100
	9	176	F	U-T**T**AAAATATGGAAAGCACCTCATG**A**	2.0
			R	H-CTCATAAACAGCAAGTCAACATATATAC**T**	200
	10	260	F	U-AGGCTGTTTCAAGAGATCAAGCCA	1.0
			R	H-CTGAC**TCCAG**T**G**C**C**T**GCGC**	100
RHCE	1	185	F	U-GCTGCCTGCCCCTCTG**C**	0.5
			R	H-TGCTATTTGCTCCTGTGACCACT**G**	50
	2	244	F	U-CTTCCCCCTC**C**TCCTTCTC**A**	0.5
			R	H-GTGATGACCACCTTCCCAG**G**	50
	3	121	F	U-CAGTC**A**TCCTGGCTCTCC**T**TCTC**A**	0.5
			R	H-TTCCCCAAGACAGCA**C**CC**G**	50
	4	222	F	U-ACTACCACATGAAC**C**TGA**G**GCAC**T**	0.4
			R	H-GCCATTCTGCTCAGCCCAAGTA**T**	40
	5	160	F	U-GCTCTGCTGAGAAGTCCAATC**C**	0.75
			R	H-TGCTCACC**A**TGCTGATCTTCC**T**	75
	6	195	F	U-TGGCTGGGCTGATCTCC**A**	1.0
			R	H-TGAAGCCAATAAGAGAATGC**A**CC**A**	100
	7	138	F	U-ATTC**A**CCACA**T**CTCC**G**TCATG**C**	0.5
			R	H-CATGCCATTGCCG**TTC**C**A**	50
	8	308	F	U-CTGGAGGCTCTGAGAGGTT**A**A**A**	0.5
			R	H-ACTGTCGGTGTCAGTAGTGCCATT	50
	9	175	F	U-**C**AAAATATGGAAAGCACCTCATG**T**	1.0
			R	H-CTCATAAACAGCAAGTCAACATATATAC**C**	100
	10	359	F	U-AGGCTGTTTCAAGAGATCAAGCCA	1.0
			R	H-**G**A**TAGCATCA**T**CC**T**A**ATG**AAACTA**A**ACAT**	100

RHD and *RHCE* sequence-specific nucleotides are bold underlined; bp: base pairs

[a]F: forward; R: reverse

[b]U and H refer to the universal primer sequence 5′-FAM-GTCGTAGTCGACGACCGTTA-3′ and the 5′-GTTTCTT-3′ nucleotide heptamer, respectively

[c]Primer concentrations for the *RHD*-QMPSF

[d]Primer concentrations for the *RHCE*-QMPSF

2.2 DNA Samples

Adjust DNA concentration up to 50–100 ng/μL with DNase-free water (*see* **Note 5**).

2.3 PCR, Capillary Electrophoresis, and Data Mining

1. QIAGEN Multiplex PCR Kit (Qiagen, Courtaboeuf, France). Store at −20 °C.
2. Thermal cycler.
3. Highly deionized Hi-Di™ Formamide (Life Technologies, Saint Aubin, France). Store at −20 °C.
4. GeneScan™ 500 ROX™ Size Standard (Life Technologies). Store at 4 °C.
5. 3130*xl* Genetic Analyzer (Life Technologies) for capillary electrophoresis.
6. POP-4® Polymer (Life Technologies). Store at 4 °C.
7. GeneMapper® Software Version 4.0 (Life Technologies).

3 Methods

All steps can be carried out at room temperature. Prepare two PCR tubes per sample (i.e., *RHD*-QMPSF and *RHCE*-QMPSF). Always include a calibrator DNA with known gender and exon copy numbers in all series for normalization.

1. In a PCR tube, add 2× QIAGEN Multiplex PCR Master Mix (1× final concentration), *F9* primer pair mix, *HFE* primer pair mix, the ten *RHD*-specific primer pair mix (at concentrations indicated in Table 1), as well as the FAM-labeled, universal primer (0.5 μM final concentration). Complete with DNase-free water up to a final volume of 9 μL.
2. Proceed the same way for the *RHCE* gene by replacing the *RHD*-specific primers with the *RHCE*-specific primers.
3. Add 1 μL genomic DNA (50–100 ng/μL) in each tube, for a reaction volume of 10 μL.
4. Carry out the PCR in a thermal cycler in the following conditions: 95 °C for 15 min, and then 28 cycles at 95 °C for 30 s, 60 °C for 90 s, and 72 °C for 90 s. Hold at 4 °C.
5. Per reaction, mix 13.7 μL Hi-Di™ Formamide and 0.3 μL GeneScan™ 500 ROX™ Size Standard in a 96-well plate for sequencing.
6. Add 1 μL QMPSF product for a total volume of 15 μL.
7. Denature at 95 °C for 5 min, and then place on ice for 5 min.
8. Run the capillary electrophoresis in the 3130*xl*Genetic Analyzer (Fig. 1).
9. Import the .fsa files within GeneMapper® Software and process the data.

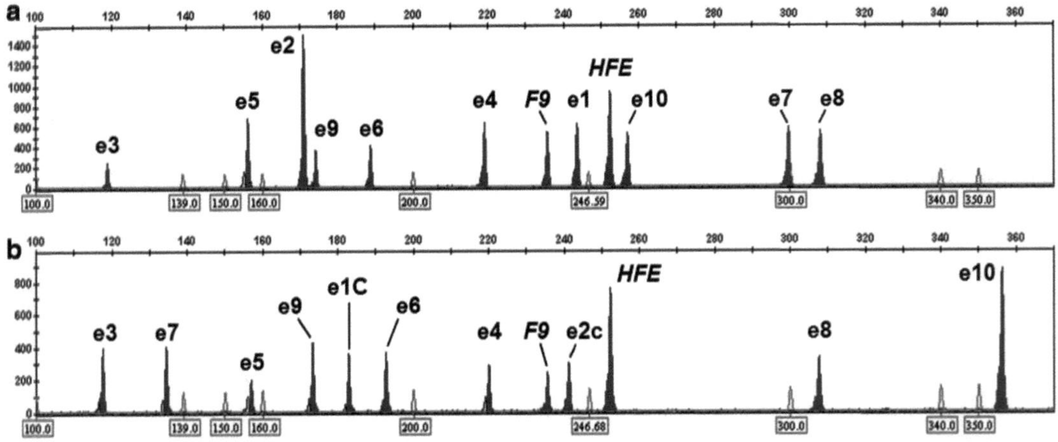

c

	HFE	F9	1	2	3	4	5	6	7	8	9	10
RHD	2	1	1	2	1	1	2	1	1	1	1	1
RHCE	2	1	1	1	2	2	1	2	2	2	2	2

Fig. 1 Male DNA sample carrying the *RHCE-D*(5)-*CE* allele as deduced from (**a**) *RHD*-QMPSF, (**b**) *RHCE*-QMPSF, and (**c**) exon calculation. (**a**) and (**b**): Marker IDs are mentioned above or next to the fluorescent peaks; e1 to e10: exon 1 to exon 10, respectively; *x*-axis: product length (bp); *y*-axis: fluorescence arbitrary unit. *F9* copy numbers ($n=1$) are identical in both analyses (i.e., *RHD* and *RHCE*), and in accordance with the known gender (male) in this sample. *RHD*-QMPSF (**c**) displays one copy per exon, except in exon 2 ($n=2$), which may be explained by the *C*/*c* heterozygous status of the sample [18], and in exon 5 ($n=2$). *RHCE*-QMPSF (**c**) results in one copy of both *RHCE**c* exon 1 and *RHCE**C* exon 2, in accordance with what predicted above concerning the *C*/*c* heterozygous status [18], and two copies of the other exons, except exon 5, which was found at one copy. Overall these analyses suggest that this DNA sample is *RHD* hemizygous (i.e., one copy of the gene), and carries two copies of the *RHCE* gene, including one allele with a *RHCE-D*(5)-*CE* hybrid gene structure

10. Select all peaks of interest and export table to an Excel datasheet.
11. Counting is carried out as previously described [24] by using the *HFE* peak area ($n=2$) of the calibrator DNA as the reference for normalization (*see* **Note 6**).

4 Notes

1. Several criteria are critical for primer design considering the high degree of similarity between these two paralogous genes, and the specificity of the multiplex PCR approach. First, include a gene-specific nucleotide at the 3′-end, when possible, to promote

gene-specific amplification. Second, homogenize theoretical primer melting temperatures to make sure that all products can be amplified in a single run of PCR at a similar annealing temperature (i.e., 60 °C ≤ Tm ≤ 66 °C in this work). Third, the theoretical length of the amplicons to be amplified is in the range of 90–350 bp, with at least a ≥4 bp difference to discriminate between two PCR products by capillary electrophoresis sizing. As exon 8 and the coding sequence of exon 10 are strictly identical between the two genes, targeting two allele-specific nucleotides within intron 7 (i.e., at positions c.1074-329 and c.1074-327) potentially allows to discriminate *RHD* exon 8 from *RHCE* exon 8, while PCR amplification of a marker with a highly divergent, reverse primer sequence within the 3′-UTR is sufficient to specifically identify either genes (Table 1). Overall, only the forward and the reverse primers of exon 8 and exon 10 markers, respectively, are not gene specific (Table 1).

2. Consider Tm and length criteria defined in **Note 1**.
3. Make sure that no variation, which may alter annealing between the primer and its target, has been reported in the primer sequences, and that primer melting temperatures are in the range of 60–66 °C.
4. Amplicon size extends 27 bp.
5. Both DNA concentration and quality are critical for proper exon dosage by QMPSF. A high-quality DNA extraction system is indeed mandatory. Qualifying DNA with a microvolume spectrophotometer, such as NanoDrop 2000 (Thermo Scientific, Courtaboeuf, France), is highly recommended before setting up the reaction. The 260/280 and 260/230 absorbance ratios, which are good indicators of nucleic acid purity, are ideally ~1.8 and in the range of 2.0–2.2, respectively. Exon copy numbering by QMPSF may be significantly altered, if not totally impaired, with template DNA exhibiting absorbance ratio(s) outside the range (±10–20 %).
6. Analysis is considered as reliable when marker *F9* copy number matches with the sample gender (i.e., $n = 1$: male; $n = 2$: female). All samples displaying a saturated fluorescence signal must be excluded from the analysis. Alternatively, dilute the QMPSF products, decrease the injection parameters, or carry out a novel PCR reaction with a reduced amount of template DNA.

Acknowledgements

This work was supported by the Institut National de la Santé et de la Recherche Médicale (Inserm) et l'Etablissement Français du Sang (EFS)—Bretagne.

References

1. Daniels G (2013) Rh and RHAG blood group systems. In: Daniels G (ed) Human blood groups, 3rd edn. Wiley-Blackwell, Chichester, pp 182–258
2. Klein HG, Anstee DJ (2005) The Rh blood group system (and LW). In: Klein HG, Anstee DJ (eds) Mollison's blood transfusion in clinical medicine, 11th edn. Blackwell Publishing, Oxford, pp 163–208
3. Avent ND, Ridgwell K, Tanner MJ et al (1990) cDNA cloning of a 30 kDa erythrocyte membrane protein associated with Rh (Rhesus)-blood-group-antigen expression. Biochem J 271:821–825
4. Chérif-Zahar B, Bloy C, Le Van Kim C et al (1990) Molecular cloning and protein structure of a human blood group Rh polypeptide. Proc Natl Acad Sci U S A 87:6243–6247
5. Colin Y, Chérif-Zahar B, Le Van Kim C et al (1991) Genetic basis of the RhD-positive and RhD-negative blood group polymorphism as determined by Southern analysis. Blood 78:2747–2752
6. Le Van Kim C, Mouro I, Chérif-Zahar B et al (1992) Molecular cloning and primary structure of the human blood group RhD polypeptide. Proc Natl Acad Sci U S A 89:10925–10929
7. Chérif-Zahar B, Mattéi MG, Le Van Kim C et al (1991) Localization of the human Rh blood group gene structure to chromosome region 1p34.3-1p36.1 by in situ hybridization. Hum Genet 86:398–400
8. Arce MA, Thompson ES, Wagner S et al (1993) Molecular cloning of RhD cDNA derived from a gene present in RhD-positive, but not RhD-negative individuals. Blood 82:651–655
9. Mouro I, Colin Y, Chérif-Zahar B et al (1993) Molecular genetic basis of the human Rhesus blood group system. Nat Genet 5:62–65
10. Flegel WA (2011) Molecular genetics and clinical applications for RH. Transfus Apher Sci 44:81–91
11. Wang D, Lane C, Quillen K (2010) Prevalence of RhD variants, confirmed by molecular genotyping, in a multiethnic prenatal population. Am J Clin Pathol 134:438–442
12. Silvy M, Simon S, Gouvitsos J et al (2011) Weak D and DEL alleles detected by routine SNaPshot genotyping: identification of four novel *RHD* alleles. Transfusion 51:401–411
13. Fichou Y, Le Maréchal C, Jamet D et al (2013) Establishment of a medium-throughput approach for the genotyping of *RHD* variants and report of nine novel rare alleles. Transfusion 53:1821–1828
14. Gassner C, Meyer S, Frey BM et al (2013) Matrix-assisted laser desorption/ionisation, time-of-flight mass spectrometry-based blood group genotyping–the alternative approach. Transfus Med Rev 27:2–9
15. Granier T, Beley S, Chiaroni J et al (2013) A comprehensive survey of both *RHD* and *RHCE* allele frequencies in sub-Saharan Africa. Transfusion 53(Suppl 2):3009–3017
16. Kappler-Gratias S, Auxerre C, Dubeaux I et al (2013) Systematic *RH* genotyping and variant identification in French donors of African origin. Blood Transfus 17:1–8
17. Maaskant-van Wijk PA, Faas BH et al (1998) Genotyping of RHD by multiplex polymerase chain reaction analysis of six RHD-specific exons. Transfusion 38:1015–1021
18. Fichou Y, Le Maréchal C, Bryckaert L et al (2013) A convenient qualitative and quantitative method to investigate *RHD-RHCE* hybrid genes. Transfusion 53(Suppl 2):2974–2982
19. Haer-Wigman L, Veldhuisen B, Jonkers R et al (2012) *RHD* and *RHCE* variant and zygosity genotyping via multiplex ligation-dependent probe amplification. Transfusion 53: 1559–1574
20. Shimizu M, Kosaka N, Shimada T et al (2002) Universal fluorescent labeling (UFL) method for automated microsatellite analysis. DNA Res 9:173–178
21. Guo DC, Milewicz DM (2003) Methodology for using a universal primer to label amplified DNA segments for molecular analysis. Biotechnol Lett 25:2079–2083
22. Fichou Y, Chen JM, Le Maréchal C et al (2012) Weak D caused by a founder deletion in the *RHD* gene. Transfusion 52:2348–2355
23. Fichou Y, Génin E, Le Maréchal C et al (2008) Estimating the age of *CFTR* mutations predominantly found in Brittany (Western France). J Cyst Fibros 7:168–173
24. Casilli F, Di Rocco ZC, Gad S et al (2002) Rapid detection of novel *BRCA1* rearrangements in high-risk breast-ovarian cancer families using multiplex PCR of short fluorescent fragments. Hum Mutat 20:218–226

Chapter 9

Microarrays in Blood Group Genotyping

Stephanie A. Boccoz, Gaëlle Le Goff, Loïc J. Blum, and Christophe A. Marquette

Abstract

Thirty-five blood group systems, containing more than 300 antigens, are listed by the International Society of Blood Transfusion (ISBT). Most of these antigens result from a single-nucleotide polymorphism (SNP). Blood group typing is conventionally carried out by serology. However, this technique has certain limitations and cannot respond to the growing demand for blood products typed for a large number of antigens. Here we describe a blood group genotyping assay, from genomic DNA extraction from whole-blood samples to results. After DNA extraction, the on-chip test is based on the hybridization of targets beforehand amplified by multiplex polymerase chain reaction, followed by a revelation step allowing the simultaneous identification of up to 24 blood group antigens and leading to the determination of extended genotypes.

Key words Blood group, DNA biochip, Microarray, Multiplex, Polymerase chain reaction

1 Introduction

Today, 35 blood group systems representing over 300 antigens are listed by the ISBT. Most of them have been cloned and sequenced [1, 2] unraveling the molecular bases of these blood group systems. The majority result from single-nucleotide polymorphism (SNP). Red blood cells (RBC) carrying a particular antigen may elicit an immune response if introduced in the blood circulation of a patient who lacks this antigen. It is the antibody produced during the immune response which is problematic and leads to donor/patient transfusion incompatibility, maternal-fetal incompatibility, and autoimmune hemolytic anemia. This immune response can be immediate or delayed and in some cases lethal. For this reason, antigen-negative blood is required for a safe transfusion. For decades the method of reference for testing blood group antigens has been the hemagglutination technique. However, this gold standard method has certain limitations (immunological reagent availability and specificity) when it comes to the determination of

Peter Bugert (ed.), *Molecular Typing of Blood Cell Antigens*, Methods in Molecular Biology, vol. 1310,
DOI 10.1007/978-1-4939-2690-9_9, © Springer Science+Business Media New York 2015

minor or rare blood group antigens, critical to fulfill a perfect matching between patient and donor [3]. Reagents are specialized and must be obtained from immunized patients or donors (polyclonal and monoclonal antibodies) or from immunized mice (monoclonal antibodies). Cost of immunological reagents keeps increasing and many antibodies are not available or weakly reactive, which is not suitable for the growing need of blood products typed for a large number of antigens. These limitations led to a relatively low number of donors typed for larger number of antigens, which limits the establishment of an antigen-negative inventory. In addition, antigen expression on the surface of the RBCs is often too weak to be detected by serology and discrepancies in serologic activity can occur between different manufacturers' reagents [4]. The identification of the molecular bases of most of the blood group systems paved the way for DNA-based assays as typing tools. One type of existing DNA-based assays uses DNA biosensors or microarrays (planar arrays or suspended bead arrays). Microarray-based genotyping tools allow testing of a large number of donors on a large number of antigens at potentially high throughput [3]. Moreover, they help overriding the limitations of serology, replacing the immunochemical reagents by synthetic and controlled probes. Here we describe a new blood group genotyping assay, from genomic DNA extraction of whole-blood samples to results analysis (Fig. 1). DNA is extracted from whole-blood samples and targets are amplified using biotinylated gene-specific primers. Then polymerase chain reaction (PCR) products are directly hybridized on the spotted microarray and labeled to produce stained positive spots which are detected and quantified using optical imaging. Images of each well are then processed in silico to produce scores useful for the sorting of the sample according to their genotypes. Examples of two multiplex PCR are presented, allowing the identification of 22 blood group antigens (KEL1/2, 3/4; JK1/2; FY1/2; MNS1/2, 3/4; in panel 1; YT1/2; CO1/2; DO1/2; LU1/2, HY+/–, JOa+/a– in panel 2), as well as two variants part of the Duffy system (*FY*Fy* and *FY*X*, in panel 1).

The purpose of this chapter is to give a protocol for implementation of blood group genotyping, with TKL (AXO Science, France) immobilization support and a colorimetric labeling. The user should adapt probe and primer panels according to his needs. The protocol described here is fully automatable with two liquid-handling systems (one for DNA extraction/PCR and the other one for hybridization). In this configuration, images taken with the Colorimetric Array Imaging Reader can be analyzed automatically on the principle that spot intensity can be directly connected to the genotype [5, 6] (Fig. 2; www.axoscience.com).

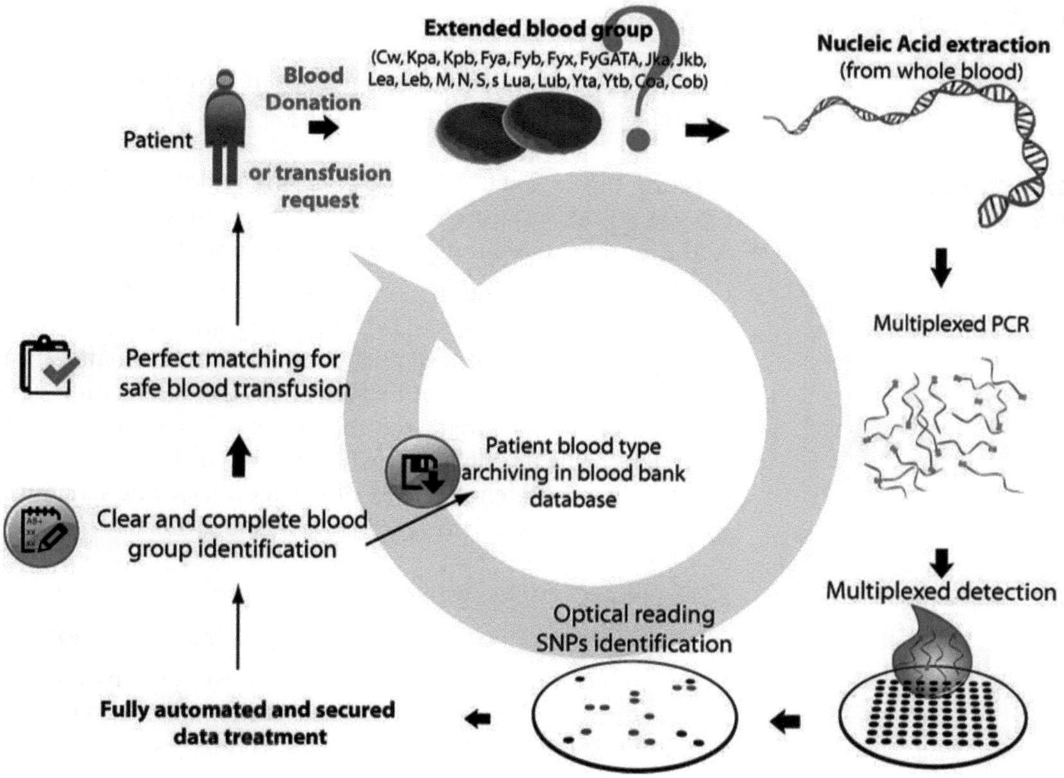

Fig. 1 RBC genotyping and transfusion safety

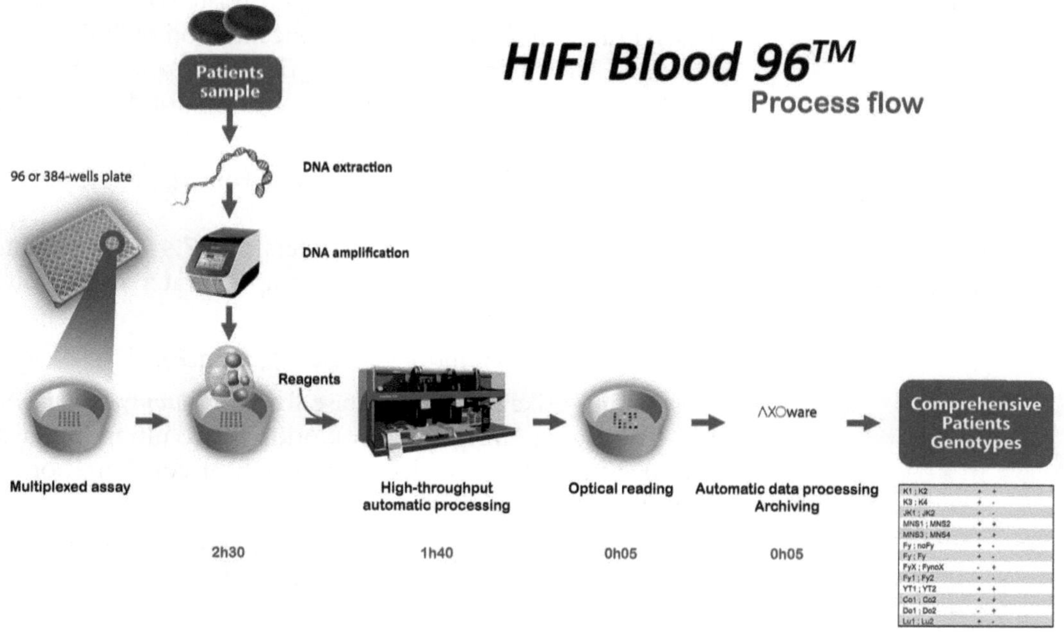

Fig. 2 Principle of *HIFI Blood 96*™

2 Materials

Use ultrapure or molecular biology-grade water (5Prime, Germany) to prepare all solutions.

2.1 Microarray Spotting

1. Spotting buffer 2×: 0.2 M NaAc, 0.2 M KCl, pH 5.5. Weight 0.6804 g sodium acetate and 0.37275 g potassium chloride. Add 25 mL water and dissolve with stirring. Store at 4 °C.
2. Oligo dT probe (positive control for spotting and hybridization composed of 16 dTs) and oligonucleotide probes (Eurogentec, Belgium). All probes carry a C6-amino modification at their 3′-end to bind to the TKL immobilization support. Add the appropriate volume of water in each probe tube to reach a final concentration of 150 μM and store at −20 °C. For confidentiality reasons, oligonucleotide sequences will not be disclosed here.

2.2 DNA Extraction

1. EDTA blood samples (with or without plasma). Store at −20 °C.
2. NucleoSpin® 96 Blood kit (Macherey-Nagel, France) (*see* **Note 1**).
3. Prepare the proteinase K solution by dissolving the lyophilized proteinase K in 3.35 mL Proteinase Buffer PB. Proteinase K solution is stable at −20 °C for at least 6 months.
4. Ethanol (>96 % grade).

2.3 Polymerase Chain Reaction

1. Oligonucleotide primers (Eurogentec): One primer in each primer pair is biotinylated. Add the appropriate volume of water in each primer tube to have a final concentration of 800 μM for primers of panel 1 and 600 μM for primers of panel 2. Store at −20 °C. For confidentiality reasons, oligonucleotide sequences will not be disclosed here.
2. GoTaq® G2 Colorless Master Mix kit (Promega, France).

2.4 Hybridization and Result Acquisition

1. Phosphate buffer saline (PBS) tablets pH 7.4 (AppliChem, France). Add one tablet for 1 L of ultrapure water and dissolve with stirring. Store at 4 °C.
2. LowCross-Buffer® (Candor Bioscience, France).
3. Streptavidin–Alkaline Phosphatase from *Streptomyces avidinii* (SAV-AP; Sigma Aldrich, France). Add 250 μL ultrapure water to 250 μg powder in order to have a final concentration of 1 mg/mL. Vortex and store at −20 °C.
4. BCIP®/NBT-Blue Liquid Substrate System for Membranes (Sigma Aldrich). Store at 4 °C (*see* **Note 2**).

2.5 Laboratory Equipment and Supplies

1. sciFLEXARRAYER S3 spotter (Scienion, Germany).
2. 384-Well microplate (Genetix, UK).
3. Microtiter sealing tape.

4. TKL immobilization support (AXO Science).
5. Bottomless 96-well plate (Dutscher, France).
6. 96-Well PCR plate (VWR, France).
7. Teleshake 95 (Inheco, Germany).
8. Falcon tubes, 15 mL.
9. Eppendorf tubes, 1.5 mL.
10. Twin.tec 96-well PCR Plate, skirted (Eppendorf).
11. Alumaseal II™ (Dutscher).
12. Thermocycler.
13. Vortex.
14. CPAC Ultraflat HT 2-TEC (heating and cooling unit; Inheco).
15. Colorimetric Array Imaging Reader (CLAIR; Sensovation, Germany).
16. HydroSpeed microplate washer (Tecan, Germany).
17. Optional: TECAN EVO 100 (liquid-handling system; Tecan).
18. Data analysis software (AXO Science).

3 Methods

Carry out all procedures at room temperature unless otherwise specified.

3.1 Microarray Spotting

1. Prepare the probe plate by dispensing 20 μL spotting buffer and 20 μL probe in each well of a 384-well microplate, according to the map plates 1 and 2 (Figs. 3 and 4). For negative control wells (T−), replace 20 μL probe with 20 μL ultrapure water. Mix by pipetting up and down in each well. Seal the plate with microtiter sealing tape and store at −20 °C until used.
2. Use a non-contact arrayer, preferably a sciFLEXARRAYER S3 spotter, to dispense arrays of probes at the bottom of a microtiter plate (350 pL per drop, 2 drops per SNP).
3. Store the printed microtiter at 4 °C.

	A	B	C	D	E	F	G	H	I	J	K	L	M	N	O	P
24	T-									dT	FynoFy	FyFy	K4	K3	K2	K1
23											JK2	JK1	MNS4	MNS3	MNS2	MNS1
22										T-	FynoX	FyX			Fy2	Fy1
21																
20																
...																
2																
1																

Fig. 3 Map plate for panel 1

	A	B	C	D	E	F	G	H	I	J	K	L	M	N	O	P
24	T-										HY+	dT	DO-2	DO-1	LU-2	LU-1
23											HY-		DI-2	DI-1	Cart-2	Cart-1
22											T-	T-	Jo(a-)	Jo(a+)	Co-2	Co-1
21																
20																
...																
2																
1																

Fig. 4 Map plate for panel 2

3.2 DNA Extraction

The protocol used here is the NucleoSpin® 96 Blood—vacuum processing. All reagents except ethanol are provided in the kit.

1. Thaw EDTA blood samples at room temperature for at least 15 min.
2. Prepare the wash buffer B5 by adding 400 mL 96–100 % ethanol (>96 % grade) in the bottle.
3. Dispense 200 μL blood and 25 μL proteinase K solution to each well of the lysis block. Add 200 μL BQ1 solution and mix three times by pipetting up and down. Incubate at 22 °C with shaking during 10 min.
4. Prepare the NucleoVac 96 Vacuum Manifold for binding/washing steps: insert spacers "MTP/MULTI-96 PLATE" in the manifold base. Place the MN Wash Plate in the manifold. Place the manifold lid on top of the manifold base. Place the NucleoSpin® Binding Plate on top of the manifold lid.
5. Add 200 μL 96–100 % ethanol in each well of the lysis block. Mix five times by pipetting up and down and transfer samples to the NucleoSpin® Blood Binding Plate (*see* **Note 3**).
6. Overlay samples with 150 μL B5 buffer in each well of the binding plate. Apply vacuum until all lysates have passed through the wells of the NucleoSpin® Blood Binding Plate (−0.2 bar for 5 min). Release the vacuum.
7. Preheat elution buffer BE to 70 °C (*see* **Note 4**).
8. Add 600 μL BW buffer to each well. Apply vacuum (−0.2 bar for 3 min) until all buffer has passed through the wells of the NucleoSpin® Blood Binding Plate. Release the vacuum.
9. Add 900 μL B5 buffer to each well. Apply vacuum (−0.2 bar for 1 min) until all buffer has passed through the wells of the NucleoSpin® Blood Binding Plate. Release the vacuum. Repeat a second time.
10. Raise the NucleoSpin® Blood Binding Plate, remove MN wash plate, and put it on a clean paper towel. Replace NucleoSpin®

Blood Binding Plate. Apply maximum vacuum (at least −0.6 bar) for 10 min to dry the membrane completely (*see* **Note 5**). Release the vacuum.

11. Prepare the NucleoVac 96 Vacuum Manifold for elution step: insert spacers "MICROTUBE RACK" in the manifold base. Place the rack of tube strips in the manifold. Place the manifold lid on top of the manifold base. Place the NucleoSpin® Binding Plate on top of the manifold lid.
12. Add 80 μL (*see* **Note 6**) BE buffer preheated at 70 °C, directly to the bottom of each well. Incubate for 5 min at room temperature. Apply vacuum for elution (-0.6 bar for 1 min). Release vacuum.
13. Close tube strips with cap strips for storage at 4 °C if used directly in multiplex PCR, or at −20 °C for a long-term storage.

3.3 Multiplex PCR

1. Equilibrate all the reagents to room temperature.
2. Prepare the primer mix for panel 1: in a 1.5 mL tube mix 6.25 μL of each primer. Mix by vortexing.
3. Prepare the primer mix for panel 2: in a 1.5 mL tube mix 6 μL of each primer. Mix by vortexing.
4. Prepare the PCR mix in a 15 mL tube: for panel 1 mix 1,400 μL 2× GoTaq® Colorless master mix, 90 μL panel 1 primer mix, and 1,310 μL nuclease-free water; for panel 2 mix 1,400 μL 2× GoTaq® Colorless master mix, 60 μL panel 2 primer mix, and 1,340 μL nuclease-free water. Mix by vortexing.
5. Dispense 25 μL PCR mix in each well of the 96-well PCR plate. Add 2 μL DNA template in each well.
6. Cover the plate with Alumaseal adhesive film.
7. Place the plate in a thermocycler and run the cycling program given in Table 1.
8. After cycling store the PCR plate at −20 °C.

Table 1
Cycling program for multiplex PCR

Step	Temperature (°C)	Time (min)	Number of cycles
Initial heat activation	95.0	15	1
Denaturation	94.0	0.5	35
Annealing	57.5	0.5	
Extension	72.0	0.5	
Final extension	72.0	10	1
	4.0	Hold	

3.4 Hybridization and Result Acquisition

1. Remove LowCross-Buffer® from the fridge 15 min before starting the protocol. Equilibrate the PCR plate and SAV-AP to room temperature.
2. Prepare PBS by dissolving 1 PBS tablet in 1 L water with stirring.
3. Prepare SAV-AP solution: dissolve 30 μL streptavidin–alkaline phosphatase (1 mg/mL) in 15 mL LowCross-Buffer®.
4. Remove protective films from the spotted plate (above and below the plate), and place it inside the CLAIR reader. Start initial imaging sequence. Once finished, remove the plate from the CLAIR.
5. Add 200 μL LowCross-Buffer® per well. Incubate at 37 °C for 10 min.
6. Wash three times with 300 μL PBS per well.
7. For each sample, dilute 27 μL PCR products with 50 μL LowCross-Buffer® and transfer onto the spotted plate. Incubate at 88 °C for 60 s, and then decrease the temperature to 55 °C.
8. Wash two times with 300 μL PBS per well.
9. Add 100 μL SAV-AP per well and incubate at 37 °C for 30 min.
10. Wash two times with 300 μL PBS per well.
11. Add 100 μL BCIP®/NBT solution per well and incubate at 37 °C for 30 min.
12. Wash two times with 300 μL ultrapure water.
13. Place the plate on the CPAC and allow the plate to dry for 10 min at 55 °C.
14. Place the plate into the CLAIR. Start final reading sequence. Once finished, remove the plate from the CLAIR (Fig. 5).

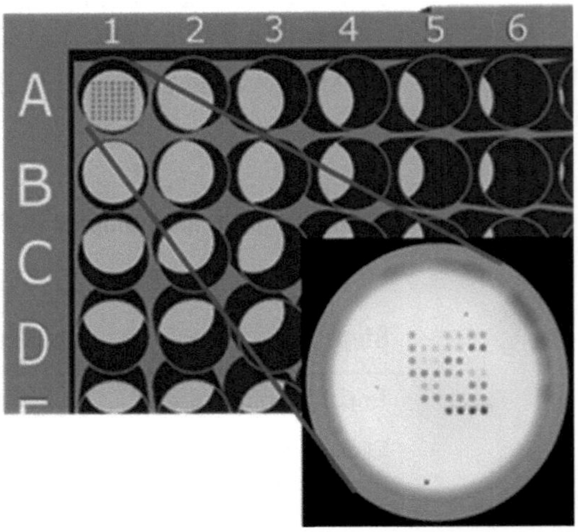

Fig. 5 Example of a result obtained at the end of the test

3.5 Results Analysis

1. Image obtained for each of the 96 wells should be analyzed using an image analysis software (for example AXOWare™) and the intensity of each spot should be quantified using 0–255 grayscale intensities.
2. Then, allele-specific spots (within one blood group system) should be compared. The easiest way to compare and sort the different genotype is to calculate a score for each biallelic system:

$$P_{\text{score}} = \left[I(A_2) - I(A_1)\right] / \left[I(A_2) + I(A_1)\right]$$

where $I(A_1)$ and $I(A_2)$ refer to the median spot intensity for a given allele, and to sort the different samples according to their P_{score}.

3. Depending on the patient's genotype, P_{score} values range in three different clusters (ideally around −1, 0, and 1).

3.6 Notes

1. Wear gloves and goggles in protection from chaotropic salts contained in BQ1 and BW buffers. All kit reagents must be stored at room temperature (18–25 °C) except proteinase K (store at 4 °C) and are stable for at least 1 year. Salts contained in buffers can precipitate. In this case, incubate for several minutes at 30–40 °C and mix until precipitate is dissolved.
2. BCIP is light sensitive. Remove from the fridge just before using.
3. Avoid moistening the edges of the wells when dispensing samples to prevent any cross-contamination.
4. Preheating BE buffer increases final yield from 10 to 15 %.
5. Ethanol contained in B5 buffer inhibits enzymatic reactions. It is very important to dry completely the columns before DNA elution.
6. A volume of 80 μL of BE allows to obtain approximately 65 μL DNA eluate.

References

1. Logdberg L, Reid ME, Lamont RE et al (2005) Human blood group genes 2004: chromosomal locations and cloning strategies. Transfus Med Rev 19:45–57
2. Logdberg L, Reid ME, Zelinski T (2011) Human blood group Genes 2010: chromosomal locations and cloning strategies revisited. Transfus Med Rev 25:36–46
3. Reid ME (2009) Transfusion in the age of molecular diagnostics. Hematology Am Soc Hematol Educ Program 171–177
4. Westhoff CM (2006) Molecular testing for transfusion medicine. Curr Opin Hematol 13: 471–475
5. Le Goff GC, Brès JC, Rigal D et al (2010) Robust, high-throughput solution for blood group genotyping. Anal Chem 82: 6185–6192
6. Boccoz SA, Bailly P, Brès JC et al (2013) Oral abstracts. Vox Sang 105:1–64

Chapter 10

Next-Generation Sequencing for Antenatal Prediction of KEL1 Blood Group Status

Klaus Rieneck, Frederik Banch Clausen, and Morten Hanefeld Dziegiel

Abstract

The KEL1 antigen can give rise to immunization of KEL2 mothers. Maternal antibodies can be transferred to the fetus and destroy fetal red blood cells and their stem cell precursors and give rise to serious fetal disease. It is important to be able to predict the fetal KEL status in order to intervene in those pregnancies where the fetus is at risk, and to ascertain when the fetus is not at risk. Technically it can be demanding to predict KEL1 status from a maternal blood sample. The KEL1 allele is based on a single SNP present in about 1–10 % of cell-free maternal DNA after gestation week 10. Here we describe our protocol for antenatal prediction of fetal KEL1 status by NGS analysis of maternal DNA on a MiSeq instrument.

Key words NGS, KEL, Antenatal, DNA, Phenotype prediction

1 Introduction

The KEL blood group can give rise to immunization of KEL2 mothers against KEL1 antigen after incompatible blood transfusion or fetomaternal hemorrhage [1, 2]. Maternal antibodies can be transferred to the fetus [3] and destroy fetal red blood cells and their stem cell precursors leading to serious disease. It is clinically important to predict fetal KEL status in order to intervene in those pregnancies where the fetus is at risk, and on the other hand to ascertain when there is no risk for the fetus.

Detecting fetal KEL1 in maternal plasma antenatally can be difficult as the fetal DNA only makes up a small proportion of the total cell-free DNA in maternal plasma [4]. We surmised that deep sequencing of PCR amplicons covering the KEL1 SNP could provide a method for reliable detection of low levels of KEL1 SNP in a background of the antithetical SNP, KEL2 [5]. Our experience is based on a small number of cases as it is rare to encounter a KEL1-negative mother carrying a KEL1-positive fetus while the mother has detectable anti-KEL1 antibodies [1]. Currently we do not

Peter Bugert (ed.), *Molecular Typing of Blood Cell Antigens*, Methods in Molecular Biology, vol. 1310,
DOI 10.1007/978-1-4939-2690-9_10, © Springer Science+Business Media New York 2015

reliably predict KEL1 status earlier than gestation week 10 and only pregnancies with one fetus have been investigated.

The method would be generally applicable for other antenatal amplicons as long as specific amplification and very deep sequencing are possible. This approach, however, is still rather costly but the price per sequenced base has historically been decreasing and this is expected to continue. It has been shown that it is possible to sequence a large proportion of the fetal genome but for antenatal diagnosis very deep sequencing is necessary surpassing the 200× coverage used for the whole fetal genome [6].

2 Materials

All reagents were of molecular biology grade including the water.

2.1 Reagents, Solutions, and Kits

1. dNTPs (Roche).
2. PAGE purified primers (Eurofins, Ebersberg, Germany).
3. Phusion hotstart DNA polymerase (New England Biolabs, Ipswich, MA, USA).
4. Bromophenol Blue (Sigma-Aldrich).
5. DNA Molecular Weight Marker V (Roche).
6. Ethidium bromide (Sigma-Aldrich).
7. Agarose (Sigma-Aldrich).
8. AMPure beads (Agencourt).
9. 70 % Ethanol.
10. Qubit high sensitivity assay kit.
11. NGS sequencing kit that includes sequencing buffer and chip (Illumina).
12. MiSeq washing solution: 0.5 % Tween 20 in water is prepared by adding 25 ml 10 % Tween 20 to 475 ml water.
13. 0.2 N NaOH (Merck) (*see* **Note 1**).

2.2 Equipment, Supplies, and Consumables

1. Vacuum collection tubes with either EDTA or citrate for anticoagulation of blood and needles for general blood sampling are used (*see* **Note 2**).
2. Automated DNA purification from 1.2 ml plasma using a Qiagen Symphony robot (Qiagen, Hilden, Germany) (*see* **Note 3**).
3. Plasma-purified DNA was PCR amplified on a PTC-200 thermocycler (MJ Research, Waterford, MA).
4. Standard gel electrophoresis equipment.
5. Gel documentation system G: Box (Syngene, Cambridge, UK).

6. Magnetic stand for 1.5 ml tubes.
7. Qubit instrument.
8. MiSeq system (Illumina).

3 Methods

For purification of PCR products, the Agencourt AMPure bead protocol from the manufacturer is followed without deviations. For DNA sequencing on the MiSeq, the on-screen guidance as well as the lab protocols are adhered to meticulously. And these protocols are described in brief here (*see* **Note 4**).

3.1 Blood Sample Handling and DNA Purification

1. Blood samples are stored at room temperature until DNA purification which should be performed as soon as possible and within 3 hours at the most.
2. Blood samples were centrifuged at 5,000 × *g* for 10 min at room temperature, and the plasma carefully removed by pipetting.
3. The plasma was stored at −20 °C until use in screw-cap tubes.
4. QiaSymphony instrument is used for DNA purification. DNA is eluted into 60 μl TE buffer (*see* **Note 5**).

3.2 DNA Amplification

1. KEL-specific PCR primers to amplify the KEL1/2 SNP are used as shown in Table 1. The primers consist of a gene-specific part, a short identity tag, and adapters used for attachment and in situ amplification in the MiSeq instrument (*see* **Note 6**) [5].
2. For the PCR 12 μl of the 60 μl purified DNA is used. We routinely set up this amplification in duplicate. The amplification is performed in a total volume of 20 μl containing 200 μM of each dNTP, 0.5 μM each of forward and reverse primers, and 0.02 U/μl Phusion hotstart DNA polymerase (*see* **Note 7**).
3. The amplification is done using the following cycling program: 98 °C, 30 s for initial denaturation; 45 cycles with denaturation at 98 °C for 5 s, annealing at 63 °C for 15 s, extension at 72 °C for 15 s. Heated lid and calculated temperature settings of the thermocycler are used during the PCR amplification.

Table 1
Primers used

Upstream primer (5′–3′)	AATGATACGGCGACCACCGAGATCTACACTCTTTCCCTACACGAC GCTCTTCCGATCTtagcGTAAATGGACTTCCTTAAACTTTAACCGA
Downstream primer (5′–3′)	CAAGCAGAAGACGGCATACGAGATCGTGATGTGACTGGAGTTCA GACGTGTGCTCTTCCGATCTCCATACTGACTCATCAGAAGTCT CAGC

3.3 Analysis of the PCR Product

1. Prepare a 2 % agarose gel containing ethidium bromide.
2. Mix 10 µl of the PCR solution with 2 µl marker containing bromophenol blue and load on the agarose gel. Also load DNA molecular weight marker.
3. Perform electrophoresis at 100 V for 30 min at room temperature.
4. Evaluate and document the PCR result using a gel documentation system.

3.4 Purification of PCR Product and Measurement of DNA Concentration

1. Purification by AMPure beads is performed by adding 10 µl PCR product to 18 µl AMPure beads after thoroughly resuspending the beads.
2. Mix the beads and PCR products carefully by pipetting ten times.
3. Incubate at room temperature for 10 min.
4. Place the mixture in the magnetic stand for 2 min and remove and discard the supernatant carefully by pipetting.
5. Wash the beads by adding 200 µl 70 % ethanol without removing the tube from the magnetic stand.
6. After 30 s, remove the ethanol and repeat the washing step once.
7. Remove the tube and resuspend the beads in water by pipetting ten times.
8. Place the tube back in the magnetic stand and after 1 min transfer the supernatant containing the purified PCR product into a new tube (*see* **Note 8**).
9. The DNA concentration of the purified PCR product is measured on a Qubit instrument using a Qubit high sensitivity assay kit.

3.5 Preparation of PCR Product for NGS Sequencing on MiSeq

The following steps are described in detail in the protocol "Preparing DNA libraries for sequencing on the MiSeq" found on the Illumina homepage (www.illumina.com).

1. First concentration of PCR product is adjusted to 4 nM. Using the equation as follows gives the volume of water that should be added to 5 µl PCR:

$$\left(\left(\left(\frac{1{,}000{,}000 \times \text{concentration of PCR product}\,(\mu\text{g}/\text{mL})}{\text{molecular weight of the PCR product}\,(\text{g}/\text{mol})}\right)\Big/4\right)\times 5\right)-5.$$

2. 5 µl of the 4 nM PCR product is mixed carefully with 5 µl 0.2 N NaOH, and incubated for 5 min at room temperature to ensure denaturation of the PCR product.
3. Cold buffer HT1 from the sequencing kit is added. This gives a 20 pM PCR product in 1 ml total volume.

4. 570 μl is combined with 30 μl likewise denatured PhiX control library resulting in 600 μl denatured PCR product with about 5 % spiked PhiX library ready for sequencing (*see* **Note 9**).

3.6 Setting Up the Sequencing Reaction on MiSeq

Before preparing the sequencing prepare a sample sheet with instructions for the MiSeq instrument. The Illumina Experiment Manager (IEM) v1.8 (or later versions) is a desktop tool that guides you in creating the sample sheet necessary for sequencing on the MiSeq. Sample sheets are files that must be created prior to starting a run and that contain the parameters for the run including the bar code number for the particular reagent kit at hand; this bar code number must also be entered into the sample sheet and is found on the Reagent Cartridge Label.

1. For automated analysis in BaseSpace a manifest file specifying the part of the genome to which alignment is wanted must be specified. For the KEL amplicon we have specified exon 6 chr7:142654980-142655039 in the manifest folder.
2. Once the sample sheet has been prepared by following the online instructions and copied into the correct folder in the MiSeq PC, the sequencing kit, e.g., the MiSeq® Reagent Kit v2 (50 cycle) (Illumina), can be thawed on a room-temperature water bath (*see* **Note 10**).
3. Load washing solution and ensure that the waste bottle is empty.
4. When the sequencing kit has been fully thawed, the 600 μl sample sitting on ice including the PhiX spike in is loaded into the sample well. The well cover is first pierced with a pipette tip.
5. The sequencing buffer is loaded, the waste container emptied, and the lever placed in the lowered position.
6. The sequencing cassette is loaded on the MiSeq and the screen instructions are followed. We routinely use upload to BaseSpace which means that the MiSeq PC must first be connected to the Internet.
7. The cluster generation and sequencing reaction are performed automatically on the MiSeq after pressing start. Finished DNA sequences will be aligned after the run.
8. After a number of cycles have been performed the software will show a number of quality parameters. Make sure to check these after the sequencing is complete.

3.7 Analysis of Sequencing

After sequencing the results can be accessed through the MiSeq reporter program that is used to process the base calls generated by the MiSeq Real Time Analysis software, and the MiSeq reporter program produces information about alignment and structural variants, for each alignment requested based on the analysis workflow specified in the sample sheet. The number of alignments is read from this result (*see* **Note 11**).

4 Notes

1. 0.2 N NaOH must be freshly prepared the same day.
2. We routinely do not trust material from earlier than gestational week 10 to yield reliable results and require that there be only one fetus. It has been estimated that about 75 copies (range 12–3,400) per ml plasma of a fetal gene are present in gestational week 25 estimated by PCR. More copies may be detectable by sequencing. Streck tubes may also be used.
3. Manual purification, e.g., with QIAamp® DNA blood midi kit does also work well.
4. The protocol is rather long but fairly straightforward once the PCR amplification has been optimized and once you have become acquainted with the MiSeq instrument which is easy to operate and very user friendly.
5. There is so little DNA at this stage that no attempts are made to measure it. The DNA can be stored at this stage but we always proceed with PCR amplification soon after DNA purification from plasma.
6. We have taken great care in designing the primers so as to avoid areas of polymorphism in the primer target area but one can never be sure, and an additional independently amplified PCR product would give extra security.
7. We used Phusion because of the low error rate. If using your own polymerase, please consult the vendor and familiarize yourself with the polymerase. We suggest using a polymerase with low error rate as the error rate will be a determinant of the highest sensitivity attainable. The 12 μl used for PCR would correspond to probing a plasma volume of 200 μl. The identity tag in the primers can be obviated if only a single PCR product is analyzed. Automated purification of plasma DNA is performed from about 1.2 ml when a nominal volume of 1 ml is desired. This extra volume allows for automated pipetting. Plasma DNA is rather stable; however, due to death of maternal leucocytes in the blood sample the percentage of fetal DNA will appear to diminish as a function of time. Thus it is advisable to purify plasma DNA soon after the blood sample has been collected [4]. The reason for choosing such long primers was to streamline the procedure which can be split into two with a primary amplification with gene-specific primers and a secondary PCR for appending the adaptors.
8. Agencourt AMPure beads should be used, not other methods for purifying PCR products; we have wasted time trying other methods. Freshly made 70 % ethanol should be used. Concentrated ethanol is hygroscopic; keep lids carefully closed.

9. It is necessary to register at the Illumina homepage to get access to protocols and supplementary software such as IEM which is necessary for preparation of sample sheets containing instructions for the sequencing as well as the alignment of the sequences. Strict adherence to the optimized protocols described in Illumina materials is highly recommended. We follow them carefully. Illumina has a well-functioning support help where competent Illumina employees can access the local MiSeq instrument and give on-screen help. The protocols as well as the kits for the MiSeq instrument are frequently updated and the latest version should be used.
10. As to choice of Sequencing kit (Illumina), we use single-pass sequencing of 75 bases. As only one of the primers is tethered to the sequencing chip the software will score a strand bias. It might be useful to consider including, in equimolar amounts, another PCR product amplified with different primers with the adaptors attached to the opposite strand from the primers shown in Table 1.
11. The result of the test is given as the number of KEL1 reads as percentage of all reads as well as the absolute number of acceptable reads. These data can be taken directly from the window of the MiSeq reporter program. We have currently set the cut-off at 0.5 % KEL1 sequences.

References

1. Nordvall M, Dziegiel M, Hegaard HK, Bidstrup M, Jonsbo F, Christensen B, Hedegaard M (2009) Red blood cell antibodies in pregnancy and their clinical consequences: synergistic effects of multiple specificities. Transfusion 49:2070–2075
2. Dziegiel MH, Koldkjær O, Berkowicz A (2005) Massive antenatal fetomaternal hemorrhage evidence for long-term survival of fetal red blood cells. Transfusion 45:539–544
3. Mathiesen L, Nielsen LK, Andersen JT, Grevys A, Sandlie I, Michaelsen TE, Hedegaard M, Knudsen LE, Dziegiel MH (2013) Maternofetal transplacental transport of recombinant IgG antibodies lacking effector functions. Blood 122:1174–1181
4. Clausen FB, Jakobsen TR, Rieneck K, Krog GR, Nielsen LK, Tabor A, Dziegiel MH (2013) Pre-analytical conditions in non-invasive prenatal testing of cell-free fetal RHD. PLoS One 8: e76990
5. Rieneck K, Bak M, Jønson L, Clausen FB, Krog GR, Tommerup N, Nielsen LK, Hedegaard M, Dziegel MH (2013) Next generation sequencing: proof of concept for antenatal prediction of the fetal Kell blood group phenotype from cell free fetal DNA in maternal plasma. Transfusion 53(Suppl 2):2892–2898
6. Lo YM, Chan KC, Sun H, Chen EZ, Jiang P, Lun FM, Zheng YW, Leung TY, Lau TK, Cantor CR, Chiu RW (2010) Maternal plasma DNA sequencing reveals the genome-wide genetic and mutational profile of the fetus. Sci Transl Med 2:61ra91

Chapter 11

454-Sequencing™ for the KEL, JR, and LAN Blood Groups

Carola Wieckhusen and Peter Bugert

Abstract

The KEL (ISBT 006), JR (ISBT 032), and LAN (ISBT 033) blood group systems are defined by a complex genetics with a large number of exons, and numerous gene variants. In order to sequence the 53 coding exons and flanking intron regions of all three blood group genes we developed a next-generation-sequencing method using 454-sequencing™ on a Genome Sequencer (GS) Junior™ system. Multiplex analysis of eight individual DNA samples was achieved using molecular identifiers.

Key words Next-generation sequencing (NGS), Pyrosequencing, Blood group antigen, Molecular blood typing, *KEL*, *ABCG2*, *ABCB6* genes

1 Introduction

Currently, there are 35 antigens known, defining the KEL (ISBT 006) blood group system. The JR (ISBT 032) and LAN (ISBT 033) blood groups are defined by one antigen, Jr^a and Lan, respectively. All three blood group systems have a complex genetics in common; that is, the three genes (*KEL*, *ABCG2*, and *ABCB6*, respectively) are characterized by a large number of exons and numerous gene variants have already been described [1, 2].

Here, we describe the primers and protocols for multiplex sequencing of the 53 coding exons of the KEL, JR, and LAN blood group systems using the 454-sequencing™ technology on a Genome Sequencer (GS) Junior™ system (Roche Applied Science, Mannheim, Germany). Compared to other next-generation sequencing (NGS) technologies the 454-sequencing enables significantly longer sequence reads of more than 500 bp. Taking this into account we designed 46 amplicons in a size range of 366–574 bp for sequencing all 53 coding exons of the KEL, JR, and LAN blood group genes. For multiplex sequencing of eight individual DNA samples we used the molecular identifiers (MIDs) developed by Roche.

Peter Bugert (ed.), *Molecular Typing of Blood Cell Antigens*, Methods in Molecular Biology, vol. 1310,
DOI 10.1007/978-1-4939-2690-9_11,

2 Materials

Prepare all solutions using ultrapure water and analytical grade chemicals. All pipetting steps should be performed using sterile filtered tips.

2.1 PCR Reagents

1. Primer mixtures (2×) for the first PCR: Primer stock solutions of 100 μM in water or 10 mM Tris–HCl pH 8.3 should be stored at −20 °C. For each amplicon a 2× primer mixture is prepared by adding 1 μL each of the primer F and R to 198 μL water giving a concentration of 0.5 μM each of the F and R primer (Table 1). The primer mixtures for all 46 amplicons could be prepared on a 96-well plate.

Table 1
Primers for the first PCR

Primer name	Sequence (5′–3′)[a]	Exon coverage	Product size
LANset1a-F LANset1a-R	aagactcggcagcatctccaAGTCCAACACCGAGCATTCC gcgatcgtcactgttctccaCCTGAAGTGTGGCCAGAAGC	1	550
LANset1b-F LANset1b-R	aagactcggcagcatctccaGGTGCTGATTCGCTGTCTTG gcgatcgtcactgttctccaCTCCCTTCTCCCTTTGCTTAG	1	496
LANset2-F LANset2-R	aagactcggcagcatctccaGCCTGTAAGTGCTGAATGTGTTC gcgatcgtcactgttctccaGGATCACGAGGTCAAGAGATC	2	498
LANset3-4-F LANset3-4-R	aagactcggcagcatctccaTGAAGGGTTTCTGGCTAGTGC gcgatcgtcactgttctccaCCTATACCTAGCAGGGTGAG	3,4	574
LANset5-F LANset5-R	aagactcggcagcatctccaCAGGCATTCCCTCAGCATCC gcgatcgtcactgttctccaTTGCCCTCTGCCCGCATTAC	5	504
LANset6-F LANset6-R	aagactcggcagcatctccaTCCATGCCTGAAGGTCTCCC gcgatcgtcactgttctccaCCCTCAGCTAGGTTAAGGTTTG	6	524
LANset7-8-F LANset7-8-R	aagactcggcagcatctccaTGTGTACATGGCAGGTAGTGG gcgatcgtcactgttctccaACCAGGCCAGGGCATTATTC	7,8	515
LANset9-10-F LANset9-10-R	aagactcggcagcatctccaAGGGCCAAGAGTGATAGTCG gcgatcgtcactgttctccaTGCTGGTTAGGACTTCTCTG	9, 10	550
LANset11-12-F LANset11-12-R	aagactcggcagcatctccaGGTTTGGCACCTACTACAGG gcgatcgtcactgttctccaGCACCTTCCATCACCAGAGC	11, 12	514
LANset13-F LANset13-R	aagactcggcagcatctccaGAAGGGCCGTATTGAGTTTGAG gcgatcgtcactgttctccaGCTGGGATTACAGGCATGTG	13	502

(continued)

Table 1 (continued)

Primer name	Sequence (5′–3′)[a]	Exon coverage	Product size
LANset14-F LANset14-R	aagactcggcagcatctccaGAGATCGCGCCATTGCACTG gcgatcgtcactgttctccaCCTTAACATGACTACTTTACTTGTG	14	366
LANset15-F LANset15-R	aagactcggcagcatctccaCCACACGGCTAGGATATGGG gcgatcgtcactgttctccaTGAGGATGGTGCGGGCAATG	15	508
LANset16-F LANset16-R	aagactcggcagcatctccaTGGTGTTGTCCTGCTAATCCC gcgatcgtcactgttctccaTGCGGTTGGCACAGACTTTG	16	495
LANset17-18-F LANset17-18-R	aagactcggcagcatctccaCAGCCTGCCTCCTTCCATTG gcgatcgtcactgttctccaGCTGCCACATGTCAGCATAC	17, 18	545
LANset19-F LANset19-R	aagactcggcagcatctccaGGACGGTAAGAGACACATAGATC gcgatcgtcactgttctccaCAAACAGGAAAGCCGTGTCAAG	19	554
JRset2-F JRset2-R	aagactcggcagcatctccaCAATGGTATGGGCCATTCATTG gcgatcgtcactgttctccaGCCCAGTTATTTCACTCCTAG	2	537
JRset3-F JRset3-R	aagactcggcagcatctccaTCAGGCAATCCTGCTTTGGTC gcgatcgtcactgttctccaGGTCAACTGCTACATGTCAATC	3	515
JRset4-F JRset4-R	aagactcggcagcatctccaGATCAGCCAATGGTGTCTTGC gcgatcgtcactgttctccaCAGATTCTCCCTGCCTTTTCAC	4	549
JRset5-F JRset5-R	aagactcggcagcatctccaGCAGAACTGCAGGTTCATCATTAG gcgatcgtcactgttctccaCCTCACTTCAGGTGCAGAATTC	5	511
JRset6-F JRset6-R	aagactcggcagcatctccaACAGGACTGGCACACGTTAG gcgatcgtcactgttctccaACACCCTCATCACAGACATC	6	441
JRset7-F JRset7-R	aagactcggcagcatctccaTGTCTGGGAAGACTGTCCTAG gcgatcgtcactgttctccaCCTTTGCTCTCCTTCAGGATTC	7	490
JRset8-F JRset8-R	aagactcggcagcatctccaCTCTAGCCTTACCTCCCTCAC gcgatcgtcactgttctccaCTGGTTGTTGCTTCCTACTATATGC	8	505
JRset9-F JRset9-R	aagactcggcagcatctccaCCTCCCAAAGTGCTGAGATTAC gcgatcgtcactgttctccaCCCAGGTGGAGTGAAGATAAC	9	547
JRset10-F JRset10-R	aagactcggcagcatctccaGGTGGTGCAATGGGAGGAAG gcgatcgtcactgttctccaCCTGGGCAACAGAGCATGAC	10	531
JRset11-F JRset11-R	aagactcggcagcatctccaCCACTGTGGAGACATAAGAG gcgatcgtcactgttctccaGGATATCAGGTCCCAAAGGC	11	550
JRset12-F JRset12-R	aagactcggcagcatctccaGTTTCCCTGGACTGAGTGTTC gcgatcgtcactgttctccaGCAACTGACTTCACCCATAGG	12	469
JRset13-F JRset13-R	aagactcggcagcatctccaACTGCCTGTAGCTCTTCATC gcgatcgtcactgttctccaGCCCCATTTACAGAATCCTC	13	525
JRset14-F JRset14-R	aagactcggcagcatctccaGTGCACATGCAGAGGAGAAG gcgatcgtcactgttctccaCTTTACTAGGAGGTATCTCCC	14	505

(continued)

Table 1
(continued)

Primer name	Sequence (5′–3′)[a]	Exon coverage	Product size
JRset15-F JRset15-R	aagactcggcagcatctccaGAAGGAGGAAGGAGCTATGG gcgatcgtcactgttctccaGCGCACAACTCACTTTATGG	15	504
JRset16-F JRset16-R	aagactcggcagcatctccaGGCTCCTTTAAGGAACAGTG gcgatcgtcactgttctccaGACCAGATTTCTTCCCCATGG	16	482
KELset1-F KELset1-R	aagactcggcagcatctccaCAAGGGCAAGATTGCTTGGG gcgatcgtcactgttctccaTATCTCGGAGCAGTGTTCCC	1	489
KELset2-F KELset2-R	aagactcggcagcatctccaGGGACAGGTTCGTTCTGAAG gcgatcgtcactgttctccaGACAGGGATGGGAAGAAGAG	2	494
KELset3-F KELset3-R	aagactcggcagcatctccaCTCCCAGGAGTTAAAGTAGG gcgatcgtcactgttctccaGGCTAGGCAAAGAACATCAG	3	497
KELset4-F KELset4-R	aagactcggcagcatctccaGAACTGTGGCCCTCGTAAGC gcgatcgtcactgttctccaGGCACAGAGTCACCCACTTG	4	497
KELset5-F KELset5-R	aagactcggcagcatctccaCAGCTTTGCAGGGCCATTTC gcgatcgtcactgttctccaGGGCATAACCATTTCCATCTCC	5	529
KELset6-F KELset6-R	aagactcggcagcatctccaAGCTGTGTAAGAGCCGATCC gcgatcgtcactgttctccaTGGCTCTGCTGCTCCATTTC	6	423
KELset7-8-F KELset7-8-R	aagactcggcagcatctccaGCCATCTCCCATGGTATATTCC gcgatcgtcactgttctccaGGTATTAAGGGCACTAGG	7, 8	529
KELset9-F KELset9-R	aagactcggcagcatctccaCAGAAGACTGTGGGCATGGG gcgatcgtcactgttctccaGTGGCAGGTTCCTCTTATCC	9	492
KELset10-F KELset10-R	aagactcggcagcatctccaTTGAAGGCTGCCTCTTCATC gcgatcgtcactgttctccaCAACTTGCCTGCTTCTATGG	10	507
KELset11-F KELset11-R	aagactcggcagcatctccaTGAGACCAGCTCTGAGGAAG gcgatcgtcactgttctccaTTTGTGGCCTGAAGCTGAAC	11	507
KELset12-13-F KELset12-13-R	aagactcggcagcatctccaAGGCCTCTCCTGATCCTGTC gcgatcgtcactgttctccaAGGAGGGTCAGAGAAGTGAC	12, 13	532
KELset14-15-F KELset14-15-R	aagactcggcagcatctccaTGGTCCCATTGGTGTTTGTC gcgatcgtcactgttctccaCCTCTTGGGAAACTCCCTAC	14, 15	518
KELset16-F KELset16-R	aagactcggcagcatctccaCCTTGGGACGTCAATGCTTAC gcgatcgtcactgttctccaTTGGTGCTGCCTAGGTGAG	16	494
KELset17-F KELset17-R	aagactcggcagcatctccaCTGGGAGGTGGGATAATAGG gcgatcgtcactgttctccaGGGATGCGAAGGGCAGAAAG	17	506
KELset18-F KELset18-R	aagactcggcagcatctccaGAATAGACGGCAACTTGGGG gcgatcgtcactgttctccaGGGTGCTGAATTAGGTAGAAG	18	525
KELset19-F KELset19-R	aagactcggcagcatctccaCCTCCTGGACTCCTATTGC gcgatcgtcactgttctccaCCAGGCATAGAACATAGCAG	19	508

[a]Each forward (F) primer and each reverse (R) primer carries universal adapter sequences (small letters) at the 5′ end

Table 2
Primers for second PCR

Name	Sequence (5′–3′)[a]
MultiplicomMID1-A	CGTATCGCCTCCCTCGCGCCATCAGACGAGTGCGTaagactcggcagcatctcca
MultiplicomMID1-B	CTATGCGCCTTGCCAGCCCGCTCAGACGAGTGCGTgcgatcgtcactgttctcca
MultiplicomMID2-A	CGTATCGCCTCCCTCGCGCCATCAGACGCTCGACAaagactcggcagcatctcca
MultiplicomMID2-B	CTATGCGCCTTGCCAGCCCGCTCAGACGCTCGACAgcgatcgtcactgttctcca
MultiplicomMID3-A	CGTATCGCCTCCCTCGCGCCATCAGAGACGCACTCaagactcggcagcatctcca
MultiplicomMID3-B	CTATGCGCCTTGCCAGCCCGCTCAGAGACGCACTCgcgatcgtcactgttctcca
MultiplicomMID4-A	CGTATCGCCTCCCTCGCGCCATCAGAGCACTGTAGaagactcggcagcatctcca
MultiplicomMID4-B	CTATGCGCCTTGCCAGCCCGCTCAGAGCACTGTAGgcgatcgtcactgttctcca
MultiplicomMID5-A	CGTATCGCCTCCCTCGCGCCATCAGATCAGACACGaagactcggcagcatctcca
MultiplicomMID5-B	CTATGCGCCTTGCCAGCCCGCTCAGATCAGACACGgcgatcgtcactgttctcca
MultiplicomMID6-A	CGTATCGCCTCCCTCGCGCCATCAGATATCGCGAGaagactcggcagcatctcca
MultiplicomMID6-B	CTATGCGCCTTGCCAGCCCGCTCAGATATCGCGAGgcgatcgtcactgttctcca
MultiplicomMID7-A	CGTATCGCCTCCCTCGCGCCATCAGCGTGTCTCTAaagactcggcagcatctcca
MultiplicomMID7-B	CTATGCGCCTTGCCAGCCCGCTCAGCGTGTCTCTAgcgatcgtcactgttctcca
MultiplicomMID8-A	CGTATCGCCTCCCTCGCGCCATCAGCTCGCGTGTCaagactcggcagcatctcca
MultiplicomMID8-B	CTATGCGCCTTGCCAGCCCGCTCAGCTCGCGTGTCgcgatcgtcactgttctcca

[a]MID sequences are underlined; sequences at the 3′ end (small letters) correspond to the adapter sequences of the primers for the first PCR

2. Primer mixtures (20×) for the second PCR: Primer stock solutions of 100 μM in water or 10 mM Tris–HCl pH 8.3 should be stored at −20 °C. For each MID adapter a 20× primer mixture is prepared by adding 10 μL each of the primer F and R to 180 μL water giving a concentration of 5 μM each of the F and R primer (Table 2).
3. For the first PCR: FastStart 10× puffer, dNTP mix, polymerase, all from *FastStart High Fidelity PCR System dNTPack* (Roche).
4. For the second PCR: HOTStar Taq Mastermix (Qiagen, Hilden, Germany).

2.2 Amplicon Library Reagents

1. 70 % ethanol.
2. AMPure beads.
3. 1× TE puffer: Mix 500 μL 1 M Tris/acetate pH 8 and 100 μL 0.5 M EDTA and fill with water to a total volume of 50 mL.

2.3 Emulsion-Based Clonal Amplification (emPCR) Reagents

1. Enzyme mix, PPiase, Amp mix, Amp primer A and B, additive, mock mix, emulsion oil, capture beads A and B, wash buffer, annealing buffer, enrich primer A and B, enhancing buffer, all from *GS Junior Titanium emPCR Kit* (*Lib-A*) (*see* **Note 1**).
2. 1× Wash buffer: Mix 0.5 mL of wash buffer with 4.5 mL water.
3. Isopropanol.
4. Melt solution: Prepare by mixing 125 μL NaOH (10 N) and 9.875 mL water.
5. Enrichment beads from *GS Junior Titanium emPCR Kit* (*Lib-A*).
6. Seq Primer A and B from *GS Junior Titanium emPCR Kit* (*Lib-A*).

2.4 454-Sequencing Reagents

1. *GS Junior Titanium Sequencing Kit* (Roche) including reagents, enzymes, buffers, packing beads, and supplement CB.
2. *GS Junior Titanium PicoTiterPlate Kit* (Roche) including PicoTiterPlate (PTP), cartridge seal, bead deposition device (BDD) gasket.

2.5 Laboratory Equipment

1. QIAxcel®Advanced system with Fast Analysis Kit (Qiagen, Hilden, Germany).
2. PCR cycler with 96-well block.
3. NanoDrop Lite (PEQLAB Biotechnologie GmbH, Erlangen, Germany).
4. Magnetic Particle Collector (MPC; Promega GmbH, Mannheim, Germany).
5. Heat block for 1.5 mL tubes.
6. Centrifuge for 1.5 mL tubes.
7. Ultra Turrax Tube Drive (UTTD; IKA GmbH, Staufen, Germany).
8. GS Junior Bead Counter (Roche).
9. GS Junior system (Roche).

3 Methods

We describe a procedure with two PCR steps, first for exon amplification and second for adapter fusion. PCR is followed by the standard procedures according to the Roche manual for amplicon library sequencing that includes amplicon library preparation, emulsion PCR, bead enrichment, and 454-sequencing (*see* **Note 2**).

Table 3
Cycling program for the first PCR

Step	Temperature (°C)	Time (s)	Number of cycles
Initial denaturation	95	180	
Denaturation	95	30	30
Annealing	60	45	
Extension	72	60	
Final extension	72	480	
	12	Hold	

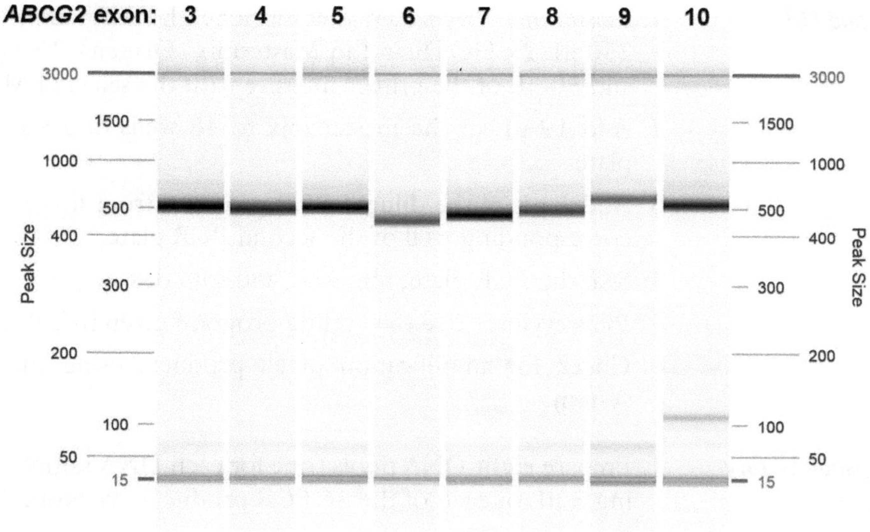

Fig. 1 Representative result from first PCR amplification of *ABCG2* exons 3–10. PCR products were analyzed using a QIAxcel® Advanced system with a Fast Analysis cartridge (Qiagen)

3.1 First PCR

1. Master mix: Prepare a master mix including 50 μL DNA (10–20 ng/μL), 100 μL FastStart 10× buffer, 20 μL dNTP mix, 10 μL FastStart polymerase, and 320 μL water.
2. Add 10 μL of each primer mixture to a 96-well PCR plate.
3. Add 10 μL of the master mix to each primer mix.
4. Seal the PCR plate, mix well, and spin down.
5. PCR cycling: Use the cycling program given in Table 3.
6. Check for amplification of all products using the QIAxcel system (Fig. 1).
7. Prepare a 1:100 dilution of each of the first PCR products by adding 2 μL PCR product to 198 μL water in a 96-well plate.

Table 4
Cycling program for the second PCR

Step	Temperature (°C)	Time (s)	Number of cycles
Initial denaturation	95	900	
Denaturation	95	30	20
Annealing	65	30	
Extension	72	60	
Final extension	72	600	
	12	hold	

3.2 Second PCR

1. Master mix: Prepare a master mix for each DNA sample including 250 μL 2× HOTStar Taq Mastermix (Qiagen), 150 μL water, and 50 μL of the primer mixture with the selected MID.
2. Add 19 μL of the master mix to 46 wells of a 96-well PCR plate.
3. Add 1 μL of the diluted PCR products from first PCR to the corresponding well of the second PCR plate.
4. Seal the PCR plate, mix well, and spin down.
5. PCR cycling: Use the cycling program given in Table 4.
6. Check for amplification of all products using the QIAxcel system.

3.3 Amplicon Library Preparation

1. Prepare eight DNA pools (one for each DNA sample) by pooling 5 μL of each of the 46 PCR products (*see* **Note 3**).
2. Follow the instructions given in the Roche manual [3]. The magnetic AMPure beads are used to purify the pooled amplicons.
3. Measure the DNA concentration of each purified amplicon pool by using a NanoDrop Lite instrument (*see* **Note 4**).
4. The mean size of all 46 amplicons in a pool is 510 bp (*see* PCR product sizes given in Table 1). Use the following equation to calculate the numbers of molecules/μL:

$$\left(\mathrm{DNA}\left(\mathrm{ng}/\mu\mathrm{L}\right)\times 6.022\times 10^{23}\right)/\left(656.6\times 1{,}000{,}000{,}000\times 510\left(\mathrm{bp}\right)\right) = \mathrm{molecules}/\mu\mathrm{L}$$

5. Dilute each DNA pool to a final concentration of 10^9 molecules/μL by using 1× TE buffer. Prepare 500 μL of each diluted amplicon pool and store aliquots of 100 μL at −20 °C.
6. Prepare the amplicon library by pooling 50 μL of each amplicon pool. Dilute the library concentration from 10^9 molecules/μL to 10^6 molecules/μL in a 10× dilution series using 1× TE buffer. Prepare 500 μL of the diluted library and store aliquots of 100 μL at −20 °C.

3.4 Emulsion-Based Clonal Amplification (emPCR)

1. The aim of the emPCR is the clonal amplification of a single-DNA molecule per bead. Follow the instructions given in the Roche manual [3] (*see* **Note 5**).
2. After the amplification reaction (in a 96-well plate) pool there is the collection of the emulsion and rinsing of the used wells of the 96-well plate with isopropanol (*see* **Note 6**).
3. Continue with the bead washes and recovery by following the instructions given in the Roche manual [4].

3.5 454-Sequencing™

1. The first step of the sequencing procedure is the pre-wash. Either use the PTP from a previous run or install a used but intact one (including a cartridge seal). Follow the instructions given in the Roche Manual [5].
2. The second step is the preparation and deposition of the different beads (4 layers) in the BDD. The first layer to be loaded is layer 1, and layer 4 is last. Each layer is prepared separately. For loading use 350 µL of each layer: layer 1, enzyme beads pre-layer; layer 2, DNA and packing beads; layer 3, enzyme beads post-layer; layer 4, PPiase beads.
3. The third part of the sequencing procedure is the priming of the instrument with reagents and buffers. Strictly follow the Roche manual instructions (*see* **Note 7**).
4. Preparing the GS Junior Instrument PTP Cartridge: Follow the given instructions (*see* **Note 8**).
5. The fourth step is the sequencing run. Stick to the given instructions from the Roche manual. You get to choose the number of cycles, depending on the number of bases (for JR, Lan, and Kel 200 cycles, approximately 500 bases). Next you can select the data processing scheme for the run (in our case: full processing for amplicon libraries). Load the PTP device into the cartridge (*see* **Note 9**) and start the sequencing run.

3.6 Result Evaluation

1. For the evaluation of sequencing results use the *GS Amplicon Variant Analyzer* software and create a project for the KEL, JR, and LAN sequencing.
2. Load the genomic reference sequences for the *KEL*, *ABCG2*, and *ABCB6* genes from the gene database.
3. Define the amplicons by entering the primer sequences used for exon amplification (*see* Table 1).
4. Load the data from the sequencing run and assign the eight MIDs to the DNA samples analyzed.
5. Start computation for variant identification with a minimum read count of 2 and a minimum read percentage of 0.25 % in the bidirectional mode.
6. Check for sequence read coverage of each amplicon in each sample. Specific variants can be further evaluated in the Global Alignment view (Fig. 2).

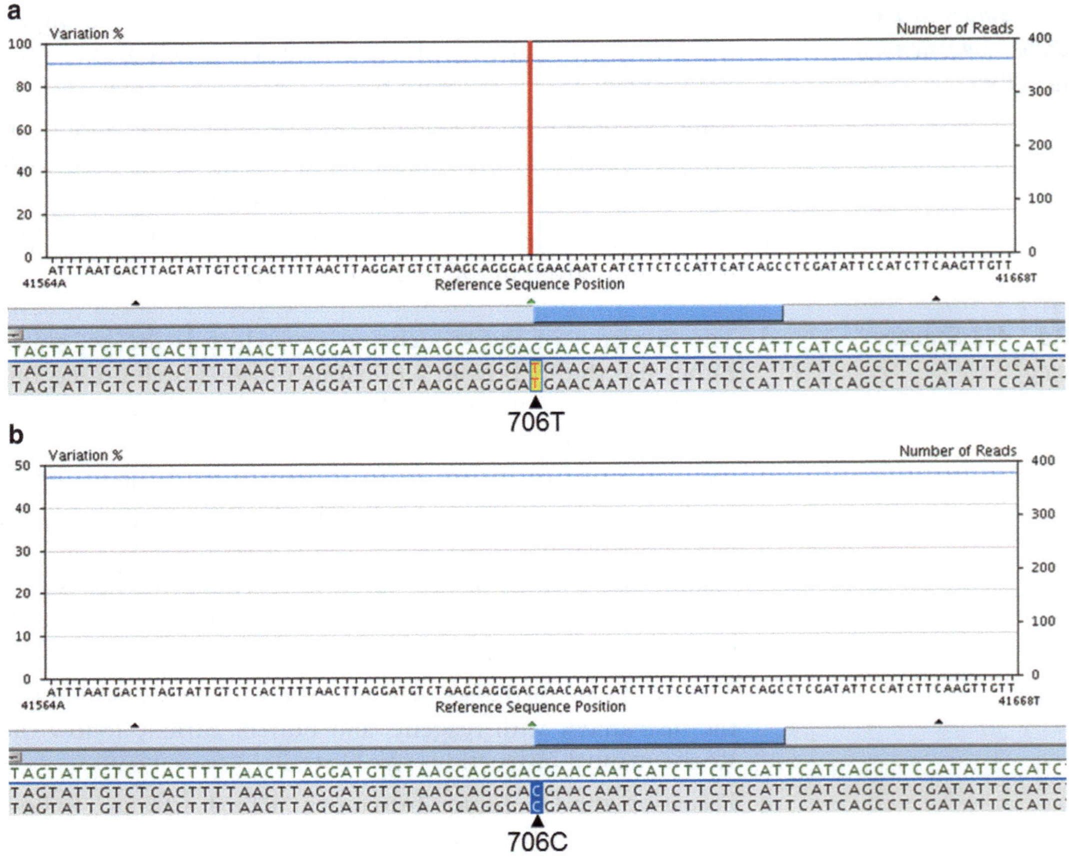

Fig. 2 Result from 454-sequencing™ of *ABCG2* exon 7. (**a**) A patient with a Jr^{a-} phenotype was homozygous for a nonsense mutation corresponding to position 706 of the coding sequence (706C>T). (**b**) Individuals that are positive for the high-frequency antigen Jr^{a} are homozygous (or heterozygous in rare cases) for the C allele at position 706

4 Notes

1. The *GS Junior Titanium emPCR Kit* (*Lib-A*) is for preparing a single emulsion. The *GS FLX Titanium MV emPCR Lib-A Kit* is for preparing eight emulsions.
2. For the establishment of the method it is advantageous to run DNA samples with known mutations as reference samples.
3. Pooling of the second PCR products followed by bead purification is less elaborately compared to purification of each PCR product and then pooling as described in the Roche manual [3]. However, concentration differences between amplicons cannot be considered for the amplicon library preparation.
4. The Roche manual quotes fluorometry using the *Quant-iT PicoGreen dsDNA Assay Kit* for the library quantitation. We rather use a NanoDrop system for measuring the DNA

concentration. Compared to fluorometry it showed a similar accuracy with less time and effort.

5. The Roche manual states a calculation for the volume of DNA library needed. Instead of calculating the volume, we used 10 μL of the 10^6 dilution of the DNA library.
6. Instead of the vacuum-assisted emulsion breaking setup, as described in the Roche manual, we collected the emulsion in a solution basin with a normal multichannel pipette and transferred it into a 50 mL tube, rinsing the solution basin with isopropanol.
7. After priming the GS Junior instrument the IDs and barcodes must be entered. Write down the ID code of the used picotiter plate before loading it.
8. For wiping the surface of the cartridge in order to remove any residues of beads and reagents, 70 % ethanol instead of 50 % ethanol should be used.
9. To clean the camera faceplate it is said to use either a Zeiss moistened cleaning tissue or Lens paper from Thorlabs. However, a simple lint-free tissue can be used as well. When loading the PTP device into the cartridge make sure that the wells face downwards.

References

1. dbRBC: http://www.ncbi.nlm.nih.gov/gv/mhc/xslcgi.cgi?cmd=bgmut/home
2. Reid ME, Lomas-Francis C, Olsson ML (2012) The blood group antigen facts book. Academic Press by Elsevier Ltd, London, UK
3. (2012) Amplicon library preparation method manual GS junior titanium series. 454 Life Sciences Corp, Branford, CT
4. (2012) Roche emPCR amplification method manual—Lib-A GS junior titanium series. 454 Life Sciences Corp, Branford, CT
5. (2012) Sequencing method manual GS junior titanium series. 454 Life Sciences Corp, Branford, CT

Chapter 12

Noninvasive Prenatal Blood Group Genotyping

Andrea Doescher and Thomas H. Müller

Abstract

Determination of fetal *RHD* from maternal plasma is increasingly used as a valuable tool for prenatal diagnosis. A remaining pitfall which hampers its use in situations with severe consequences is the following: (a) The reliability of negative results, however, is limited by difficulties to distinguish true negative results from false negative results due to insufficient amounts of free fetal DNA (ffDNA). False negative results can result in severe complications for the fetus and have to be reliably excluded. Large studies were performed in the last 10 years to investigate the reliability of noninvasive fetal *RHD* typing with real-time PCR. The majority of the assays were performed without internal controls. We present a protocol for inclusion of standards to assess the presence of adequate amounts of ffDNA for prenatal genotyping in maternal blood.

Key words Free fetal DNA, Noninvasive prenatal *RHD* genotyping, Single base extension

1 Introduction

The co-amplification of specific markers of fetal genes and blood group sequences in the same tube offers an attractive option to avoid false negative results, provided that the sensitivity for the detection of blood group sequences is higher than the sensitivity for the internal control [1]. Detection of *Y*-specific sequences (e.g., *SRY* and *AMEL*) multiplexed with blood group markers provides the opportunity to control the presence of ffDNA in blood of mothers pregnant with a male fetus. Large studies were performed in the last 10 years to investigate the reliability of noninvasive fetal *RHD* typing with real-time PCR. The majority of the assays were performed without internal controls [2–12]. Several methods have been published for the co-amplification of *SRY* and *RHD* sequences in a real-time PCR setting [13–17]. The proof for the presence of ffDNA in maternal blood samples from pregnancies with a female fetus is more complex. The hypermethylated promoter region of the *RASSF1A* gene in fetal DNA, different STR loci (short tandem repeats), and insertion/deletion polymorphisms have been tested for their suitability as gender-independent internal control [18, 19].

Peter Bugert (ed.), *Molecular Typing of Blood Cell Antigens*, Methods in Molecular Biology, vol. 1310,
DOI 10.1007/978-1-4939-2690-9_12, © Springer Science+Business Media New York 2015

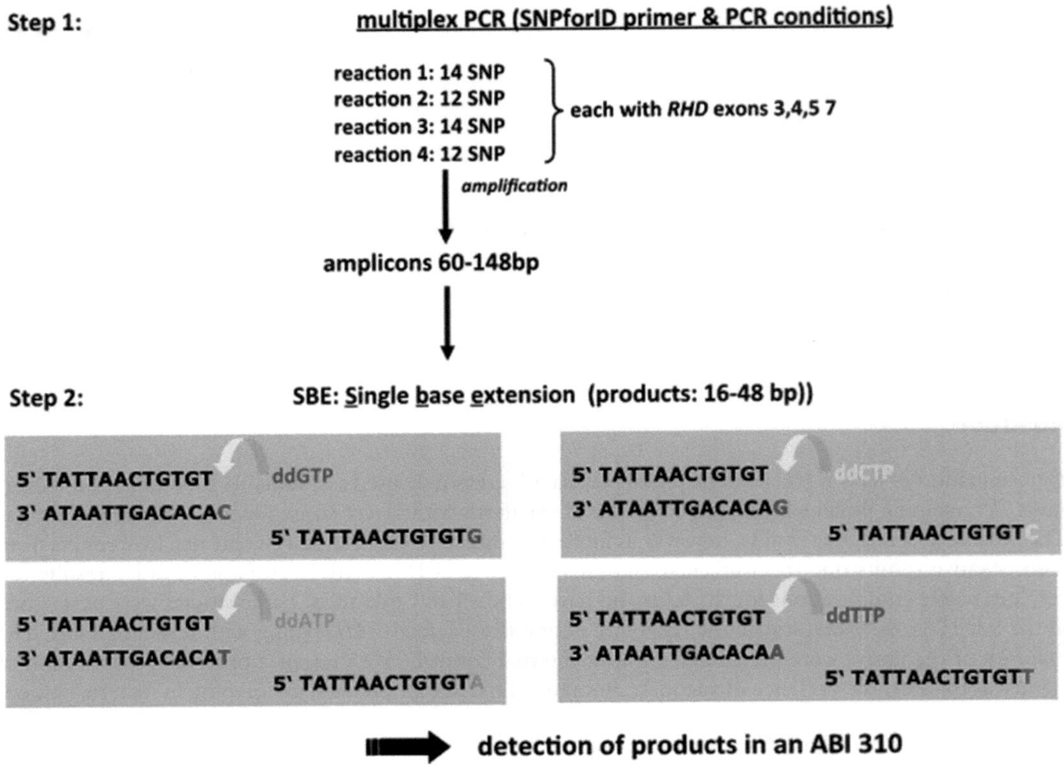

Fig. 1 Schematic presentation of the principle of the SNaPshot method

Sanchez and colleagues [20] have published a method with 52 SNPs established for identification of individuals with a calculated power of discrimination about 99.98 %. By decreasing the number of primer pairs per mix to 16–18 and including the co-amplification of *RHD* sequences, we increased the sensitivity from 500 to 10 pg. The amplification primers have been designed to generate small PCR products (59–115 bp) essential for forensic applications with more or less degraded DNA. Free fetal DNA in maternal blood is also in highly degraded state with reported sizes from 190 to 313 bp. This SNP approach was therefore chosen to detect the presence of a sufficient amount of ffDNA in the maternal blood. The method is based on the extension of a dideoxy single nucleotide to the unlabeled primer at its 3′ end (Fig. 1).

2 Materials

2.1 Isolation of DNA

MagnaPure Large Volume Kit (DNA from plasma, MagnaPure compact, Roche Diagnostics GmbH, Mannheim, Germany).

2.2 Real-Time PCR

1. TaqMan Buffer A.
2. 2× Genotyping Master mix (ready to use, Applied Biosystems, Foster City, USA).

Table 1
Primers and probes for the detection of *RHD* exons 3 and 10

Gene	Primer and probe sequences (5′ ⇒ 3′)
RHD	*Exon 3* Forward: GGCCACCATGAGTGCTTTG Reverse: CTCCACCAGCACCATCACC Probe: FAM-TGCTGATCTCAGTGGATGCTGTCTTGG-TAMRA *Exon 10* Forward: ATTTGTACGTGAGAAACGCTCAT Reverse: CCTCAAAGAGTGGCAGAGAAAG Probe: FAM-AGTCTCCAATGTTCGCGCAGGC-TAMRA
Y-AMEL	*Amelogenin Y specific* Forward: CCCTGGGCTCTGTAAAGAATAGTG Reverse: ATCAGAGCTTAAACTGGGAAGCTG Probe: VIC-CCAAATAAAGTGGTTTCTCAA-TAMRA

3. 200 μM each dNTP.
4. 5 mM $MgCl_2$.
5. AmpliTaq Gold.
6. Primer and probes for *RHD* exons 3 and 10 (Table 1).
7. Real-Time PCR System 7900 HT Fast.

2.3 Multiplex PCR

1. TaqGold buffer without $MgCl_2$.
2. 200 μM each dNTP.
3. 5 mM $MgCl_2$.
4. Primer pool (Tables 2 and 3).
5. AmpliTaq Gold.
6. ExoSAP.

2.4 Single Base Extension

1. SNaPshot Multiplex Kit (Applied Biosystems).
2. Primer for single base extension (SBE) (Tables 4 and 5).
3. Rapid alkaline phosphatase.

2.5 Capillary Electrophoresis

1. Matrix Standard FAM, HEX, NED, ROX, LIZ.
2. GeneScan LIZ 120 size standard.
3. Formamide.
4. Peak detection software (e.g., GeneMapper, Peak Scanner).

Table 2
SNP primer for preparation of 1 mL reaction mix 1–4 for use in multiplex PCR

Internal ID	NCBI NO	Forward primer (5′ ⇒ 3′)	Reverse primer (5′ ⇒ 3′)	µL	Final conc. [nM]
Primer pool 1					
SNP_20	rs2056277	CCAAACTGGGTGTTAGGGAGAC	TCATTATCTCGTCATACTTCCCTGT	25	661
SNP_10	rs914165	AGCAGCAGAGCCTGGATG	AGACCAGTCACCTCTTTTGCACT	12.5	331
SNP_6	rs2111980	AGCATCTTGGCAGCATCC	AGCAAGATCTTTGCCAGTGAGT	25	661
SNP_12	rs737681	ACATGTGAGGCCATCTCCAC	CCTTACTGTGATGTAGGCACTGTTC	25	661
SNP_13	rs735155	GGAGAAAACCGGAGAGCTG	GAGTGTCACCGAATTCAACG	25	661
SNP_1	rs717302	CTTTAGAAAGGCATATCGTATTAACTGTG	AACACAGAAAGAGGTTCATATGTTGG	12.5	331
SNP_19	rs1528460	TCCTGGAGATCAATATTTAGCCTTA	GGGTGACCAGTAGTTCTATGAGC	25	661
SNP_8	rs8037429	TTCACTTTGCTACACCTCCATAGTA	TGCTACGTAAGAGGTCATTGCTATC	25	661
SNP_9	rs2831700	GGCTAAACTATTGCCGGAGA	TTCCCTAGAACCACAATTATCTGTC	25	661
SNP_16	rs727811	GTGTTTCTTTTTCTCTTACCGGAAC	GTGAATGAAATCATGAGATTGCTG	25	661
SNP_29	rs1005533	TAACAGAAATCTGTAGACTTCAGAATCAGATA	GAGACAGGATTTTGCCATGTTAGTC	12.5	331
SNP_15	rs729172	CATTAATATGACCAAGGCTCCTCT	ACATTTCCCTCTTGCGGTTAC	25	661
SNP_7	rs354439	GGCTTCTCTTTCCCTTATGTATCTC	CAGGTTGCGATAGAAAACAGTGAAT	25	661
SNP_30	rs873196	TCCTAGTCTGTGTTCGGATTTGGTAA	TAATTTCCCAGCAAAAACTTCTTTTCTC	12.5	331
H_2O				250	
Primer pool 2					
SNP_21	rs907100	CCCCCAAACCTGGAATGATG	TCTCTTAGAAGGACACTGGTCAGAGT	25	661
SNP_26	rs876724	AATCAGAGTGGATGCTGGCTTG	GCGTGTTCAAATGTTCTCCCC	25	661
SNP_23	rs901398	GATAGGAATCTTTTGACTTAACCGAGG	AGGCTCTGGTCTTTGCTTCTGGAC	25	661
SNP_25	rs917118	AGCAAGACCAGGGGTGAATGAG	TCTGACGAAAAGGTGAAACCAGTC	12.5	331
SNP_18	rs719366	CCACAGCATCTTTTAACTCTTTTATTATCC	GTAAGGACTTATAGTGAGTAAAGGACAGG	25	661
SNP_17	rs722098	GGAAGTACACATCTGTTGACAGTAATGA	GGGTAAAGAAATATTCAGCACATCC	25	661
SNP_2	rs763869	ATCAAGTGCTTTCTGTTGACATTTG	GGCTACTCCCTCATAATGTAATGC	25	661
SNP_27	rs891700	CACCATGGAATGTGTCTTAGAGACC	CAAGTTGATTCTTTCCTTGTGTTTTCT	12.5	331
SNP_28	rs938283	TTAGGGGAGAGAGCACAAAACG	ACAAGGGGGAACCAAGGCTATG	25	661
SNP_3	rs1463729	ACTATCAGTCTCTGCCCTTATTCTG	CACATGTGCATGCTTTTGG	12.5	331
SNP_14	rs733164	GGAAGTACACATCTGTTGACAGTAATGA	GGGTAAAGAAATATTCAGCACATCC	12.5	331
SNP_5	rs2076848	GCCTCACCACCAGAAATCAG	GACATCAGAAACTCCCATGAAACT	25	661
H_2O				350	

Primer pool 3					
SNP_31	rs1024116	CCATGTGTTCTAATAAAAAGGATTGC	TGGGAAGTGAGCAAAAGTAAATACA	25	661
SNP_32	rs1028528	ACAGCTGATGCCTCCCTGA	GAGGATGAAGGTTAGAGCCAGAC	25	661
SNP_33	rs1029047	CATAACGTGGATTTGTCAGCA	GGAATAAACTGAAGGCTAAAGAAAAG	25	661
SNP_34	rs1031825	CTTATCTTTCCCACATTATGGTCCT	AAGATATAATCACTGCTTTCAAGTATGC	25	661
SNP_35	rs1335873	GTGGATGATATGGTTTCTCAAGG	TTCAACAAACGTGTGATGCTCT	25	661
SNP_36	rs1355366	CCATGATTTTCTTGTGGTGAGA	CACATGTGCTTAGGCCACAAC	25	661
SNP_37	rs1357617	AGCTGATGCAGACCACTTCAC	GGATAGCTGATAAGAAACATGACCA	25	661
SNP_38	rs1360288	AGACTCTCTGTGTGTGGCTTTG	GAGGGGGCATCTGTTGAG	25	661
SNP_39	rs1382387	ACGAAGGAGAAACACCTGAACT	TGGAGTACTTAATAAGACGCTGCAT	25	661
SNP_40	rs1413212	AACCTCCTTTGGAAACACTGAC	CAACATTCCATTATCCAGGAGAC	25	661
SNP_4	rs964681	GTACCTGGAGGTGATTTCTGTGAG	GTTATGGAGGATTGGTAAGAACCAG	25	661
SNP_11	rs740910	GTATAACAGTTTGCTAAGTAAGGTGAGTG	AGATAGGTTCGAGTTTTGGCTTTA	25	661
SNP_22	rs826472	CTGGGATAGTCAAGGATAACCTGC	GAGAGAAAGTGTATTTGACGATAGCGT	25	661
SNP_24	rs1015250	TCCCCTTCTCCTCACTTTCTAACTC	GTGTTCCAAGACCAACCAGAGC	25	661
H_2O				500	
Primer pool 4					
SNP_41	rs251934	AGAGGGCAGTGAGGCTTTTAAGTAG	TGCTAGAATCCAGACTTAACTACCAG	25	661
SNP_42	rs1454361	AGGGAAATACACCCTGAGCTG	AGCTGTCCATCATCAGTAAGACAC	25	661
SNP_43	rs1490413	GTGTGGACTGGGCTGATGT	TTCTCACTAGTGTCCCTGCTCTG	25	661
SNP_44	rs1493232	CTATTCTCTCTTTTGGGTGCTAGG	CAAACTGTTTATTGTGAGGCCTGT	25	661
SNP_45	rs1886510	GTCCTTGTCAATCTTTCTACCAGAG	GGATTTTCACAACAACACTTGC	25	661
SNP_46	rs1979255	TCAGAGACTATGGATGGTATTTAGGTC	CATGGAACGTTGGAACTCTTG	25	661
SNP_47	rs2016276	TGCATCCCAGCCTCCACT	ATTGTACCTTGCCACTTTGTGTG	25	661
SNP_48	rs2040411	TCTGGAATGCCAGTTCTTTTGT	CAGAACGCCTATGAAAACCAGT	25	661
SNP_49	rs2046361	CCTATTTGTATGTATCTATTGTCTATGAACG	GTCATTGTTGACACTTCACCTTCTA	25	661
SNP_50	rs2107612	GAGCATTCTCTTCTGTTAAAATTGC	TGAGTACATTATTCAACTGTTTTGGAG	25	661
SNP_51	rs2830795	CACTTCTATAGACATAGGACACACCAT	ATCTAGGCTCTGAATCAGGATGAG	25	661
SNP_52	rs1049540	AGATCTCCACTTCCTCTTGGTTG	CTCCCAAATTTACATTGCCACT	25	661
H_2O				550	

Table 3
***RHD* primer added in primer mix 1–4 for use in multiplex PCR**

RHD	Forward primer (5′ ⇒ 3′)	Reverse primer (5′ ⇒ 3′)	μL	Final conc [nM]
D-exon 3	GGCCACCATGAGTGCTTTG	CTCCACCAGCACCATCACC	25	661
D-exon 4	ATGATGCACATCTACGTGTTCGCA	CGGGTAGAGGCTTTGGCAGGC	12.5	331
D-exon 5	TGTTCTGGCCAAGTTTCAACTCTG	TTGCTGATCTTCCCTTGGGGGTGAGCCAAG	25	661
D-exon 7	GTTGTAACCGAGTGCTGGGGATTC	TATCAAGCACCAGCAGCACAA	12.5	331
H_2O			425	

Table 4
SBE primer for preparation of 500 μL reaction mix 1–4

Internal ID	Primer for single base extension (5′ ⇒ 3′)	Nonspecific sequence	Variation	SBE product (bp)	SBE strand	μL	Final conc. [nM]
Primer pool 1							
SNP_20	GGAGACAGGCATGAATGAGA	None	C/T	20	Upper	10	200
SNP_10	ATGGGCACCAAAGAGGGC	1× (GATC)	A/G	22	Upper	5	100
SNP_6	AGCATCTTGGCAGCATTCTTC	1× (GATC)	A/G	25	Upper	4	80
SNP_12	CATGTGAGGCCATCTCCACC	1× (GATC)	C/T	24	Upper	20	400
SNP_13	CACCGAATTCAACGGGAAG	2× (GATC)	A/G	27	Lower	30	600
SNP_1	GGCATATCGTATTAACTGTGT	2× (GATC)	A/G	29	Upper	30	600
SNP_19	TGGAGATCAATATTTAGCCTTAACATATTT	None	C/T	30	Upper	10	200
SNP_8	GCTACACCTCCATAGTAATAATGTAAGAGTTA	None	C/T	32	Upper	20	400
SNP_9	ATTTGGCTAAACTATTGCCGGAGAT	2× (GATC)	A/G	33	Upper	10	200
SNP_16	TTACCGGAACTTCAACGACTTA	3× (GATC)	A/G	34	Upper	10	200
SNP_29	GCAAGAGCCGTGGAATT	5× (GATC)	A/G	37	Upper	4	80
SNP_15	ATGACCAAGGCTCCTCTGCAGAC	4× (GATC)	A/C	39	Upper	2.5	50
SNP_7	ATATGTATCTCTCTCATGTATCACATTCCT	3× (GATC)	A/T	42	Upper	20	400
SNP_30	AATCAGGCATGTTCACATTACAA	5× (GATC)	A/G	43	Upper	2.5	50
H_2O						224.5	
Primer pool 2							
SNP_21	CCAGTTGGAGCCTTCTTT	None	C/G	18	Lower	10	200
SNP_26	CACTGCACTGAAGTATAAGTA	None	C/T	21	Upper	10	200
SNP_23	ACTAGCTGAATATCAGCCC	× (GATC)	C/T	23	Upper	20	400
SNP_25	TGACTGAGGTCAACGAGC	2× (GATC)	C/T	26	Lower	10	200
SNP_18	GCTTTTCCTCCTCCCATTCTAG	1× (GATC)	C/T	26	Upper	10	200
SNP_17	CTGTTGACAGTAATGAAATATCCTTG	1× (GATC)	A/G	30	Upper	5	100
SNP_2	TGTTTGTTTATATTATTTCTAACTCAA	1× (GATC)	C/T	31	Upper	10	200
SNP_27	TCCATTCTTTTTTTTTTGAAGCCT	2× (GATC)	A/G	32	Upper	5	100
SNP_28	CTAGTACGTTAGATGTGACCG	3× (GATC)	C/T	33	Upper	10	200
SNP_3	GGCAGCATACACTCATAGCCAC	4× (GATC)	A/G	38	Upper	10	200
SNP_14	CAACAGGCCATCCCACTTGGAAA	5× (GATC)	A/G	43	Upper	10	200
SNP_5	CTCACCACCAGAAATCAGGGC	7× (GATC)	A/T	49	Upper	10	200
H_2O						290	

(continued)

Table 4 (continued)

Internal ID	Primer for single base extension (5′ ⇒ 3′)	Nonspecific sequence	Variation	SBE product (bp)	SBE strand	μL	Final conc. [nM]
Primerpool 3							
SNP_31	TGTTCTAATAAAAAGG	5× (GATC)	A/G	36	Upper	15.2	304
SNP_32	GAAAGGTCCTTACTCGACATC	11 (dC)	A/G	32	Upper	15.2	304
SNP_33	GTAAGAATTCAAGATGGTATTT	11 (dC)	A/T	28	Upper	15.2	304
SNP_34	TTTCAAGTATGCTCGGGG	6 (dC)	A/C	18	Lower	15.2	304
SNP_35	AGGTACCTAGCTATGTACTCAGTAT	9 (dC)	A/T	34	Lower	15.2	304
SNP_36	CTGGCTTTGGCAAGTCC	5 (dC)	A/G	22	Lower	15.2	304
SNP_37	TGATAAGAAACATGACCAAGC	4 (dC)	A/T	25	Lower	15.2	304
SNP_38	AGGGGATGCAGCCAGT	11 (dC)	C/T	27	Lower	15.2	304
SNP_39	GAGAAACACCTGAACTTTCAA	9 (dC)	G/T	30	Upper	15.2	304
SNP_40	AGACATTTGTTCATATAAGTGAAATG	6 (dC)	A/G	32	Lower	15.2	304
SNP_4	ATTTCTGTGAGGAACGTCGACA	1× (GATC)	C/T	26	Upper	15.2	304
SNP_11	GCTAAGTAAGGTGAGTGGTATAATCATAT	1× (GATC)	A/G	33	Upper	15.2	304
SNP_22	GACTAATTAATCTGCTATCCTG	2× (GATC)	C/T	30	Upper	15.2	304
SNP_24	ATGAAAAATCACTGGGACAG	1× (GATC)	C/G	24	Upper	15.2	304
H_2O						187.2	
Primer pool 4							
SNP_41	TAGTAGATATCTGGCTGTCCC	None	C/T	21	Lower	15.2	304
SNP_42	AAATACACCCTGAGCTGC	None	A/T	18	Upper	15.2	304
SNP_43	TCTGAGGCCAGCCAGTT	4 (dC)	A/G	21	Lower	15.2	304
SNP_44	TTGTGAGGCCTGTTTATTTTG	16 (dC)	C/A	37	Lower	15.2	304
SNP_45	GATTTTCACAACAACACTTGC	6 (dC)	C/T	27	Lower	15.2	304
SNP_46	GAACGTTGGAACTCTTGCT	None	C/G	19	Lower	15.2	304
SNP_47	TGAGAGAGAGAAAAATGTGC	5 (dC)	A/G	25	Lower	15.2	304
SNP_48	CTCTGTATTTTCTTACTCTAAGTGC	10 (dC)	A/G	35	Upper	15.2	304
SNP_49	TTGTTGACACTTCACCTTCTA	18 (dC)	A/T	39	Lower	15.2	304
SNP_50	GTGTTTTTTCTAAATCATATTGTCT	7 (dC)	A/G	32	Upper	15.2	304
SNP_51	GGACACACCATTTTATTGTCTAAAG	None	A/G	25	Upper	15.2	304
SNP_52	GAAAAACAACAGAATGGAATAGGA	4 (dC)	A/G	28	Lower	15.2	304
H_2O						207.6	

3 Methods

3.1 Extraction of DNA

1. Centrifuge 1 mL EDTA-Plasma for 10 min at 3,000 × *g*, transfer the supernatant into a new tube, and centrifuge for 5 min at 10,000 × *g* (*see* **Note 1**).
2. Extract 1 mL plasma with the MagnaPure compact large volume protocol (elution volume: 50 μL) (*see* **Note 2**).

3.2 Real-Time PCR

3.2.1 Real-Time PCR for the Detection of RHD Exon 3

1. Prepare a PCR master mix including (final concentrations): 1× Genotyper master mix, 3.5 mM $MgCl_2$, 300 nM *RHD* exon 3 primer, 300 nM *AMEL* primer, 50 nM *RHD* exon 3 probe, 200 nM *AMEL* probe in a final volume of 15 μL.
2. Perform amplification with 5 μL plasma DNA and 15 μL master mix.
3. PCR conditions (7900 HT with 9600 emulation): Pre-PCR step 95 °C for 10 min; 45 cycles with 95 °C for 15 s and 61 °C for 1 min.

3.2.2 Real-Time PCR for the Detection of RHD Exon 10

1. Prepare a PCR master mix including (final concentrations): 1× TaqMan buffer A, 5 mM $MgCl_2$, 200 μM each dNTP, 300 nM *RHD* exon 10 primer, 300 nM *AMEL* primer, 50 nM *RHD* exon 10 probe, 200 nM *AMEL* probe in a final volume of 15 μL.
2. Perform amplification with 5 μL plasma DNA and 15 μL master mix on a TaqMan plate.
3. PCR conditions (7900 HT with 9600 emulation): Pre-PCR step 95 °C for 10 min; 45 cycles with 95 °C for 15 s and 55 °C for 1 min.

3.3 Multiplex PCR

According to the workflow depicted in Fig. 2, the following steps are only necessary in samples, where a D-negative female fetus is suspected.

1. Prepare 100 μM stock solutions of all primers (*RHD*- and SNP-specific primer) (*see* **Note 3**).
2. Prepare mixes for primer pool 1–4 (Table 1, *see* **Note 4**).
3. Dilute the maternal DNA from leucocytes to 100 pg/5 μL.
4. Add PCR master mix for each primer pool: 1× TaqGold buffer (without $MgCl_2$), 8 mM $MgCl_2$, 250 μM dNTP, 6.6 μL primer pool, 2 U TaqGold.
5. Add 5 μL from each sample (DNA from plasma, maternal DNA from leucocytes, positive and negative control, no-template control) per well and add 20 μL PCR master mix.
6. PCR conditions: 95 °C for 5 min; 35 cycles with 95 °C for 30 s, 60 °C for 30 s, 65 °C for 30 s; 65 °C for 7 min; hold at ≤10 °C.
7. Mix 2 μL ExoSAP and 10 μL PCR product and incubate for 15 min 37 °C and 15 min at 80 °C and hold at ≤10 °C.

Table 5
***RHD* primer added in primer mix 1–4 for use in single base extension**

RHD	Primer for single base extension (5′ ⇒ 3′)	Nonspecific sequence	Variation	SBE product (bp)	SBE strand	μL	Final conc. [nM]
D-exon 3	GACCTTCCCCAAGACAGCA	None	T	19	Upper	30	600
D-exon 4	AGCCTATTTTGGGCTG	None	T	16	Upper	20	400
D-exon 5	TGTTCAACACCTACTATGCT	8 (dC)	G	28	Blue	30	600
D-exon 7	CAGACCCAGCAAGCTGAAG	7 (dC)	T	27	Upper	30	600
H_2O						390	

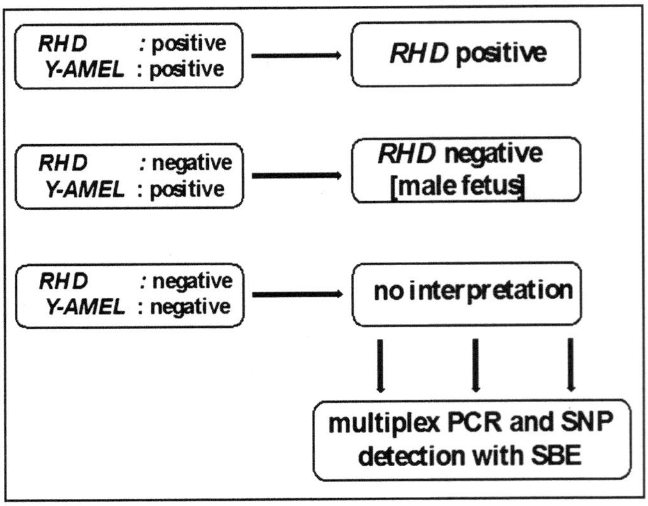

Fig. 2 Work flow for fetal *RHD* detection: Use of internal controls with single base extension can be restricted to pregnancies with a female *RHD*-negative fetus

3.4 Single Base Extension

1. Prepare 50 μM stock solutions of all primer (*RHD*- and SNP-specific primer).
2. Prepare mixes for primer pool 1–4 (Table 2).
3. Reaction mix for SBE includes 2 μL primer pool, 3 μL ExoSAP-treated amplicons from multiplex PCR, and 5 μL SNaPshot Multiplex Mix (ready to use) (*see* **Note 5**).
4. Cycler conditions for SBE: 25 cycles with 96 °C for 10 s, 58 °C for 5 s, 60 °C for 30 s; hold at ≤10 °C.
5. Add 2 μL rapid alkaline phosphatase to the reaction plate and incubate for 15 min at 37 °C and 15 min at 70 °C and hold at ≤10 °C (*see* **Note 6**).

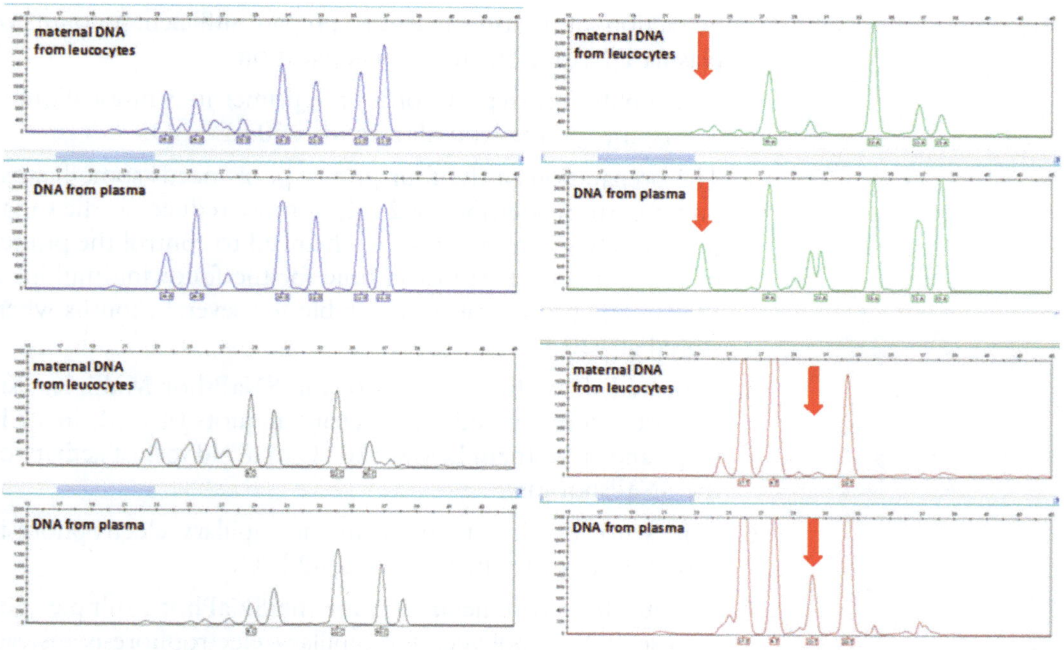

Fig. 3 Single base extension of maternal DNA from leucocytes and cell-free DNA from plasma: Differences in SNP patterns as proof for the presence of fetal DNA are indicated with *arrows*

3.5 Capillary Electrophoresis

1. Mix 2 µL of each sample with 1 µL LIZ size standard and 10 µL formamide, and denature the samples at 95 °C for 5 min.
2. Setup of the instrument: module: GS STR POP 6 (1 mL) E5; run voltage: 15 kV; injection voltage: 15 kV; injection time: 5 s; temperature: 60 °C; collection time: 24 min (*see* **Note 7**).

3.6 Data Analysis

1. Open a new SNaPshot project in the GeneMapper program (*see* **Note 8**).
2. Load the samples in the GeneMapper program.
3. Import the data from factory-provided LIZ 120 standard.
4. Define the peak position of the SBE products using the panel manager.
5. Compare the peaks of maternal DNA from leucocytes with the DNA from plasma (Fig. 3).

4 Notes

1. The DNA extraction should be performed at the same day; otherwise store the plasma at −70 °C.
2. Automated DNA extraction is a good choice for standardization of the procedure. Nevertheless, the use of extractions kits based on column technique, e.g., QIAgen mini or midi

extraction kit, is also suitable to prepare sufficient amounts of plasma DNA for downstream application.

3. To simplify this step, we order the primer in 5 nmol aliquots and resuspend the lyophilisates with 50 μL H_2O.
4. The preparation of the four primer pools needs some hands-on time; stock solutions of 2 mL or more reduce (a) the variation between primer pools, (b) the need to control the primer mixes, and (c) the hands-on time for the following multiplex PCRs. The primer mixes are stable for several months when stored at −20 °C.
5. Repeated thaw/freeze cycles of the SNaPshot Multiplex Kit are not recommended. We prepare aliquots of 5 μL in PCR strips and store them below −20 °C to avoid loss of activity of the SNaPshot mix.
6. If it is not possible to perform the capillary electrophoresis within 24 h, store the samples at −20 °C.
7. Despite the recommendation for the SNaPhot Multiplex Kit we use POP-6 polymer for capillary electrophoresis instead of POP-4. Thus, the detected base pairs of the SBE products differ slightly from the calculated sizes.
8. It is not necessary for data analysis to use the GeneMapper program. Peak Scanner software, for example, also ensures sufficient size-calling. This software is available for download from Life Technologies' homepage.

References

1. Daniels G, Finning K, Martin P, Massey E (2009) Noninvasive prenatal diagnosis of fetal blood group phenotypes: current practice and future prospects. Prenatal Diagn 29:101–107
2. Bischoff FZ, Nguyen DD, Marquez-Do D, Moise KJ Jr, Simpson JL, Elias S (1999) Noninvasive determination of fetal RhD status using fetal DNA in maternal serum and PCR. J Soc Gynecol Investig 6:64–69
3. Brojer E, Żupanska B, Guz K, Orzińska A, Kalińska A (2005) Noninvasive determination of fetal RHD status by examination of cell-free DNA in maternal plasma. Transfusion 45: 1473–1480
4. Clausen FB, Krog GR, Rieneck K, Nielsen LK, Lundquist R, Finning K, Dickmeiss E, Hedegaard M, Dziegiel MH (2005) Reliable test for prenatal prediction of fetal RhD type using maternal plasma from RhD negative women. Prenatal Diagn 25:1040–1044
5. Finning K, Martin P, Summers J, Massey E, Poole G, Daniels G (2008) Effect of high throughput RHD typing of fetal DNA in maternal plasma on use of anti-RhD immunoglobulin in RhD negative pregnant women: prospective feasibility study. BMJ 336:816–818
6. Gassner C, Schmarda A, Kilga-Nogler S, Jenny-Feldkircher B, Rainer E, Müller TH, Wagner FF, Flegel WA, Schönitzer D (1997) RHD/CE typing by polymerase chain reaction using sequence-specific primers. Transfusion 37:1020–1026
7. Hromadnikova I, Vechetova L, Vesela K, Benesova B, Doucha J, Vlk R (2005) Noninvasive fetal RHD and RHCE genotyping using real-time PCR testing of maternal plasma in RhD-negative pregnancies. J Histochem Cytochem 53:301–305
8. Legler TJ, Lynen R, Maas JH, Pindur G, Kulenkampff D, Suren A, Osmers R, Köhler M (2002) Prediction of fetal Rh D and Rh CcEe phenotype from maternal plasma with real-time polymerase chain reaction. Transfus Apher Sci 27:217–223

9. Minon JM, Gerard C, Senterre JM, Schaaps JP, Foidart JM (2008) Routine fetal RHD genotyping with maternal plasma: a four-year experience in Belgium. Transfusion 48: 373–381
10. Müller SP, Bartels I, Stein W, Emons G, Gutensohn K, Köhler M, Legler TJ (2008) The determination of the fetal D status from maternal plasma for decision making on Rh prophylaxis is feasible. Transfusion 48: 2292–2301
11. Van der Schoot CE, Soussan AA, Koelewijn J, Bonsel G, Paget-Christiaens LGC, de Haas M (2006) Non-invasive antenatal RHD typing. Transfus Clin Biol 13:53–57
12. Zhang J, Fidler C, Murphy MF, Chamberlain PF, Sargent IL, Redman CW, Hjelm NM, Wainscoat JS, Lo YM (2000) Determination of fetal RhD status by maternal plasma DNA analysis. Ann N Y Acad Sci 906:153–155
13. Hyland CA, Gardener GJ, Davies H, Ahvenainen M, Flower RL, Irwin D, Morris JM, Ward CM, Hyett JA (2009) Evaluation of non-invasive prenatal RHD genotyping of the fetus. Med J Aust 191:21–25
14. Randen I, Hauge R, Kjeldsen-Kragh J, Fagerhol MK (2003) Prenatal genotyping of RHD and SRY using maternal blood. Vox Sang 85:300–306
15. Tounta G, Vrettou C, Kolialexi A, Papantoniou N, Destouni A, Tsangaris GT, Antsaklis A, Kanavakis E, Mavrou A (2011) A multiplex PCR for non-invasive fetal RHD genotyping using cell-free fetal DNA. In Vivo 25: 411–417
16. Tynan JA, Angkachatchai V, Ehrich M, Paladino T, van den Boom D, Oeth P (2011) Multiplexed analysis of circulating cell-free fetal nucleic acids for noninvasive prenatal diagnostic RHD testing. Am J Obstet Gynecol 204:e1–e6
17. Zhong XY, Holzgreve W, Hahn S (2000) Detection of fetal Rhesus D and sex using fetal DNA from maternal plasma by multiplex polymerase chain reaction. BJOG 107:766–769
18. Chan KCA, Ding C, Gerovassili A, Yeung SW, Chiu RWK, Leung TN, Lau TK, Chim SSC, Chung GTY, Nicolaides KH, Lo YMD (2006) Hypermethylated RASSF1A in maternal plasma: a universal fetal DNA marker that improves the reliability of noninvasive prenatal diagnosis. Clin Chem 52:2211–2218
19. Page-Christiaens GC, Bossers B, van Der Schoot CE, de Haas M (2006) Use of bi-allelic insertion/deletion polymorphisms as a positive control for fetal genotyping in maternal blood. Ann N Y Acad Sci 1075:123–129
20. Sanchez JJ, Phillips C, Børsting C, Balogh K, Bogus M, Fondevila M, Harrison CD, Musgrave-Brown E, Salas A, Syndercombe-Court D, Schneider PM, Carracedo A, Morling N (2006) A multiplex assay with 52 single nucleotide polymorphisms for human identification. Electrophoresis 27:1713–1724

Chapter 13

Genotyping of Human Platelet Antigens by BeadChip Microarray Technology

Gerald Bertrand and Fabiana Conti

Abstract

Human platelet antigen (HPA) typing plays a critical role in the diagnosis of fetal/neonatal alloimmune thrombocytopenia, and the prevention of posttransfusion purpura and refractoriness to platelet transfusions. The recent development of high-throughput genotyping methods, allowing simultaneous genotyping of as many as 17 HPAs, is of utmost interest for saving time and money. Here, we describe a microarray technology named "BeadChip," designed for HPA-1 to -9, -11, and -15 genotyping of up to 96 individuals, in approximately 5 h. This technology was used to study allele frequencies in Brazilian blood donors, considering the heterogeneous ethnic composition.

Key words Human platelet antigens, Genotyping, BeadChip, Fetal/neonatal alloimmune thrombocytopenia, Posttransfusion refractoriness, Posttransfusion purpura

1 Introduction

1.1 Role of HPA Genotyping in Platelet Immunology

Platelet immunology investigations are essential for the diagnosis and therapy of alloimmune disorders such as fetal/neonatal alloimmune thrombocytopenia (FNAIT), platelet refractoriness, and posttransfusion purpura. FNAIT results from maternal immunization against fetal platelet antigen(s) inherited from the father. This syndrome may be regarded as the platelet counterpart of hemolytic disease of the fetus and newborn (HDFN). In contrast to HDFN, FNAIT frequently occurs during first pregnancies. The incidence of FNAIT has been estimated to be about 1 in 1,000 live births among Caucasians [1]. FNAIT is the most common cause of isolated severe fetal and neonatal thrombocytopenia in maternity wards. The most feared complication of this disorder is the occurrence of intracranial hemorrhage, or ICH, as a result of severe thrombocytopenia, leading to death (10–20 % of the cases in retrospective studies) or neurological sequelae (20–30 %) [2]. Contrary to HDFN, there is no systematic screening of at-risk pregnancies.

Peter Bugert (ed.), *Molecular Typing of Blood Cell Antigens*, Methods in Molecular Biology, vol. 1310,
DOI 10.1007/978-1-4939-2690-9_13, © Springer Science+Business Media New York 2015

Another alloimmune disorder is platelet transfusion refractoriness, defined as two consecutive failures to achieve platelet increments after platelet transfusions. Its incidence in onco-hematologic patients varies from 7 to 34 % depending on study populations [3]. Alloimmune refractoriness is mostly associated with sensitization to foreign class I human leukocyte antigens (HLA) and, less frequently, to human platelet antigens (HPAs).

Posttransfusion purpura is a rare syndrome occurring 7–14 days after transfusion of blood products. It is characterized by severe thrombocytopenia and bleeding caused by patient alloimmunization against transfused platelet antigens, which paradoxically destroy their own platelets. The incidence is estimated at 1:50,000 to 1:100,000 transfusions, most often occurring in multiparous women.

Whatever the clinical context, diagnosis of alloimmunization relies on (1) the detection of the antibodies, and (2) the identification of the offending antigen. Thus far, 28 HPAs have been discovered [4]. Most of them are located on the platelet glycoprotein (GP) complexes GPIIb/IIIa, GPIa/IIa, and GPIb/IX. Platelet typing can be determined either with serological methods or by molecular biology. The first method requires human reference sera containing anti-HPA antibodies, which restricts phenotyping to the most frequent antigens. Moreover, it is not suitable for severe thrombocytopenic patients or recently transfused individuals. With the progresses in molecular biology, genotyping is the routine method for most laboratories. Platelet genotyping is commonly performed by polymerase chain reaction (PCR)-sequence-specific primers (SSP), faster than the historical method of PCR-restriction fragment length polymorphism (RFLP). However, the implementation of miniaturized and high-throughput methods based on new technologies allows saving time and biological material. It also opens new fields of investigations in platelet immunology, such as HPA allele frequency studies, towards the direction of prevention of alloimmunization.

1.2 HPA Frequencies in Human Populations, and Prevention of Alloimmunization

The risk of alloimmunization depends largely on antigen frequencies, which vary in different populations worldwide (Table 1). Knowledge of HPA frequencies is important for diagnosis and to guide platelet transfusion in those patients. For example, FNAIT caused by anti-HPA-4b is more prevalent in the Japanese population and anti-HPA-2b has been described in platelet refractoriness in Japan, but not in European countries.

Such studies could be time consuming when using conventional methods such as PCR-SSP. However, it can be easily performed with high-throughput methods, like DNA microarray technology, first described for blood group genotyping by Hashmi et al. in 1989 [5] and later for HPA genotyping [6]. One example is the BeadChip array (BioArray, Immucor) that is based on (a) a

Table 1
Summary of HPA allele frequencies in several populations worldwide [7]

	HPA gene frequencies													
Population	*n*	**1a**	**1b**	**2a**	**2b**	**3a**	**3b**	**4a**	**4b**	**5a**	**5b**	**15a**	**15b**	**Reference[a]**
Central Europe														
UK	134	0.840	0.161	0.925	0.075	0.627	0.373	1.000	0.000	0.914	0.086	0.602	0.398	Jones et al. (2003)
Norwegian	105	0.867	0.133	0.943	0.057	0.471	0.529	1.000	0.000	0.929	0.071	0.495	0.505	Randen et al. (2003)
Danish	557	0.831	0.169	0.917	0.083	0.626	0.374	1.000	0.000	0.921	0.079	0.532	0.468	Steffensen et al. (1996)
French	800	0.800	0.200	0.940	0.060	–	–	–	–	0.800	0.200	–	–	Mérieux et al. (1997)
German	126	0.820	0.180	0.920	0.080	0.630	0.370	–	–	0.900	0.100	–	–	Chen et al. (1997)
Austrian	900	0.852	0.148	0.918	0.082	0.612	0.388	–	–	0.892	0.108	–	–	Holensteiner et al. (1995)
Dutch	200	0.846	0.154	0.934	0.066	0.555	0.445	1.000	0.000	0.902	0.098	–	–	Simsek et al. (1993)
Finn	200	0.860	0.140	0.910	0.090	0.590	0.410	0.976	0.024	0.950	0.050	–	–	Kekomaki et al. (1995)
Eastern Europe														
Croatian	219	0.854	0.146	0.890	0.110	0.575	0.425	0.895	0.105	–	–	–	–	Pavic et al. (2009)
Croatian	279	–	–	–	–	–	–	–	–	–	–	0.530	0.470	Tomicic et al. (2006)
Polish	30	0.874	0.126	0.898	0.102	0.592	0.408	1.000	0.000	0.937	0.063	–	–	Drzewek et al. (1998)
Slovenian	152	0.809	0.191	0.891	0.109	0.591	0.407	0.997	0.003	0.934	0.066	–	–	Rozman et al. (1999)
Macedonian	122	0.865	0.135	0.852	0.148	0.578	0.422	–	–	0.909	0.091	–	–	Pavkovic et al. (2005)
Africa														
Benin	154	0.896	0.104	0.708	0.292	0.679	0.321	1.000	0.000	0.818	0.182	0.646	0.354	Halle et al. (2005)
Cameroon	118	0.907	0.093	0.763	0.237	0.614	0.386	1.000	0.000	0.746	0.254	0.691	0.309	
Congo	125	0.904	0.096	0.776	0.224	0.596	0.404	1.000	0.000	0.732	0.268	0.701	0.299	
Pygmies	111	1.000	0.000	0.607	0.393	0.500	0.500	1.000	0.000	0.595	0.405	0.698	0.302	

(continued)

Table 1
(continued)

	HPA gene frequencies													
Population	*n*	**1a**	**1b**	**2a**	**2b**	**3a**	**3b**	**4a**	**4b**	**5a**	**5b**	**15a**	**15b**	**Reference**[a]
Arab countries														
Saudi Arabians	84	0.800	0.200	0.805	0.195	0.881	0.119	0.964	0.036	0.839	0.161	–	–	Al-Sheikh et al. (2000)
Pakistani	593	0.885	0.115	0.920	0.080	0.690	0.310	1.000	0.000	0.900	0.100	0.590	0.410	Bhatti et al. (2010)
Bahraini Arabs	194	0.760	0.240	0.767	0.233	0.568	0.432	0.932	0.068	0.861	0.132	–	–	Al-Subaie et al. (2007)
Tunisian	116	0.780	0.220	0.860	0.140	0.750	0.250	1.000	0.000	0.800	0.200	0.510	0.490	Hadhri et al. (2010)
Southeast Asia														
Indonesian	107	0.991	0.009	0.940	0.060	0.505	0.495	1.000	0.000	0.995	0.005	–	–	Liu et al. (2002)
Indonesian	107	0.991	0.009	0.940	0.060	0.505	0.495	1.000	0.000	0.995	0.005	–	–	Liu et al. (2002)
Thai	137	0.985	0.015	0.938	0.060	0.507	0.493	1.000	0.000	0.963	0.037	–	–	Liu et al. (2002)
Vietnamese	120	0.986	0.014	0.953	0.047	0.486	0.514	1.000	0.000	0.972	0.028	0.523	0.477	Halle et al. (2004)
Asia														
Korean	200	0.990	0.010	0.920	0.080	0.550	0.450	0.990	0.010	0.980	0.020	–	–	Seo et al. (1998)
Japanese	331	0.998	0.002	–	–	–	–	0.989	0.011	–	–	–	–	Tanaka et al. (1996)
Chinese	750	0.991	0.009	0.948	0.052	0.558	0.442	0.998	0.002	0.988	0.012	0.547	0.453	Xu et al. (2011)
Chinese	112	1.000	0.000	0.955	0.045	0.588	0.412	1.000	0.000	0.977	0.023	0.582	0.418	Xu et al. (2009)
Chinese	300	0.997	0.003	0.960	0.040	0.575	0.425	0.998	0.002	0.985	0.015	–	–	Lyou et al. (2002)
Chinese Han	1000	0.994	0.006	0.952	0.048	0.595	0.405	0.995	0.005	0.986	0.014	0.532	0.468	Feng et al. (2006)

North America														
Canadian	750	0.850	0.150	0.830	0.170	0.700	0.300	1.000	0.000	0.930	0.008	0.600	0.400	Shehata et al. (2011)
US Caucasian	100	0.890	0.110	0.920	0.090	0.670	0.330	1.000	0.000	0.890	0.110	–	–	Kim et al. (1995)
African Americans	100	0.920	0.080	0.820	0.180	0.630	0.370	1.000	0.000	0.790	0.210	–	–	Kim et al. (1995)
South America														
Argentinian	384	0.878	0.122	0.875	0.125	0.612	0.388	1.000	0.000	0.927	0.073	0.511	0.489	De La Vega et al. (2008)
Chilean	604	0.880	0.120	–	–	–	–	1.000	0.000	–	–	–	–	Pereira et al. (1992)
Parakana Indians	70	1.000	0.000	0.821	0.190	0.757	0.243	1.000	0.000	1.000	0.000	–	–	Castro et al. (1999)
Amazon Indians	95	1.000	0.000	0.963	0.037	0.708	0.292	1.000	0.000	0.963	0.037	–	–	Chiba et al. (2000)
Xicrin Indians	106	–	–	–	–	–	–	–	–	–	–	0.780	0.220	Cardone et al. (2004)
Amazon Indians	120	–	–	–	–	0.679	0.321	–	–	–	–	–	–	Kunyoshi et al. (2010)
Caucasian patients	0.837	0.163	0.830	0.170	0.700	0.300	1.000	0.000	0.887	0.113	–	–	0.457	Bianchi et al. (2012)
Oceania														
Australian	1000	0.858	0.003	1.000	0.000	0.932	0.068	1.000	0.000	0.754	0.246	–	–	Bennett et al. (2002)

[a]For detailed references *see* Conti et al. [7]

multiplex PCR amplification of DNA fragments containing ten HPA polymorphisms, and (b) the identification of HPAs with a glass slide, where a monolayer of colored microbeads is fixed. DNA probes specific of each HPA polymorphism are coated onto the beads (Fig. 1).

This method was used to investigate allele frequencies in Brazilian blood donors, considering the heterogeneous ethnic composition of the Brazilian population due to European, African,

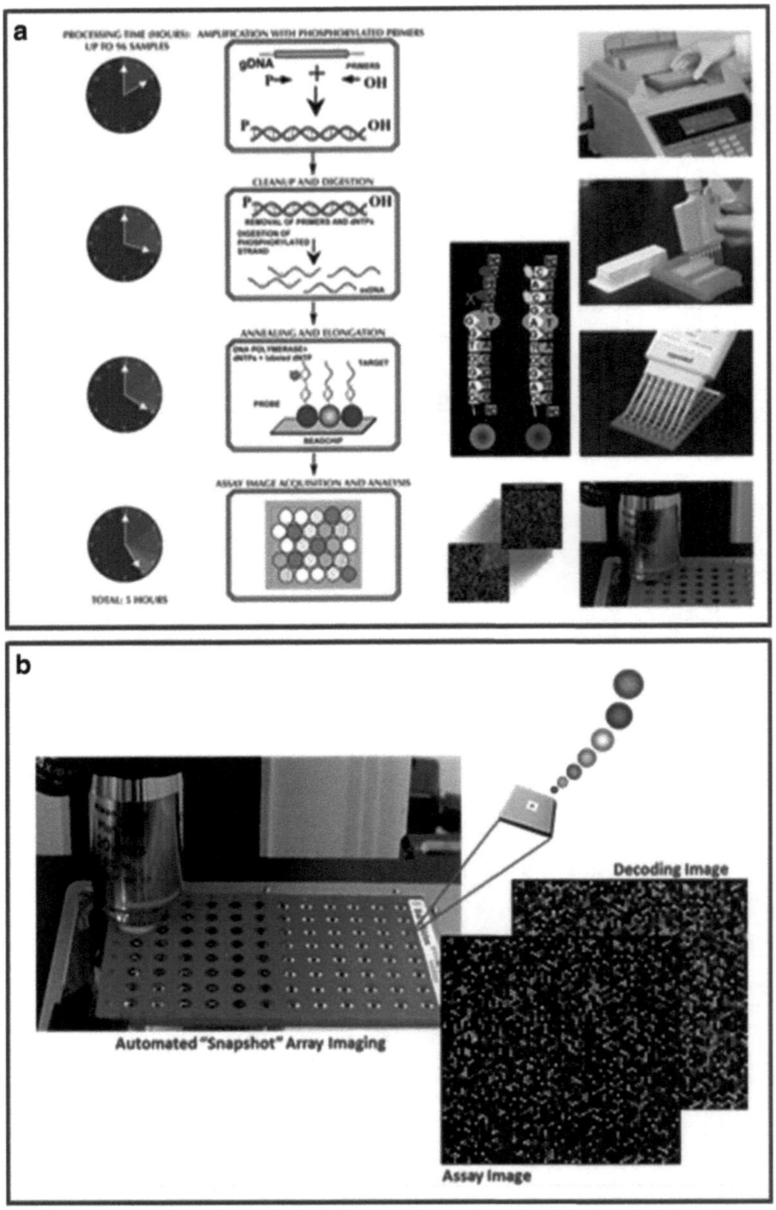

Fig. 1 HPA genotyping using the BeadChip array. (**a**) Main steps of the method, (**b**) Interpretation by overlapping of the decoding and array images

and Asian immigrations, mixed with the local native Amerindians. The goal was to determine the frequencies of HPA alleles, both common and rare, in Brazilian donors with the microarray technology, and provide basic information for further studies in platelet immunology that may guide decision making in platelet transfusion [7].

A total of 158 blood donors were enrolled in the study. Classification according to ethnicity showed that 96.3 % belonged to the same ethnic group as determined by two independent observers. A third observer was necessary to sort out the 3.7 % of discrepancies (six cases). There were 83.8 % Caucasians, 13.6 % Afro-descendants (including mulattos and blacks), 2.6 % Asians, and no indigenous donors. The results for genotypes, allele frequencies, and Hardy-Weinberg chi-square analyses of HPA-1 to -9, -11, and -15 obtained by microarray are presented in Table 1. All tested allele frequencies followed the Hardy-Weinberg equilibrium. The *a* allele was clearly predominant for HPA-1 to -9 and -11. HPA-3 and HPA-15 showed a higher prevalence of the heterozygous *ab* genotypes (44.30 and 46.84 %, respectively), as opposed to the other systems in which the *aa* genotype prevails. No *b* alleles were found for HPA-6, -7, -8, or -11, neither were homozygous *bb* genotypes detected for HPA-4, -6, -7, -8, -9, and -11. Some rare phenotypes were identified, such as two cases of heterozygosity for HPA-9 (*9abw*) and one case of heterozygosity for HPA-4 (*4ab*). One BeadChip reaction out of 158 samples yielded an inconclusive result (IC, *indeterminate call*) for HPA-2 (2aIC/2b), meaning a precise identification of the HPA-2 allele could not be performed. The light intensity charts were reviewed, but the signal obtained for HPA-2a was not informative. Microarray was repeated for that sample, which typed HPA-2*bb*. Two consecutive PCR-SSP procedures with the same sample typed HPA-2*ab*. The discrepancy found was solved after sequencing and revealed a novel silent mutation near the HPA-2 polymorphism [8].

HPA genotyping has been used to screen pregnant women for HPA-1 to identify those at risk of bearing an infant affected with NAIT. In a large Norwegian trial, after prenatally screening 100,488 pregnancies for HPA-1bb, there was a 75 % risk reduction in NAIT incidence [9], which was calculated to potentially save 210–230 quality-adjusted life years and reduce up to US$2.2 million in healthcare costs [10]. Mass-scale prenatal screening programs for NAIT will soon become available.

1.3 The BeadChip Genotyping Technology

The HPA BeadChip is used to determine platelet antigens through DNA analysis in order to predict the phenotype using a multiplex assay. Eleven HPA polymorphisms are included in the BeadChip (Table 2).

Table 2
Platelet antigens genotyped by the BeadChip array

System	Antigen	Glycoprotein	SNP localization	Nucleotide
HPA-1	HPA-1a HPA-1b	GPIIIa	176	T C
HPA-2	HPA-2a HPA-2b	GPIba	482	T C
HPA-3	HPA-3a HPA-3b	GPIIb	2621	T G
HPA-4	HPA-4a HPA-4b	GPIIIa	506	G A
HPA-5	HPA-5a HPA-5b	GPIa	1600	G G
HPA-6	HPA-6a HPA-6b	GPIIIa	1544	G A
HPA-7	HPA-7a HPA-7b	GPIIIa	1297	C G
HPA-8	HPA-8a HPA-8b	GPIIIa	1984	C T
HPA-9	HPA-9a HPA-9b	GPIIb	2602	G A
HPA-11	HPA-11a HPA-11b	GPIIIa	1976	G A
HPA-15	HPA-15a HPA-15b	CD109	2108	C A

The BeadChip kit uses the PCR technology to detect alleles associated with a particular phenotype. After an initial step of multiplex PCR amplification, there is a phase of digestion using Lambda exonuclease. The remaining single-DNA strands are incubated with the BeadChip array, leading to the annealing of the corresponding probes. In the subsequent elongation reaction, fluorescent-labeled dCTP molecules are incorporated in the strand where the 3′ end matches the hybridized oligonucleotide. The elongation products from A and B alleles are simultaneously detected using a computerized image analyzer.

Each probe is attached to microbeads through covalent bonds, which can be distinguished into different types by color spectrum, thus forming a library of several individual types. This library contains internal positive, negative, and system controls and is immobilized in the chip to form the array, so that different polymorphisms can be detected in the same reaction.

The image analyzer system (AIS400) captures the fluorescent signal emitted by individual microbeads and determines the microbead type by its spectral characteristics and signal intensity, the intensity variation coefficient, and the number of particles measured for each probe. The BASIS software imports the data with the measured intensities, verifies the internal controls for validation, and releases the results.

Laboratory investigation for common HPA is no longer sufficient to evaluate maternal immunization or the potential for alloantigen sensitization among high-risk patients. The availability of reliable techniques now makes genotyping possible for routine platelet typing that does not require reference sera or large number of platelets. The development of BeadChip arrays and automation has the potential to routinely screen each sample for multiple polymorphisms. However, because the true genotype can be masked by a small percentage of unknown polymorphisms [8], diversification of techniques remains important to ensure accurate HPA antigenic system typing.

2 Materials

2.1 Reagents, Solutions, and Kits

1. HPA BeadChip Kit containing HPA eMAP®PCR mix, Reagent Clean-Up, Lambda exonuclease, eMAP elongation Mix, and HPA eMAP 8-BeadChip carrier or 96-BeadChip carrier (Fig. 2) (*see* **Note 1**).
2. HotStar Taq DNA Polymerase PCR Kit (Qiagen, Hilden, Germany).
3. DNA Extraction Kit (Qiagen).
4. Nuclease-free water.
5. DNA cleaner.

2.2 Equipment, Supplies, and Consumables

1. AIS400 Array Imaging System (Immucor) (Fig. 3).
2. Hybridization oven.
3. Thermal cycler (Applied Biosystems Veriti or equivalent).
4. Vortex mixer with tube and flat adaptors.
5. Tube centrifuge.
6. Microplate centrifuge.
7. Precision pipettes capable of delivering 2–1,000 μL.
8. 8-Channel precision pipettes capable of delivering 2–20 μL.
9. PCR Workstation hood with UV light.
10. Unfiltered disposable pipette tips (covering the range 1–1,000 μL).
11. Filtered (aerosol resistant) disposable pipette tips (covering the range of 1–1,000 μL).

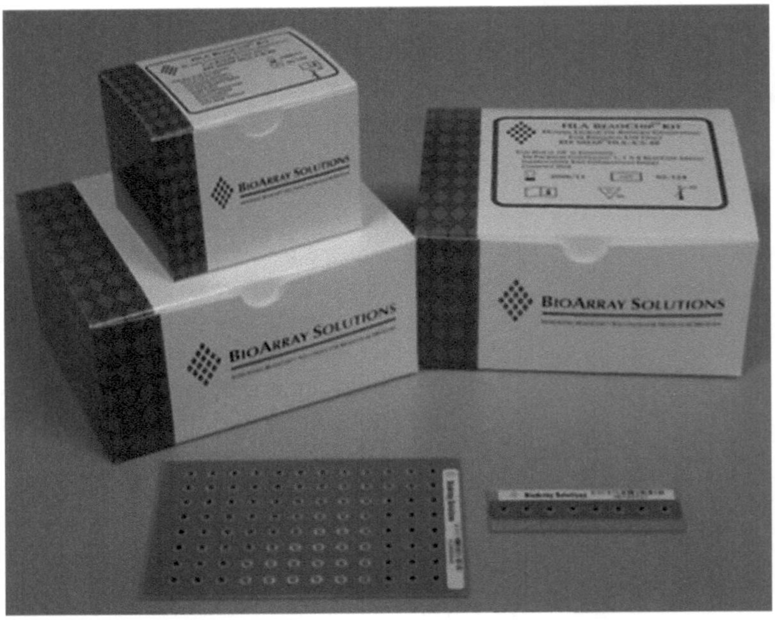

Fig. 2 The components included in the BeadChip kit

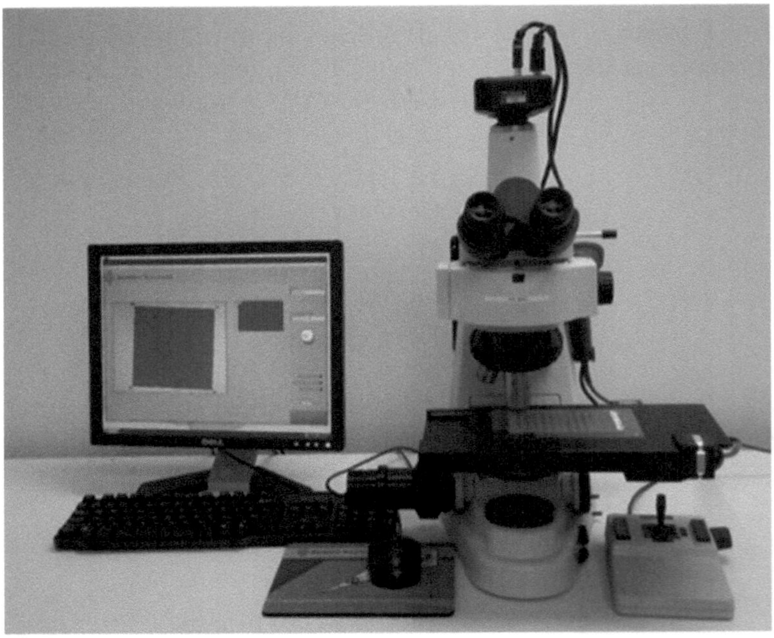

Fig. 3 Setup of the AIS400 Array Imaging System

12. 8-Tube strip 0.2 mL thin-wall thermal cycler tubes including caps.
13. 96-Well thin-walled PCR plates and plate seals.
14. 1.5 mL reaction tubes.
15. Canned air (oil free).

3 Methods

Cross-contamination of samples and reagents may lead to erroneous results. In order to prevent cross-contamination between BeadChip wells, pipetting, rinsing, and removing fluids should be performed with care and filtered tips, which is extremely important for accurate results.

3.1 Sample Preparation

1. The BeadChip platform requires a genomic DNA concentration ≥20 ng/μL (ideally between 10 and 80 ng/μl), with A_{260}/A_{280} ratio (purity quotient) of 1.50–1.95 for optimal PCR amplification.
2. Samples should be collected in EDTA anticoagulant tubes, as PCR inhibitors such as citrate, heparin, hemoglobin, and ethanol can interfere with the PCR reaction.
3. Genomic DNA should be stored at −20 to 80 °C in a d freezer until use. Avoid multiple freeze/thaw cycles.

3.2 Reagent Preparation and PCR Setup

1. Determine the total number of samples and controls to be run.
2. Check reagent name, lot, expiry dates, and manufacturer. BeadChip carrier and reagents must belong to the same lot number.
3. Cool reagents down in ice for 5–10 min before use (except for Clean-Up, which must be kept in the freezer and thawed immediately before use) (*see* **Note 2**).
4. Prepare the PCR master mix according to Table 3.
5. Aliquot the PCR master mix into an 8-tube strip slide following Table 4 (*see* **Note 3**).
6. Dispense 17 μL of PCR master mix into an appropriately labeled thin-wall PCR plate.
7. Seal plate and transfer to DNA addition area, outside of the pre-PCR hood.
8. Pipette 8 μL of prepared DNA into each of the PCR wells and mix three times by pipette aspiration.
9. For the negative control, pipette 8 μL of nuclease-free H_2O into the appropriate well and mix three times by pipette aspiration.
10. Carefully seal the plate, mix gently (vortex), and centrifuge (spin).
11. Place the plate in thermal cycler and run the specific PCR profile. For example, if using Applied Biosystems Veriti or 9700 models: 15 min at 94 °C; 35 cycles with 30 s at 94 °C (60 % ramp), 30 s at 62 °C (50 % ramp), 50 s at 72 °C (35 % ramp); 8 min at 72 °C; 4 °C until removal (*see* **Note 4**).

Table 3
Volumes of the PCR master mix according to the number of samples

Number of samples	1	8	16	24	32	40	48	56	64	72	80	88	96
HPA eMAPPCR mix (μL)	16	150	304	432	592	720	880	1,008	1,168	1,296	1,456	1,584	1,744
HotStar Taq DNA polymerase (μL)	1	9.4	19	27	37	45	55	63	73	81	91	99	109

Table 4
Volumes of the PCR master mix aliquots according to the number of samples

Up to sample	8	16	24	32	40	48	56	64	72	80	88	96
Master mix volume (μL) per tube in strip	17	38	56	76	92	112	128	148	164	188	200	224

3.3 Amplicon Treatment

1. Mix the PCR product vigorously and centrifuge (vortex and spin).
2. Transfer 7 μL from each PCR product to the new strip.
3. Aliquot the Clean-Up reagent using the single-channel pipette: 2 μL aliquots for single samples; 18 μL aliquots for 8 samples; 36 μL aliquots for 16 samples. If performing test with over 16 samples, use the multichannel pipette according to Table 5.
4. Add 2 μL of Clean-Up reagent in each well and mix three times with the pipette. Discard reagent that was not used (*see* **Note 5**).
5. Seal plate securely and vortex to mix thoroughly. Briefly centrifuge to bring solution to the bottom of the wells.
6. Place the plate in thermal cycler and run the following profile: 15 min at 37 °C; 8 min at 85 °C; 4 °C until removal (*see* **Note 6**).

3.4 Single-Strand DNA Generation (Lambda Exonuclease Treatment)

1. Vortex and spin the microtubes containing PCR products to bring the solution to the bottom of the wells.
2. Aliquot Lambda exonuclease reagent to run tests in an 8-tube strip: 2 μL aliquots for single samples; 18 μL aliquots for 8

Table 5
Volumes of the Clean-Up reagent aliquots according to the number of samples

Up to sample	8	16	24	32	40	48	56	64	72	80	88	96
Clean-Up reagent volume (μL) per tube in strip	2	6	9	12	14	16	18	20	22	24	26	28

Table 6
Volumes of the Lambda exonuclease reagent (LER) aliquots according to the number of samples

Up to sample	8	16	24	32	40	48	56	64	72	80	88	96
LER volume (μL) per tube in strip	2	6	9	12	14	16	18	20	22	24	26	28

samples; 36 μL aliquots for 16 samples. If performing test with over 16 samples, use the multichannel pipette according to Table 6 (*see* **Note 7**).

3. Add 2 μL of Lambda exonuclease reagent in each well and mix three times with the pipette. Store unused reagent at ≤−20 °C for up to 16 h.
4. Seal plate securely and vortex to mix thoroughly. Briefly centrifuge to bring solution to the bottom of the wells.
5. Place the plate in thermal cycler and run the following profile: 15 min at 37 °C; 8 min at 85 °C; 4 °C until removal (*see* **Note 6**).

3.5 Hybridization

1. Turn on the AIS4000 light source and the computer. Open and initialize the BASIS—AISR program (*see* **Note 8**).
2. Turn on and prepare the Hybridization (Boekel) oven. Ensure that the hybridization oven is at the correct temperature (55 °C).
3. Identify the BeadChip carriers and leave them at room temperature for 15 min.
4. Load files from the HPA carrier data CD to the computer (*see* **Note 9**).
5. Mix and centrifuge (vortex and spin) the PCR products.
6. Aliquot the Elongation eMAP® reagent to run tests in 8- or 16-microtube strips. Pipette carefully to avoid foam formation. Aliquots: 10 μL aliquots for single samples; 90 μL aliquots for 8 samples; 180 μL aliquots for 16 samples. If performing test

Table 7
Volumes of the eMAP® elongation mix aliquots according to the number of samples

Up to sample	8	16	24	32	40	48	56	64	72	80	88	96
eMAP® elongation Mix volume (μL) per tube in strip	18	25	37	47	60	70	80	90	100	114	125	135

with over 16 samples, use the multichannel pipette according to Table 7 (*see* **Note 10**).

7. Add 10 μL from eMAP® elongase in each tube and mix three times. Discard unused reagent.
8. Transfer 18 μL from elongation mix to the corresponding BeadChip.
9. Place the BeadChip carriers on the hybridization oven and incubate for 20 min at 22 °C.
10. Remove the carriers from the oven and wash with distilled water while keeping the slide in the upright position.
11. Rinse each BeadChip individually with distilled water under constant flow pressure. The water flow must form a straight angle with the slide and be approximately 2.5 cm away. Rinse each BeadChip for about 3 s.
12. Remove remaining water using the compressed/canned air. Do not shake the canned air. Wipe off any excess water from the back of the slide with a disposable cleaning tissue.
13. Read the BeadChip slides using the AIS400 Imaging System. Process captured images using the HPA analysis in the BASIS system.

3.6 Test Validation and Result Analysis

1. Positive and negative controls must be included in each test run. The negative control should be nuclease-free water. DNA samples with known genotypes are recommended as positive controls at least in the first run for each kit.
2. The negative control helps identify contamination by genomic DNA. Less than 11 results for the negative control sample on the phenotype report indicates possible contamination, so that results of all samples are considered invalid and the tests must be repeated (*see* **Note 11**).
3. The test is quantitative. The BASIS software calculates the data from the intensity of the array signal in each oligonucleotide, detecting specific alleles to determine the presence or absence of each allele (*see* **Note 12**).

4 Notes

1. The HPA BeadChip kit is shipped on dry ice. It is important to verify if the dry ice remains in the package. If dry ice is absent or below the expected level, please contact the supplier. All kit liquids (mix, primers, and enzymes) must be stored at −20 to −80 °C until use. Cryo racks must be used when performing reactions on bench top. Frozen reagents and samples must be thawed immediately before use. Shake vigorously and then centrifuge before use. Reagents or carriers from different lots must not be used. Enzymes and the master mix must be kept in the cool rack at all times during use. When mixing, avoid the formation of foaming. BeadChip carriers must be stored in the refrigerator at 2–8 °C until use. Unused carriers must be returned immediately to the refrigerator at 2–8 °C in their original packaging. BeadChip carriers should be removed from the refrigerator and kept at room temperature for 15 min before use.
2. After thawing, all the reagents must be mixed (vortex and spin) before use.
3. If applicable, use an alternative cuvette for multichannel pipetting. Remove all foam at the bottom of the strip before dispensing reagents. This step is critical.
4. Due to differences among thermal cyclers, each instrument must be validated with known samples. Centrifuged samples and controls must be used immediately, but can be stored at ≤−20 °C for 4 weeks for future use.
5. Perform procedure carefully to assure accurate results when pipetting small volumes. Centrifuged post-Clean-Up reagent products may be stored at −20 °C or below in a freezer for later processing in 24 h (if frozen, thaw, mix, and centrifuge before use).
6. Resting time should not exceed 3 h.
7. Return unused reagent to storage and keep working reagents on ice.
8. The AIS400 Array Imaging System and hybridization oven should be turned on at least 30 min before operation.
9. This step must be performed whenever a new kit is being used.
10. Remove all foam from the bottom of the wells before dispensing reagents.
11. If the following warnings appear in the final report, the test must be repeated: (a) HB (high background, means the background intensity is too high for the individual BeadChip), repeat the analysis paying particular attention to reagent

handling, pipetting technique, and BeadChip rinsing; (b) CV (coefficient of variation, means the intensity variance at certain probes is to high and no results are reported for this specimen),repeat the analysis paying particular attention to reagent handling and pipetting technique; (c) LS (low signal, means the signal intensity for a specific allele is too low and the analysis for this allele cannot be completed); (d) IC (indeterminate call, means the status of the specific antigen cannot be determined due to equivocal signal), repeat the test from strand generation process; if warning continues, repeat the test from PCR amplification.

12. Test limitations are as follows: (a) As with any other molecular method, in some cases the antigen might not be expressed due to a splicing mechanism, frameshift mutation, or deletion of part of the gene that does not include the primer or SNP site, so that the phenotype result will be a false positive; likewise, a rare and unexpected mutation at the oligonucleotide binding sites may result in a false negative phenotype; (b) assay failure may be due to global, systemic causes or specifically to causes related to the sample (whenever this takes place, the test should be repeated; the DNA material can also be assessed by electrophoresis); (c) microbial contamination of samples or reagents may cause erroneous results; (d) insufficient or excessive DNA may lead to low signal and/or indeterminate call results (the recommended amount of DNA is 80–640 ng); (e) inadequate DNA purity may also affect the process and the results (DNA purity should range from 1.50 to 1.95); (f) heparin and/or citrate may inhibit the PCR reaction (these substances must be absent from the PCR reaction to avoid false negative results).

Acknowledgments

The authors are indebted to Dr. Cécile Kaplan for helpful discussions and thank Dr. Mariza Mota and Marcia Dezan for their invaluable help with the technique procedure.

References

1. Dreyfus M, Kaplan C, Verdy E et al (1997) Frequency of immune thrombocytopenia in newborns: a prospective study. Immune Thrombocytopenia Working Group. Blood 89:4402–4406
2. Spencer JA, Burrows RF (2001) Feto-maternal alloimmune thrombocytopenia: a literature review and statistical analysis. Aust N Z J Obstet Gynecol 41:45–55
3. Hod E, Schwartz J (2008) Platelet transfusion refractoriness. Br J Haematol 142:348–360
4. Metcalfe P, Watkins NA, Ouwehand WH et al (2003) Nomenclature of human platelet antigens. Vox Sang 85:240–245
5. Hashmi G, Shariff T, Seul M et al (2005) A flexible array format for large-scale, rapid blood group DNA typing. Transfusion 45: 680–688

6. Bertrand G, Kaplan C (2011) Human Platelet Antigen genotyping and diagnosis of antiplatelet alloimmunization. In: Ness PM, Sloan SR, Moulds JM (eds) BeadChip molecular immunohematology: toward routine donor and patient antigen profiling by DNA analysis. Springer, New York, pp 73–81
7. Conti F, Bertrand G, Dezan M et al (2014) Molecular HPA genotyping by microarray in Brazilian blood donors. Transfusion 54:405–411
8. Nogués N, Muñiz-Díaz E, Bertrand G (2013) A new mutation in the platelet GPIbα gene interfering with HPA-2 genotyping approaches: a case report. Transfusion 53:1375–1377
9. Kjeldsen-Kragh J, Killie MK, Tomter G et al (2007) A screening and intervention program aimed to reduce mortality and serious morbidity associated with severe neonatal alloimmune thrombocytopenia. Blood 110: 833–839
10. Killie MK, Kjeldsen-Kragh J, Husebekk A et al (2007) Cost-effectiveness of antenatal screening for neonatal alloimmune thrombocytopenia. BJOG 114:588–595

Chapter 14

Sequence-Based Typing for Platelet alloantigens

Shun-Chung Pai and Liang-In Lin

Abstract

Human platelet antigen (HPA) typing is largely performed by use of DNA-based techniques in patients that require assessing the risk of HPA alloimmunization. In this chapter, HPA typing by sequencing-based typing (SBT) techniques is described.

Key words Human platelet antigen (HPA), Sequence-based typing (SBT)

1 Introduction

Human platelet antigens (HPAs) are polymorphic structures located on platelet membrane glycoproteins. HPA alloimmunization is responsible for clinically relevant immune-mediated platelet disorders including fetal/neonatal alloimmune thrombocytopenia (FNAIT), posttransfusion purpura (PTP), and platelet transfusion refractoriness (PTR) [1–3]. To date, a total of 33 HPAs have been completely characterized [4]; nevertheless, more novel low-frequency alleles continue to be emerged and identified. HPAs are found on platelet glycoproteins involved in platelet activation, most commonly GPIIb/IIIa [5]. The antigenic nature of these HPAs is mostly as a result of amino acid substitutions developing from some kinds of single-nucleotide polymorphisms [6]. The risk of alloimmunization depends largely on antigen frequencies, which vary in different populations worldwide. Knowledge of HPA frequencies in different populations is important for diagnosis and to guide platelet transfusion in those patients.

Genotyping for HPA systems is required in the investigation of patients with suspected HPA antibodies and for the provision of compatible platelet products from HPA-typed donors. A variety of different platforms have been applied to HPA genotyping throughout the years [7–11]; the most commonly used methods are sequence-specific primer-polymerase chain reaction (PCR-SSP) [9, 11], restriction fragment length polymorphism-PCR (PCR-RFLP)

Peter Bugert (ed.), *Molecular Typing of Blood Cell Antigens*, Methods in Molecular Biology, vol. 1310,
DOI 10.1007/978-1-4939-2690-9_14, © Springer Science+Business Media New York 2015

[11, 12], and TaqMan real-time PCR [11, 13, 14]. Recently, several novel high-throughput methods were developed [14, 15]. However, these methods for platelet genotyping are not without limitations. An uncovered SNP located within the antisense primer designed for genotyping with PCR-SSP, PCR-RFLP, and TaqMan real-time PCR was reported to prevent annealing to the primers and caused false-negative results [16]. In addition, several rare and silenced HPA alleles which were not compatible with known HPA genotypes were not detected with those methods and were consequently reported to produce discrepant results between genotype and phenotype [17, 18]. These uncommon alleles subsequently should be identified by using sequence-based method.

Accurate genotyping is important for genetic testing. Sanger sequencing-based typing is the gold standard for genotyping, but it has been underused for HPA genotyping, due to its high cost and low throughput. Some PCR-SBT (sequencing-based typing) for HPA genotyping had been reported [19–21]. In this chapter, we describe the detailed procedure of SBT protocol used in our laboratory examinations for the genotypes of HPA-1, -2, -3, -4, -5, -6, and -15 systems.

2 Materials

2.1 Polymerase Chain Reaction

1. Sterile work area such as biological safety cabinet or hood.
2. Oligonucleotide primers used for HPA genotyping (Table 1): 0.5 μM each.
3. TBG Taq polymerase (5 units/μL) and respective reaction buffer (*see* **Note 1**).
4. Electronic or mechanical pipettes (1–20 μL range, 20–200 μL range, 100–1,000 μL range), or multichannel pipettes (8-channel).
5. Filtered (aerosol resistant) disposable pipette tips.
6. Thin-wall thermal cycling reaction tray (0.2 mL; 8-well strips or 96-well trays).
7. Tabletop centrifuge for 96-well PCR plates.
8. PCR cycler: Different thermal cyclers are available from multiple suppliers. The thermal cycler profiles used have to be user validated.

2.2 Agarose Gel Electrophoresis and Purification of PCR Products

1. Agarose, molecular biology grade.
2. Ethidium bromide stock solution, 10 mg/mL.
3. Loading buffer: 0.5× Tris-borate-EDTA; TBE buffer.
4. TBG DNA Ladder: Tri-Band indicator at 100, 250, and 600 bp.

Table 1
Primers used for sequencing-based typing of HPA-1, -2, -3, -4, -5, -6, and -15

HPA system	CD marker	Glycoprotein	Primer sequences (5′–3′)	Amplicon size (bp)
HPA-1	CD61	GPIIIa	F:TTTATGCTCCAATGTACGGGGTAAAC R:GATTCTGGGGCACAGTTATCCTTCAGC	189
HPA-2	CD42B	GPIba	F:GGCTGACCTCGCTGCCTCTTGGTG R:GGAGGAGAAGGGTGTCGAGATTCTC	207
HPA-3	CD41B	GPIIb	F:CTGGGCCTGACCACTCCTTTGC R:TCACTACGAGAACTGGATCCTGAAG	160
HPA-4	CD61	GPIIIa	F:AAGAATTTCTCCATCCAAGTGCG R:GGTGGGGAGATATACATGTAT	218
HPA-5	CD49B	GPIa	F:ATGAGTGACCTAAAGAAAGAGG R:GAAATGTAAACCATACTATCTGTGC	178
HPA-6	CD61	GPIIIa	F:TGGGATCCCAGTGTGAGTGCTCA R:AGAAGTCGTCACACTCGCAGTAC	180
HPA-15	CD109	CD109	F:ATTTTGGCTTATTTCAAAATGTATCAGT R:ACTGGAGTAGTTGTTAGTCCAAGAC	183

The primers were used for both PCR amplification and sequencing analysis for both forward and reverse directions; *F* forward primer, *R* reverse primer

5. Agarose gel electrophoresis apparatus containing power supply.
6. UV transilluminator for visualization of the amplification products.
7. ExoSAP: Exonuclease I and Shrimp Alkaline Phosphatase (SAP).

2.3 Sequencing Reaction and Purification of Sequencing Reaction Products

1. Big Dye™ Terminator Cycle Sequencing Kit (Life Technology, Carlsbad).
2. BigDye™ Direct Sequencing Master Mix (Life Technology, Carlsbad).
3. Sequencing Primers (Table 1).
4. 1.5 M NaOAc/250 mM EDTA pH 8.0.
5. Absolute ethanol.
6. Freshly prepared 80 % ethanol.

2.4 Denaturation and Electrophoresis of Sequencing Reaction Products

1. Hi-Di™ Formamide (Life Technology, Carlsbad).
2. Automated DNA Sequencer and accessories including data collection and software.

3 Methods

3.1 Blood Sample Collection

1. Peripheral blood samples collected in blood tubes with sodium citrate or EDTA as anticoagulants should be used (*see* **Note 2**).
2. After centrifuging at 3,000 × *g* for 10 min, the buffy coat located between plasma and red cell layers is collected for further DNA isolation.

3.2 DNA Preparation

1. Genomic DNA is obtained from buffy coat isolated from peripheral blood.
2. DNA isolation should be performed by any validated protocol that produces DNA with adequate quality and quantity.
3. The DNA sample should be resuspended in sterile distilled water or appropriate buffer solution at a concentration of 10–40 ng/μL (*see* **Note 3**).

3.3 PCR Amplification

1. Calculate the total number of amplification reactions to be carried out.
2. Remove the amplification primers and Taq polymerase from freezer and thaw on ice.
3. Prepare the amplification master mix (under biological safety cabinet or hood) as given in Table 2. Keep the mix on ice and mix before use.
4. Add 6 μL of amplification master mix to the bottom of each well on a 96-well PCR tray.
5. Add 3 μL of genomic DNA (10–40 ng/μL) to the lower rim of each reaction well.
6. Add 3 μL of paired amplification primers to the upper rim of each reaction well.

Table 2
Volumes of the PCR master mix components in accordance to the number of reactions

Number of reactions	Amplification buffer (μL)	Taq polymerase (μL)
1	6	0.07
10	60	0.7
20	120	1.4
30	180	2.1

7. Cover the typing tray with PCR plate cover membrane. Make sure that all tubes are properly covered by the membrane to prevent evaporative loss during PCR process. Make sure that the dispensed solutions are mixed.
8. Place a pressure pad on top of PCR plate cover membrane and close heated thermal cycler lid. Start the amplification program as follows: 40 cycles of 96 °C for 20 s, 55 °C for 30 s, 72 °C for 90 s; hold at 4 °C (*see* **Note 4**).

3.4 Purification of the Amplification Products

The ExoSAP-IT method is a one-step enzymatic cleanup of PCR products that eliminates unincorporated primers and dNTPs.

1. Add 4 μL of Exonuclease I/Shrimp Alkaline Phosphatase to each reaction well containing PCR product.
2. Incubate in the thermal cycler: 37 °C for 15 min, 80 °C for 15 min; hold at 4 °C.

3.5 DNA Sequencing Reaction

1. Add 1.5 μL of BigDye® Direct Sequencing Master Mix to each reaction well.
2. Add 2.5 μL of each sequencing primer (Table 1) to each reaction well.
3. Add 1 μL of purified PCR product to each reaction well.
4. Briefly centrifuge, seal with PCR sealing membrane.
5. Start the sequencing program as follows: 25 cycles of 96 °C for 20 s, 55 °C for 50 s, 60 °C for 2 min; hold at 4 °C.

3.6 Purification of Sequencing Products and Preparation for Capillary Electrophoresis

In this section the ethanol precipitation to remove excess master mix and primers is described.

1. Add 5 μL of ddH_2O to each reaction well and then briefly spin down.
2. Add 2 μL of 1.5 M NaOAc/250 mM EDTA to each well slowly.
3. Briefly centrifuge to collect the contents.
4. Add 25 μL of absolute ethanol to each sequencing mixture and apply PCR cover membrane.
5. Vortex the mixture briefly but vigorously.
6. Centrifuge at 2,000 × *g* for 30 min.
7. Remove PCR cover membrane; upside down the PCR tray onto a paper towel, and then centrifuge at 100 × *g* for 10 s.
8. Add 100 μL of freshly prepared 80 % ethanol to each sequencing reaction.
9. Centrifuge at 2,000 × *g* for 5 min.
10. Remove supernatant as in **step 8**.

3.7 Performance of Capillary Electrophoresis

1. Prepare sequencing reactions for loading onto the capillary DNA fragment analysis by adding 15 μL of HiDi formamide to each sequencing reaction.
2. Centrifuge briefly to collect the liquid at the bottom of the wells, and denature in a thermal cycler for 2 min at 95 °C
3. Load the reactions directly on the capillary electrophoresis instrument.

3.8 Sequence Data Interpretation

1. Perform data collection according to the instrument-specific parameters and use any sequence alignment software to identify SNP position for final genotype assignment.
2. The sequences in NCBI accession number NG_008332, NG_008767, NG_008331, NG_008332, NG_008330, NG_008332, and NC_000006 for HPA-1, -2, -3, -4, -5, -6, and -15, respectively, should be used for comparison.
3. Figure 1 illustrates the chromatogram of sequencing results of HPA-1, -2, -3, -4, -5, -6, and -15 by Sanger's dideoxy sequencing methods (*see* **Note 5**).

4 Notes

1. Any Taq polymerase and respective reaction buffer can be used according to the manufacturer's instruction.
2. Contamination of the DNA by heparin can result in interference with the PCR reaction. For this reason, heparinized blood should not be used as a starting material for DNA isolation.
3. The DNA sample should have an A_{260}/A_{280} ratio between 1.65 and 1.8. DNA samples may be used immediately after isolation or stored at −20 °C or below for extended periods of time (over 1 year) with no adverse effects on the HPA typing results.
4. After PCR process is completed, you may proceed to gel electrophoresis immediately or store the tray at −20 °C and continue to gel electrophoresis at a later time.
5. HPA-6 is more complicated to genotype because of a 1545G>A (rs4634) polymorphism adjacent to the 1544G>A SNP (rs13306487) [22]. The sequencing data should be read carefully.

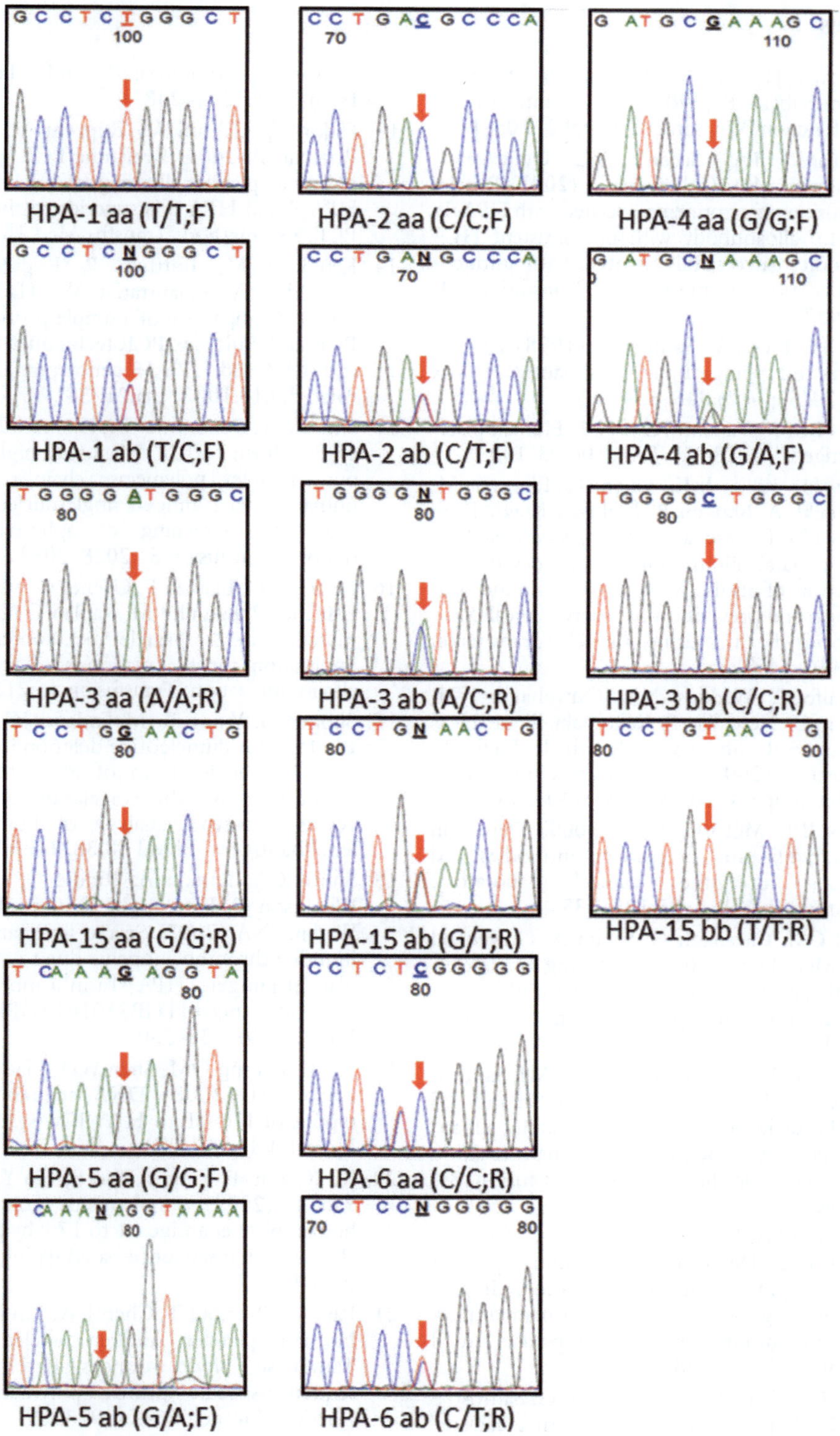

Fig. 1 Partial DNA sequencing chromatograms of HPA-1, -2, -3, -4, -5, -6, and -15 systems. The *arrows* indicated the single-nucleotide polymorphism (SNP) for each HPA system. *F* forward reading, *R* reverse reading

References

1. Deckmyn H, Ulrichts H, van de Walle G, Vanhoorelbeke K (2004) Platelet antigens and their function. Vox Sang 87(Suppl 2):105–111
2. Pappalardo PA, Secord AR, Quitevis P, Haimowitz MD, Goldfinger D (2001) Platelet transfusion refractoriness associated with HPA-1a (Pl(A1)) alloantibody without coexistent HLA antibodies successfully treated with antigen-negative platelet transfusions. Transfusion 41: 984–987
3. Kroll H, Kiefel V, Santoso S (1998) Clinical aspects and typing of platelet alloantigens. Vox Sang 74(Suppl 2):345–354
4. Curtis BR, McFarland JG (2014) Human platelet antigens - 2013. Vox Sang 106:93–102
5. Tiller H, Killie MK, Chen P, Eksteen M, Husebekk A, Skogen B, Kjeldsen-Kragh J, Ni H (2012) Toward a prophylaxis against fetal and neonatal alloimmune thrombocytopenia: induction of antibody-mediated immune suppression and prevention of severe clinical complications in a murine model. Transfusion 52:1446–1457
6. Metcalfe P, Watkins NA, Ouwehand WH, Kaplan C, Newman P, Kekomaki R, de Haas M, Aster R, Shibata Y, Smith J, Kiefel V, Santoso S (2003) Nomenclature of human platelet antigens. Vox Sang 85:240–245
7. Curtis BR, McFarland JG (2009) Detection and identification of platelet antibodies and antigens in the clinical laboratory. Immunohematology 25:125–135
8. Hurd CM, Cavanagh G, Schuh A, Ouwehand WH, Metcalfe P (2002) Genotyping for platelet-specific antigens: techniques for the detection of single nucleotide polymorphisms. Vox Sang 83:1–12
9. Skogen B, Bellissimo DB, Hessner MJ, Santoso S, Aster RH, Newman PJ, McFarland JG (1994) Rapid determination of platelet alloantigen genotypes by polymerase chain reaction using allele-specific primers. Transfusion 34: 955–960
10. Arinsburg SA, Shaz BH, Westhoff C, Cushing MM (2012) Determination of human platelet antigen typing by molecular methods: importance in diagnosis and early treatment of neonatal alloimmune thrombocytopenia. Am J Hematol 87:525–528
11. Sachs UJ, Kiefel V, Kroll H, Bein G, Santoso S (2012) Report on the 15th International Society of Blood Transfusion platelet immunology workshop. Vox Sang 103:343–351
12. Liu TC, Shih MC, Lin CL, Lin SF, Chen CM, Chang JG (2002) Gene frequencies of the HPA-1 to HPA-8w platelet antigen alleles in Taiwanese, Indonesian, and Thai. Ann Hematol 81:244–248
13. Ficko T, Galvani V, Rupreht R, Dovc T, Rozman P (2004) Real-time PCR genotyping of human platelet alloantigens HPA-1, HPA-2, HPA-3 and HPA-5 is superior to the standard PCR-SSP method. Transfus Med 14:425–432
14. Kengkate M, Butthep P, Kupatawintu P, Srisuddee A, Chantratita W, Hathalang O (2014) Comparison of a simple-probe real-time PCR and multiplex PCR techniques for HPA-1 to HPA-6 and HPA-15 genotyping. J Clin Lab Anal. doi:10.1002/jcla.21734
15. Shehata N, Denomme GA, Hannach B, Banning N, Freedman J (2011) Mass-scale high-throughput multiplex polymerase chain reaction for human platelet antigen single-nucleotide polymorphisms screening of apheresis platelet donors. Transfusion 51:2028–2033
16. Bertrand G, Bianchi F, Chenet C, Martageix C, Blanchet P, Baumler M, Kaplan C (2006) New mutation in the platelet beta3-integrin gene: implication for the diagnosis of fetomaternal alloimmunization. Transfusion 46:2138–2141
17. Skogen B, Wang R, McFarland JG, Newman PJ (1996) A dinucleotide deletion in exon 4 of the PlA2 allelic form of glycoprotein IIIa: implications for the correlation of serologic versus genotypic analysis of human platelet alloantigens. Blood 88:3831–3836
18. Smith GA, Rankin A, Riddle C, Cheetham-Wilkinson C, Ranasinghe E, Ouwehand WH, Watkins NA (2007) Severe fetomaternal alloimmune thrombocytopenia due to anti-human platelet antigen (HPA)-1a in a mother with a rare and silenced ITGB3*0101 (GPIIIa) allele. Vox Sang 93:325–330
19. Wu GG, Tang QM, Shen WD, Liao Y, Li HC, Zhao TM (2008) DNA sequencing-based typing of HPA-1 to HPA-17w systems. Int J Hematol 88:268–271
20. Xu X, Zhu F, Ying Y, Tao S, Liu Y, Hong X, Yan L (2009) Simultaneous genotyping of human platelet antigen-1 to 17w by polymerase chain reaction sequence-based typing. Vox Sang 97:330–337
21. Pai S-C, Burnouf T, Chen J-W, Lin L-I (2013) Human platelet antigen alleles in 998 Taiwanese blood donors determined by sequence-specific primer polymerase chain reaction. Biomed Res Int 973789
22. Wang R, McFarland JG, Kekomaki R, Newman PJ (1993) Amino acid 489 is encoded by a mutational "hot spot" on the beta 3 integrin chain: the CA/TU human platelet alloantigen system. Blood 82:3386–3391

Chapter 15

Miniaturized Technology for DNA Typing: Cassette PCR

Dammika P. Manage and Linda M. Pilarski

Abstract

With the smaller size, low cost, and rapid testing capabilities, miniaturized lab-on-a-chip devices can change the way medical diagnostics are currently performed in the health-care system. We have demonstrated such a device that is self-contained, simple, disposable, and inexpensive. It is capable of performing DNA amplification on an inexpensive instrument suitable for near point of care settings. This technology will enable on the spot evaluation of patients in the clinic for faster medical decision-making and more informed therapeutic choices. Our device, a gel capillary cassette, termed cassette PCR, contains capillary reaction units each holding a defined primer set, with arrays of capillary reaction units for simultaneously detecting multiple targets. With the exception of the sample to be tested, each capillary reaction unit holds all the reagents needed for PCR in a desiccated form that can be stored at room temperature for up to 3 months and even longer in colder conditions. It relies on capillary forces for sample delivery of microliter volumes through capillaries, hence avoiding the need for pumps or valves. In the assembled cassette, the wax architecture supporting the capillaries melts during the PCR and acts as a vapor barrier as well as segregating capillaries with different primer sets. No other chip sealing techniques are required. Cassette PCR accepts raw samples such as urine, genital swabs, and blood. The cassette is made with off-the-shelf components and contains integrated positive and negative controls.

Key words Miniaturization, Point of care, Lab-on-a-chip, Self-contained, Gel-PCR, Rapid diagnostics, Molecular testing, Clinical samples

1 Introduction

Medical diagnosis based on lab-on-a-chip devices provides an example of emerging applications of miniaturized technologies where biological materials and processes are performed in microscale, starting from single molecules or cells [1, 2]. The intention for this chip technology is to perform rapid sample diagnosis, most probably in a doctor's office or a clinic. Ideally, such miniaturized and automated diagnostics should be feasible with minimally trained operators and should require only minimal sample manipulation prior to testing. Such technology would avoid the need to ship samples for processing in central laboratories where the turnaround time would take much longer. Fast on-site diagnosis would allow

Peter Bugert (ed.), *Molecular Typing of Blood Cell Antigens*, Methods in Molecular Biology, vol. 1310, DOI 10.1007/978-1-4939-2690-9_15, © Springer Science+Business Media New York 2015

reduced wait times and hence better outcomes in treatments, improving the entire health-care system. Chip devices can analyze samples one at a time, or many samples simultaneously.

We have developed a lab on a chip device (cassette) that can detect multiple pathogens or genetic markers simultaneously for multiple samples [3–6] by performing PCR amplification of DNA followed by melt curve analysis (MCA). Cassette PCR involves assembly of premade and desiccated capillary reaction units that contain all reagents needed for PCR with the exception of the sample itself. Capillary reaction units are embedded in the wax architecture of the cassette. The assembled cassette can be stored for an indefinite period of time. When ready to use, sample is added which rehydrates the gel-based reaction mixture and PCR cycling begins. These ready-made cassettes, which can be assembled in a large variety of different configurations, contain integrated positive and negative controls and hold cold-chain transportation and storage capabilities. They are able to accept raw urine [3], unprocessed tissue swabs [3], and whole blood [4] without any preliminary preparation of the sample. We also demonstrated use of cassette PCR for DNA genotyping of genomic DNA from buccal swabs, requiring only minimal sample preparation [6].

The cassette contains short glass capillaries (6 mm length, 1.1 mm diameter each = 6 μL volume) that hold polymerized acrylamide gel with all the reagents required for the PCR reaction except the DNA template. These gel-filled capillaries are then desiccated for storage. To begin with, glass capillaries (Fig. 1a) are filled with gel reagents–PCR reaction mix by capillary forces, and the gel is polymerized inside the capillaries by exposing them to UV light (Fig. 1b), and finally the capillaries with polymerized gels are placed in a vacuum oven to desiccate the gel, creating a dried gel in the shape of a "noodle" inside the capillary (Fig. 1c). The space created in the capillary by drying the gel allows the sample to be delivered by capillary forces to hydrate the gel at the time of testing. The gel–reaction mix also contains a DNA intercalating dye for monitoring the reaction with a fluorescent signal. Different capillaries can contain different

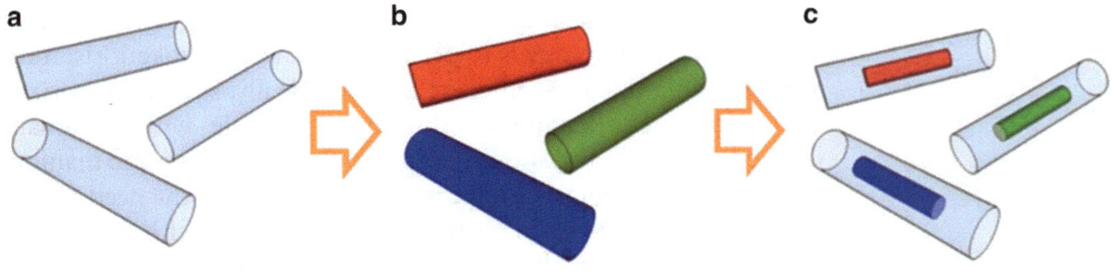

Fig. 1 Steps for making capillaries (revised from ref. [5]): (**a**) capillaries are cut to 6 mm in length, (**b**) filled with PCR/gel reaction mix and exposed to the UV light for photo-polymerization, and (**c**) desiccated to create a dried gel "noodle" inside the capillaries

primer sets for different targets. These capillary reaction units are arranged in wax trenches on a metal pan, with capillaries having different primer sets assembled next to each other in one trench. In most cases, one sample per trench is ultimately tested for multiple targets. The cassette design is extremely flexible and can accommodate a wide variety of capillary configurations. Positive and negative controls are included in the cassette. All cassette components are commercially available and low-cost. As indicated above, the entire cassette can be vacuum-sealed and stored at room temperature, in the refrigerator or in a freezer for later use [5].

When ready to use, the sample can be delivered from one end of the capillary to an individual capillary or to the entire lane of capillaries, each detecting different targets, thereby hydrating the gel (s) with a single sample. Multiple samples can be tested at once, each in a different trench on the same cassette. The cassette is then ready for PCR and MCA performed on a Peltier element that provides thermal cycling. When the PCR begins, the wax trenches that hold the capillary reaction units melt and then serve as a vapor barrier for all the reaction units in the cassette. Melted wax also forms barriers between adjacent capillaries preventing cross-contamination among primers or amplicons.

As the PCR progresses and the number of double-stranded amplicons increases, the fluorescent dye present in the gel intercalates with the double-stranded DNA resulting an increase in the fluorescence. MCA provides product verification. During MCA, the fluorescent signal drops sharply at the temperature where the double-stranded amplicon denatures/melts into single-stranded DNA, releasing the intercalated dye molecules. The melting temperature (T_m) depends on factors such as the GC-content, size of the amplicon and the salts present in the reaction. A series of fluorescence images taken through a CCD camera during the PCR and MCA, is analyzed to visualize the amplification status and to detect the products in each capillary. Upon the completion of the PCR/MCA, wax solidifies to enclose the capillaries, providing for safe disposal of biological products.

2 Materials

2.1 Reagents and Solutions

1. 1 M Tris-sulfate pH 8.6: weigh 12.1 g of tris-base (Fisher Scientific, Fair Lawn, NJ) into a 100 mL beaker. Add 80 mL of water (*see* **Note 1**) and a stir bar. Place the pH meter (calibrated) into the beaker while stirring. Stir until dissolved (pH is about 11.35). Add H_2SO_4 acid drop by drop until the pH reached 8.6. Pour into a measuring cylinder and fill up to 100 mL. Filter with 0.22 μm filter connected to a 10 mL pressure-driven plastic syringe to a 100 mL bottle and store at room temperature.

2. 1 M $(NH_4)_2SO_4$: weigh 13.2 g of $(NH_4)_2SO_4$ (Sigma, St. Louis, MO) into a 100 mL beaker. Add 80 mL of water and a stir bar. Stir until dissolved. Pour into a measuring cylinder and fill up to 100 mL. Filter with 0.22 μm filter connected to a 10 mL pressure-driven plastic syringe to a 100 mL bottle and store at room temperature.
3. PCR buffer (5×): 333 mM Tris-sulfate pH 8.6, 83 mM $(NH_4)_2SO_4$, and 40 % sucrose. Weigh 40 g of sucrose (Sigma) into a 100 mL beaker. Add 33.3 mL of 1 M Tris-sulfate. Add 8.3 mL of 1 M $(NH_4)_2SO_4$. Add a stir bar and stir until dissolved which takes about 30 min. Pour into a measuring cylinder and fill to 100 mL. Filter with 0.22 μm filter connected to a 10 mL pressure-driven plastic syringe to a 100 mL bottle (*see* **Note 2**). Store at 4 °C.
4. 40 % Trehalose solution: weigh 4 g of trehalose (Cargills Inc. Toronto, ON) and put in a 15 mL plastic conical tube. Add water to a total volume of 10 mL (*see* **Note 3**). Vortex to dissolve. Filter with 0.22 μm filter connected to a 10 mL pressure-driven plastic syringe to a 15 mL conical plastic tube and store at 4 °C (*see* **Note 2**).
5. Concentrated sulfuric acid (ca. 96 %, Anachemia, Montreal, QC).
6. 50 mM $MgCl_2$ (Fluka, Buchs).
7. 10 mM each dNTP (Sigma).
8. 1 % bovine serum albumin (BSA) solution: dilute the 2 % BSA stock (Sigma) with the same amount of water. Vortex and store at 4 °C (*see* **Note 2**).
9. Ultra pure distilled water (Invitrogen, Grand Island, NY).
10. 10 mM primer solution (Integrated DNA technologies, San Diego, CA) for each of the two primers.
11. 10× LCGreen Plus+ intercalating dye (Idaho Technology Inc., Salt Lake City, UT).
12. 20 units/μL Taq polymerase.
13. Acrylamide solution (40 % acrylamide with 4 % bis-acrylamide): in a 15 mL plastic conical tube, mix 200 mg of bis-acrylamide (*N,N*-methylene bisacrylamide, Bio-Rad, Hercules, CA) and 5 mL of 40 % acrylamide solution (Fisher Scientific). Vortex well. Filter with 0.22 μm filter connected to a 10 mL pressure-driven plastic syringe to a 15 mL conical tube (*see* **Note 2**) and store at 4 °C.
14. 3 % Azobis solution: weigh 30 mg of azobis powder (Wako, Richmond, VA) into a 1 mL eppendorf tube and add 970 μL of water (*see* **Note 4**). Vortex to dissolve. Filter with 0.22 μm filter connected to a 1 mL pressure-driven plastic syringe to an opaque (brown or black) 1 mL eppendorf tube (*see* **Note 2**) and store at 4 °C.

15. 10 % TEMED solution: mix 450 μL water and 50 μL of TEMED (*N,N,N',N'*-tetramethylethylenediamine; Sigma) in an opaque (brown or black) eppendorf tube and vortex (*see* **Note 5**). Store at 4 °C (*see* **Note 2**).
16. Filter (syringe driven, 0.22 μm; Millipore, Bedford, MA).
17. 1 and 10 mL plastic syringes (Fisher Scientific).

2.2 Capillary/ Cassette Preparation

1. Glass capillaries: Glass hematocrit tubes (Plain, Blue Tip-Fisher Scientific). The inner diameter of the capillary is 1.1 mm while the outer diameter is 1.5–1.6 mm. Cut to 6 mm in length (*see* **Note 6**) and heated (*see* **Note 7**).
2. Aluminum pans (23.5 mm × 32 mm × 4 mm) (custom-ordered, makeup powder press pans; Feldware Inc, Brooklyn, NY).
3. Microscope slides (Fisher Scientific).
4. UV lamp (Hand held, UVL-21, 4 W, 365 nm) (UVP, Upland, CA).
5. Vacuum oven (Isotemp Vacuum Oven 281A, Fisher Scientific).
6. Heater block (Isotemp, Fisher Scientific).
7. Wax pellets (Surgipath Paraplast X-tra, Leica Microsystems GmbH).
8. Silica Gel (particle size: 100–200, Selecto Scientific, Suwanee, GA).
9. Pyrex® Buchner funnel with fritted disc, capacity 600 mL, 10 mm diameter, 36060 (Fisher Scientific).
10. Vacuum sealer (generic food storage vacuum).
11. Polydimethylsiloxane (PDMS) (Bisco Silicons, Elk Grove, IL).
12. Aluminum mold (custom made to the required design for making a PDMS stamp to create wax imprints in the pan).
13. Weight ~500 g (e.g., a piece of metal).

2.3 Samples and Primers Required for DNA Amplification

Example: HSV-1 and HSV-2 (*see* **Note 8**).

1. Genital swab samples stored in universal transport media (UTM; Copan Diagnostics Inc., CA, USA) at −20 °C for detecting herpes simplex virus 1 and 2 (HSV-1 and HSV-2). (Or other sample types and targets.)
2. Forward and reverse primer sequences for detecting HSV-1 and HSV-2 (Table 1).

2.4 DNA Amplification

1. GelCycler (contains a Peltier element for performing thermocycling, a laser for exciting the LCGreen dye molecules that intercalate with double-stranded DNA and a CCD camera for taking serial images of LCGreen emissions from the cassette during the PCR and MCA—*see* Subheading 3.8).
2. Laptop computer for controlling the GelCycler as well as for acquiring, storing, and analyzing the CCD images.

Table 1
Primers used for amplification of HSV-1 and HSV-2 targets

Target (PCR product size)	Prime sequence (5′–3′)
HSV-1 (147 bp)	F-GGGCCATTTTACGAGGAGGA R-GGAACGCACCACACAAAAGA
HSV-2 (150 bp)	F-GTTTGGCGTGTGTCTCTGAA R-CTTTTATCCCCGGCACACAG

F forward, *R* reverse

3 Methods

3.1 PCR/gel Reaction Preparation

1. Dissolve primers (Table 1) to a final concentration of 10 μM according to the primer weight.
2. For the reagent mix used to fill capillaries for sample testing as well as for those to serve as negative controls: each separate reaction mix is put in an eppendorf tube (total volume: 100 μL), add 20 μL of 5× PCR buffer, 30 μL of 40 % trehalose, 4 μL of 50 mM $MgCl_2$, 2 μL of 10 μM each dNTP, 2 μL of 1 %BSA, 4 μL the 10 μM primer solution for each of the two primers, 10 μL of 10× LCGreen Plus+ and 4 μL of Taq polymerase, 10 μL of the acrylamide solution, 2 μL of 3 % azobis solution, 1 μL of 10 % TEMED, and 8 μL of water. Separate negative control reaction units are required for each primer set.
3. For the reagent mix for making capillary reaction units those serve as positive controls: 4 μL of raw sample is added, replacing 4 μL of water (*see* **Note 9**). Separate positive control reaction units are required for each primer set.
4. Repeat **steps 2** and **3** above for capillary reaction units holding the second or any subsequent primer set(s).
5. Each reaction mix (in a separate eppendorf tube for each primer set and each of the related sets of positive and negative controls) is vortexed for 5 s, then centrifuged for 2 min at 3000 × *g* (8,000 rpm) to remove any air bubbles (*see* **Note 10**).

3.2 Preparation of Glass Capillary Reaction Units

1. Glass capillaries (~6 mm each) are arranged on 4 mm wide and 2 mm thick PDMS strips (9:1 ratio with standard PDMS protocol) (*see* **Note 11**) attached to a microscope slide (Fig. 2a) (*see* **Note 12**) such that they are elevated and capillary ends are extended over the edge of the strip for easy filling of capillaries with the gel–reaction mix.
2. Pipette 100 μL gel–reaction mix to a 1,000 μL pipette tip and detach from the pipette carefully such that the liquid is not disturbed and no air bubbles are introduced, by holding the pipette tip horizontally while gently twisting off the tip.

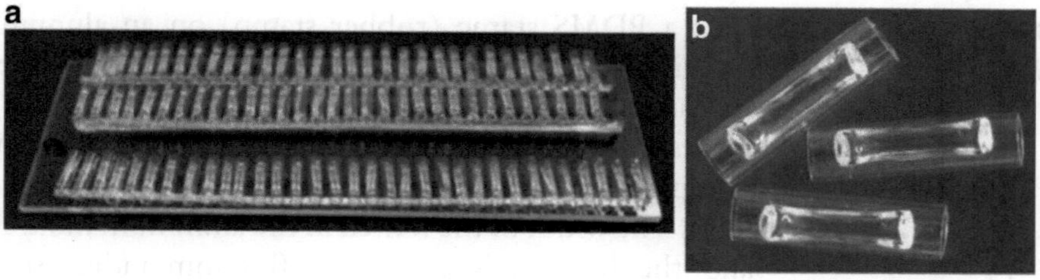

Fig. 2 Photographs of capillaries after desiccation: (**a**) the arrangement of capillaries on PDMS strips on the microscope slide for easy processing, and (**b**) desiccated gel noodles inside the capillaries

3. Hold the pipette tip at an angle (~25° to the length of the capillary) next to the end of the capillary which is laid on a the PDMS strip attached on a microscope slide and fill the capillary by simply touching the tip of the liquid filled pipette tip to the end of each capillary. The liquid fills by capillary forces (*see* **Note 13**). About 14–15 capillaries can be filled with 100 μL of reaction mix (*see* **Note 14**). To fill capillaries with a different reaction mix, have another set of capillaries assembled on the PDMS strip, load a fresh pipette tip with the required reaction mix and fill with the pipette tip as above.
4. Place the microscope slide with loaded capillaries under the UV light (the distance between the capillaries and the light is ~1.5 cm) and expose them for 30 min to polymerize the gel.
5. Then transfer the microscope slide with capillaries containing polymerized gels to the vacuum oven and leave them under 24 in. pressure of Hg overnight (~18–20 h) (*see* **Note 15**).
6. For quality control, once the gel is desiccated, briefly inspect reaction units under a microscope to see whether the gel is desiccated to ensure that a noodle shape inside the capillary creates a path for the sample to be delivered (Fig. 2b), and that both ends of the capillary are open.
7. Transfer capillary reaction units to the cassettes as explained in Subheading 3.4.

3.3 Wax Filtration

1. Pack the silica gel (~500 mL) into the Buchener funnel with a glass filter.
2. Add wax pellets on top of the silica gel and place the funnel on top of a tall 500 mL glass beaker.
3. Place the funnel–beaker assembly in the oven heated to 85 °C.
4. Let the wax melt and filter through to the glass beaker.
5. Empty the filtered wax to a clean flask and store at room temperature (*see* **Note 16**).
6. Add more wax pellets to the funnel (*see* **Note 17**).
7. Repeat the **steps 4** and **5**.
8. Repeat the **step 6** maximum of two more times (*see* **Note 18**).

3.4 Cassette Preparation

1. Cast a PDMS stamp (rubber stamp) on an aluminum mold (specifications identical to the design required for the particular cassette, i.e., Figs. 3b and 4b). Different physical arrangements of capillary reaction units require different PDMS stamps. The PDMS is made with standard protocols with 7:1 ratio. The width of the trench in the aluminum mold is 1.6 mm and the bottom is curved to 0.8 mm radius so that the imprinted trench snugly fits the capillary reaction units. Depth of the trench can be close to the height of the pan. It must not be higher or when it melts during PCR cycling, wax will overflow and flood the Peltier platform.
2. Melt the filtered wax flask or 10 mL tube in a heater block.
3. Warm up the PDMS stamp (Fig. 4a) (fins facing up) and the pan (Fig. 3a) on the heater block (*see* **Note 19**).
4. Pipette 750 μL of molten wax to the pan on the heater block.

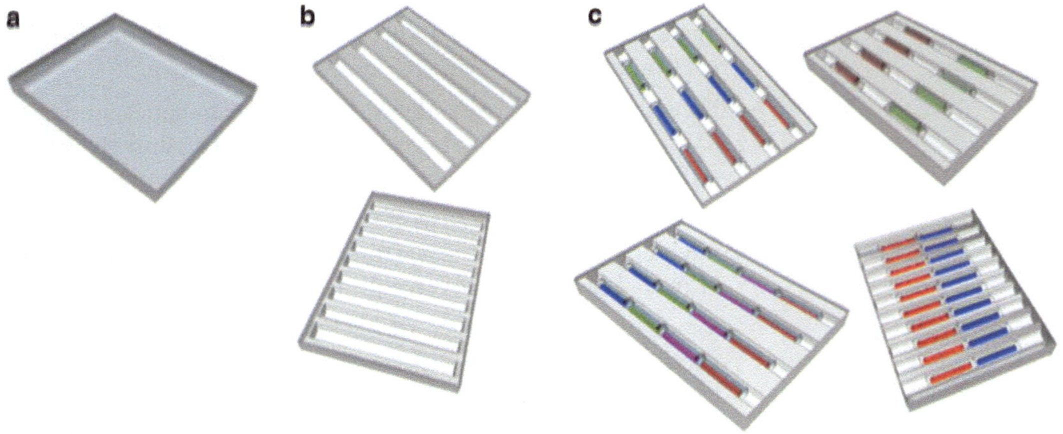

Fig. 3 Steps for the preparation of the cassettes: (**a**) aluminum pan, (**b**) different wax imprints in the pan, and (**c**) different capillary arrangements for the desired test. Capillary reaction units are colored to represent different primer sets

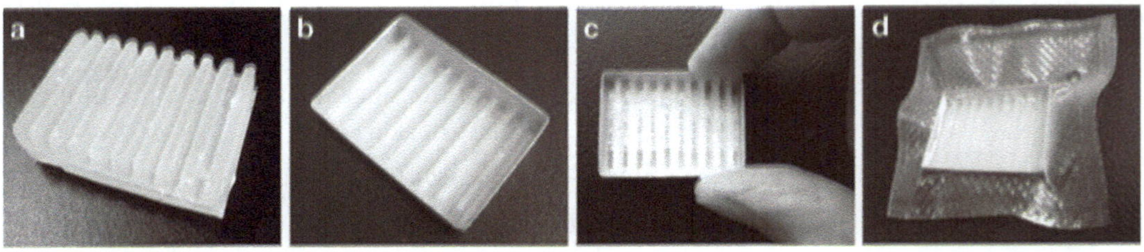

Fig. 4 Photographs showing the preparation of the cassette with the design shown in the lower right hand corner of Fig. 3c for testing eight samples of HSV-1 and HSV-2: (**a**) PDMS stamp for imprinting trenches in the wax when making the cassette, (**b**) pan with the solidified wax trenches for placing capillaries (**c**) capillaries are placed in the trenches: the last row contains capillaries made with DNA polymerized inside them, that serve as positive controls, and (**d**) a vacuum-packed cassette for storage until they are needed for use

5. Pipette another 750 μL of molten wax to the PDMS stamp carefully such that no bubbles are created between the fins of the PDMS stamp and also not allowing any wax to run off the stamp. Dispense the remainder of wax that is left in the pipette tip into the pan. Allow the wax to slightly solidify on the PDMS stamp (*see* **Note 20**).
6. Invert the wax topped PDMS stamp into the pan with the molten wax. Push the stamp to the bottom of the pan by placing a weight (~500 g, e.g., a piece of metal) on the stamp to keep it pressed to the bottom.
7. Carefully move the pan with the stamp and weight to a colder surface (preferably metal).
8. Let it reach the room temperature which takes about 10 min.
9. Carefully squeeze the PDMS stamp in order to detach it from the wax and then lift the stamp completely, leaving the pan with wax imprinted trenches for arranging capillaries (Figs. 3b and 4b).
10. Arrange the capillaries with the design required for the particular test panel being assembled, including trenches for the positive and negative control capillaries (Figs. 3c and 4c). Negative capillary reaction units are replicates of the testing set holding the same primer pair, but do not receive sample (*see* **Note 21**).
11. The cassette is now ready to be used or to be vacuum-sealed for storage (Fig. 4d). Store in a dark container.

3.5 Sample Preparation

1. Thaw the genital swab sample, or other sample type, when ready to add to the cassette (or use fresh samples) (*see* **Note 8**).
2. Dilute with water (10 %): For genital swabs, mix 2.5 μL of the sample in UTM and 22.5 μL of water. Vortex.
3. Repeat **steps 1** and **2** for all samples to be tested, in this example we show eight samples.

3.6 Sample Loading

1. Retrieve the cassette with the capillary layout shown in Fig. 5a (and also in Fig. 4c) from the vacuum-sealed plastic bag (for other cassette variations, *see* **Note 22**).
2. Deliver 11 μL of sample to both capillary reaction units in each trench by dispensing the sample to one end of the capillary (Fig. 5b) (*see* **Note 23**). Use an eppendorf pipette or a small pressure bulb pipettor (*see* **Note 24**).
3. Deliver 11 μL of water each to the trenches with positive and negative capillaries.
4. Let the gel rehydrate with sample or water for ~10 min.
5. The cassette is now ready for PCR.

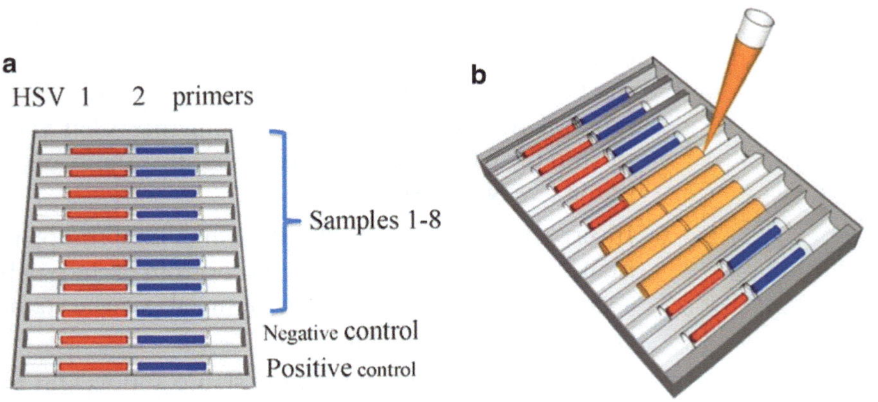

Fig. 5 Cassette layout and sample delivery: (**a**) cartoon of gel capillary cassette for detecting eight samples for HSV-1 and HSV-2 where the ninth trench is a negative control and the tenth trench is the positive control (revised from ref. [3]) (**b**) sample delivery with a pipette to each trench of the cassette from one end of the trench. The sample flows smoothly through the entire trench and hydrates the gel in the capillaries. It is essential that both ends of the capillary reaction units remain open during sample loading, to allow air movement and capillary flow to occur

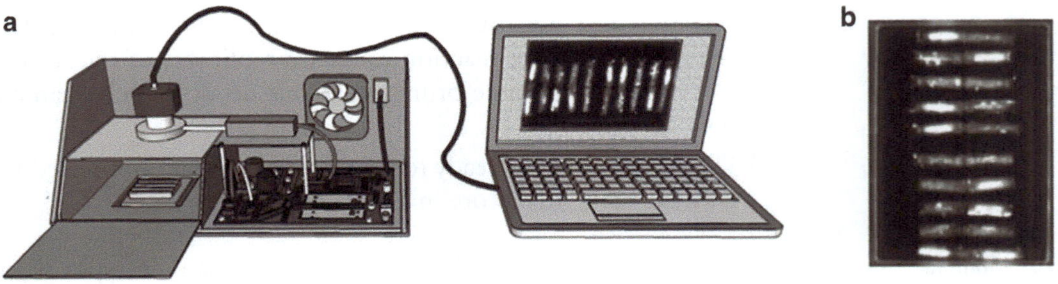

Fig. 6 GelCycler instrumentation for DNA amplification: (**a**) diagram of a PCR/MCA instrument (GelCycler) (revised from ref. [3]); (**b**) CCD image of the cassette after 31 PCR cycles are completed

3.7 PCR/MCA

1. Set the PCR and MCA parameters on the GelCycler (Fig. 6) (*see* **Note 25**) or adapt them to an alternate instrument setup. Set the PCR parameters with a pre-denaturation step of 180 s at 94 °C, 35 cycles with 94 °C for 5 s, 60 °C for 10 s, and 72 °C for 10 s, followed by a final extension step of 120 s at 72 °C. During the PCR, CCD images are to be taken at 5 s during each extension step. Set the MCA to heat from 70 to 95 °C and CCD images are to be taken at every 0.2 °C. If different primers sets are used, parameters may need to be adjusted to optimize PCR. All primer sets in a given cassette should be optimized to use the same cycling and temperature parameters.
2. Create a directory for the data (CCD images and the log file containing all the parameters) to be saved.

3. Place the cassette with hydrated capillary reaction units on the Peltier element in the GelCycler.
4. Start the PCR program which should be set up to seamlessly move onto the MCA program once the PCR is completed.

3.8 Data Analysis

1. During the PCR, if the sample template matches the primers present in a given capillary, fluorescence increases as more dye molecules are intercalated to the increasing number of double-stranded DNA amplicons. If the PCR progresses and the correct PCR product was formed, a sharp drop of the fluorescence is observed during the MCA at the melting temperature of the PCR product, due to the release of the dye molecules. This T_m is used to evaluate the sample (*see* **Note 26**).
2. With the ImageJ program (National Institutes of Health, USA), import the full set of the MCA images (or PCR images), place a grid/array of rectangle shapes (MicroArray Rectangular Plug-in: Dr. Robert Dougherty, OptiNav Inc., Redmond, WA), on each capillary reaction unit recorded on one of the CCD images (*see* **Note 27**). An example of a CCD image is shown in Fig. 6b.
3. Then use the program to extract intensities of all the CCD images during MCA (125 images taken at each 0.2 °C increment) (or for example the 35 images taken during 35 PCR cycles). Save the data with fluorescent intensities as a single text file for MCA (or PCR) containing information from all of the capillaries on the cassette at all of the time points.
4. Use Microsoft Excel (or any other program) to export the data with intensities of all the capillaries and calculate the derivative of the intensities of all the MCA data. Obtain the melt peak of the product in each capillary by plotting the negative derivative of the intensity versus the temperature as shown in Fig. 7.
5. Use the positive control capillaries to locate the peak positions and negative control signal to identify the level of the background noise. Evaluate and decide the diagnosis of the sample (yes/no) based on the presence or the absence of a peak corresponding to the capillary reaction unit(s) where the sample was delivered (*see* **Note 28**).
6. Analysis of CCD images taken during the PCR can be used to view the real-time PCR data as well. In order to obtain C_p values, custom built analysis programs can be used (*see* **Note 29**).

4 Notes

1. Water used throughout the procedure is Ultra pure distilled water (DNAs, RNAs free).
2. 500 μL or lesser aliquots can be made before storing to reduce the risks of contaminating the whole volume upon use.

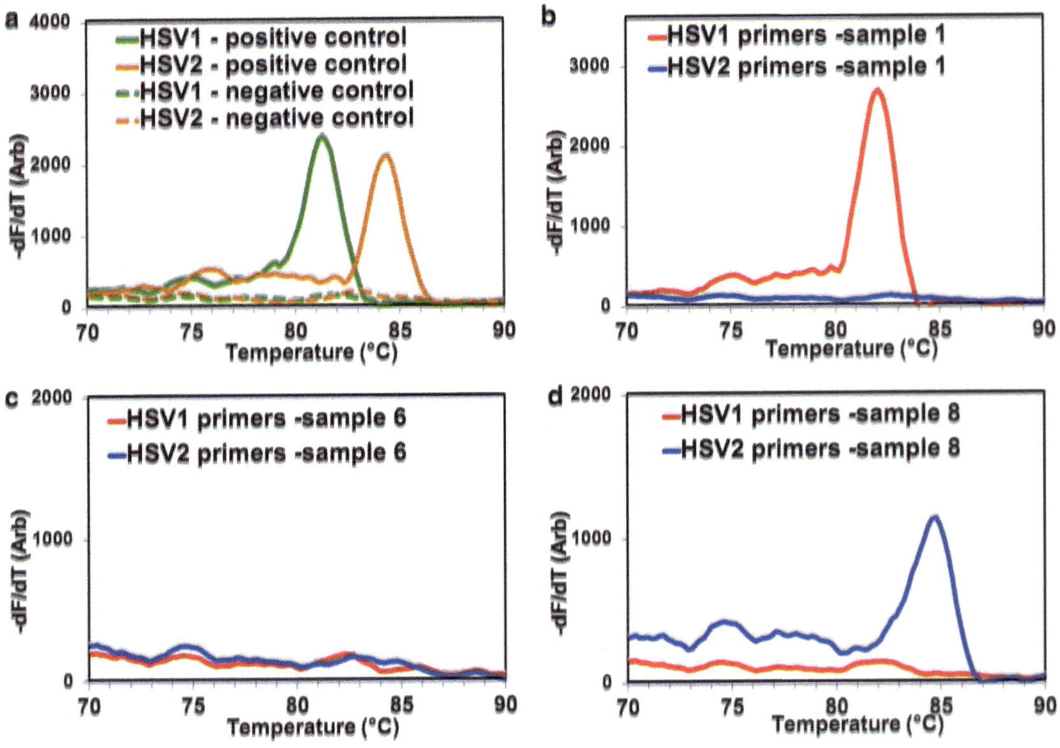

Fig. 7 Representation of MCA data for simultaneous detection of HSV-1 and HSV-2 from three different patient samples out of eight in total performed on the same cassette (revised from ref. [3]): (**a**) positive and negative controls, (**b**) sample 1 (HSV-1+), (**c**) sample 6 (Negative), and (**d**) sample 8 (HSV-2+)

3. First add only about 4 mL of water and vortex well until the powder dissolves. Then add extra water to a total of 10 mL. Vortex again.
4. Since weighing exactly 30 mg is not very practical, weigh approximately 30 mg and add a volume of water to the actual measured weight, calculated to make a final concentration of 3 %.
5. TEMED has a very strong smell. This step is best done in a fumehood.
6. Glass can be cut with a diamond cutter or commercially custom cut. The edges should be straight as much as possible such that two capillaries can be placed in proximity with a minimum gap.
7. We found that different batches of capillaries or capillaries from different manufacturers have different surface properties probably due different chemical treatments during manufacturing. These treatments interfere with the PCR process and can sometimes cause the PCR to fail completely. Heating the capillaries to ~550 °C for several hours inactivates or removes any surface treatment.

8. Raw urine samples (ten times diluted) [3] and minimally processed buccal swabs [6] can also be directly added to the gel capillary cassettes. However, in order to test blood samples, gel is used in a different format other than in capillaries. If the blood (ten times diluted) is added to the capillary with desiccated gel, the gel inside the capillary is hydrated by the blood similar to the other samples. However, when the capillary is heated during the PCR, cellular matter in blood solidifies in the boundary between the gel and the capillary walls. These randomly created patches of opaque substances block the incident laser light reaching the gel and also block the fluorescent light emitted inside the gel from reaching the CCD camera during the PCR and MCA, resulting in an uneven fluorescent image of the capillary. In order to avoid the light blockade by the solid components in the blood, the gel is used in a gel strip format that does not involve glass capillaries [4]. In this alternate method, whole blood (ten times diluted) is delivered to a capillary channel underneath the gel strip, thereby allowing unimpeded monitoring of fluorescence at the upper side of the gel strip.
9. Instead of the raw sample as the positive control, one could also use purified DNA that has the required template sequence and polymerize it into the gel.
10. Degasing the mix works similarly, however we find degasing sprays liquid droplets on the tube surface and also sprays outside causing loss of the total volume.
11. For handling capillaries, instead of PDMS strips, thick double sided tape can be used as well. However, we find that the tape sometimes leaves sticky glue on the capillary surface that would fluoresce during the PCR/MCA.
12. PDMS sticks to the glass surface of the microscope slide as well as temporarily to the glass capillaries, which is sufficient and ideal for this purpose as the user should be able to pick and retrieve the capillaries once the gels inside them are desiccated. Be sure to keep the PDMS clean and dust free and use clean glass surfaces. PDMS strips can be attached to the two edges of the microscope slide lengthwise for easy accessing when filling the capillaries with reagent mix. A slightly thicker (~3 mm) third strip can also be placed in the middle of the microscope slide for making more capillaries in one batch as shown in the Fig. 2. This strip should be placed closer to one of the strips at the edge for easy accessing from one side when loading the reagent mix to the capillaries placed on it. The extra 1 mm height in the middle strip also helps when loading the reagent mix. The width of the microscope slide is the ideal size that can be illuminated by the UV lamp used here.

13. Capillaries can also be filled by simply dipping one end of each capillary into the liquid and then placing them onto a microscope slide. However, we find that this causes some reagents to stick to the outside of the capillary. This material becomes highly fluorescent upon drying, causing the CCD images of the capillaries to have localized fluorescence spots. These dried reagents sometimes delaminate from the outside of the capillary during the thermal cycling and can drift through wax causing random fluorescent spots in the CCD images. Therefore, we found that making a PDMS assembly strip and delivering the reagents just by touching the end of the capillary is the best and cleanest way to efficiently make capillary reaction units in bulk.
14. If the liquid-filled pipette tip is held at a greater angle to the capillary, the liquid flows without control. Otherwise, the liquid flows only until the capillary is filled, without spilling any around the capillary. The method is to hold the microscope slide in one hand (steadied by either holding up or holding down to the bench) while holding the pipette tip with reagent mix in the other during the filling of the capillaries. Up to 400 μL of reagents can be taken to the pipette tip at once to fill as many as 60 capillaries. Larger amounts of liquid reagents in the pipette tip will cause the liquid to flow uncontrollably due to gravity.
15. Vacuum should be turned on very slowly as with rapid suction the gel can be damaged, resulting in a nonuniform or broken gel noodle. Taking about 5 min to reach the 24 in. Hg is a safe speed. We noticed that the vacuum should not be disturbed at least during the first hour of the desiccation to get the best shaped gel noodles.
16. To save time when melting the filtered wax, it is recommended to store smaller volumes ~50–200 mL and, at the time of use, further aliquot into 10 mL glass tubes that can be heated in a heating block.
17. To expedite the process, wax pellets can be melted ahead in the oven and the melted wax can be poured evenly over the silica in the funnel.
18. If the filter is used more than four times, the fluorescent particles present in the wax pass through and the wax begins to produce background fluorescence.
19. If the pans have a very thin plastic coating, as happens with this manufacturer, the coating can delaminate and release gas bubbles upon heating. To avoid this, with a sharp blade, make several cuts to the plastic layer throughout the inside of the pan.
20. Sometimes capillaries can roll on the pan during the melting of the wax and touch the capillary on the next row. Although DNA contamination of the samples does not happen between

them, the light bleeding from one bright capillary can create false positives on the other if they are touching each other on the side. In order for the glass capillaries remain in a stable position, barriers can be placed between the rows of capillaries at the time when the wax architecture was made, e.g., brad nails (Micropins, Bostitch, 23 ga). Brad nails can be placed and pushed down between the fins of the PDMS stamp after the wax is pipetted onto it and after the wax has slightly solidified. When the PDMS stamp with wax and the brad nails is placed upside down in the pan, the brad nails are transferred to the pan and are embedded inside the wax architecture between the trenches. These brad nails serve as barriers to the capillaries that keep them in place when the wax melts during the thermal cycling. If an alternate source of barrier is used, ensure that it does not fluoresce and does not inhibit the PCR.

21. If two or more capillaries in a trench are to be filled with the same sample loading, ensure that the capillary ends are touching one another so that capillary force continuously fills all reaction units in a given trench.

22. If two different sample types from one patient are to be tested for different targets present in them, e.g., urine and genital swabs for testing different sexually transmitted diseases [3], both sets of sample types can be tested on the same cassette. If there are many targets, two sample types can be added to two different rows of capillaries. If there are only few targets for each sample type (e.g., two), four capillaries can be placed in one trench (trenches made lengthwise in the pan), two together from each end of the trench with a gap in the middle to halt the capillary flow. This way the two types of sample can be independently delivered to the two pairs of capillaries, one sample from each end. If multiple patients are to be tested for just one target, individual capillaries can be placed in trenches with gaps such that each sample can be delivered to only one capillary reaction unit.

23. To a single capillary reaction unit, deliver 5 μL of sample with a pipette by dispensing the sample to one end of the capillary. If there are for example four capillaries in a row, deliver 24 μL allowing for sample loss, unavoidable due to the gaps between the capillaries.

24. A small transfer pipette can also be used to deliver the sample. Dispense the sample until it flows through the first capillary to the end of the last capillary. Since the wax is hydrophobic, the sample does not overflow beyond the last capillary but rather floods the opening of the capillary, where it is dispersed if extra sample is dispensed much beyond the needed volume. Such overflow is likely to cause serious problems. Therefore, for better control in the loading step, it is recommended to work with only the volume of sample needed for each trench.

25. The Gelcycler is basically a thermocycler that is connected to a light source (a laser) programmed to be to be switched on and a CCD camera programmed to take images at given times or/and temperatures during the thermal cycling. The thermal cycling is performed with a Peltier element controlled by a microprocessor which also controls the laser and the CCD camera. One could envision a simple setup with a laser that could be mounted on a chemistry clamp from the side and shining light through a diffuser to the cassette with even illumination throughout the pan and a CCD camera with an optical filter to stop the incident laser light, both of which could be mounted above the Peltier element with a chemistry clamp. A heat sink under the Peltier element will provide faster cooling during PCR cycling.
26. The T_m is dependent on the GC content and the length of the PCR product as well as the salt concentration which can change from the sample to sample especially when unprocessed samples are being used, e.g., urine. This can cause the T_m to fluctuate around the expected T_m. However, presence of a clear peak above the background noise level with about ±1 °C around the expected T_m confirms the amplification of the right product and hence the presence of the correct target. In order to further confirm product identity with a PCR performed with a new set of primers, the gel noodle can be pushed out of the capillary using a metal wire and be placed in a well on an agarose gel for size separation. The extruded gel can also be placed in ~25 μL of weak PCR buffer (1 %) to allow diffusion of amplicons into a buffer that then can be used for sequencing the product.
27. Once the grid/array of rectangles are placed on the CCD images taken during MCA (or PCR), it is possible to save the grid and export it to analyze the images during PCR (or MCA) on the same cassette, to maintain consistency and save time.
28. A custom-written Excel VBA program can be used to do the analysis without human intervention. A custom written Java based program can also be used to locate the capillaries in the CCD images and then perform the data processing and decision making based on the presence or absence of a melt peak.
29. The increase in the fluorescence during non-probe based PCR can be a combination of the expected PCR product as well as any nonspecific products that are formed during the PCR (e.g., primer dimers). Because of this, evaluating the PCR based on the C_p value, although useful for verifying that PCR has amplified to the anticipated levels, is not reliable as the sole measure of the reaction. It is therefore recommended to use the presence or absence of the melt peak for decision making

on the status of the sample. Although feasible, use of C_p values for quantifying template numbers, in the context of MCA verification, would require additional standards and controls which have not yet been implemented on cassette PCR.

Acknowledgement

Technical support for this work by Ms. Jana Lauzon is greatly appreciated. Use of wax was pioneered by Dr. Alexey Atrazhev. This work was funded by the AHFMR Interdisciplinary Team Grants Program managed by Alberta Innovates Health Solutions, and an operating grant funded by Alberta Innovates Bio Solutions, the Alberta Livestock and Meat Agency, Genome Canada and Genome Alberta.

References

1. Sackmann EK, Fulton AL, Beebe DJ (2014) The present and future role of microfluidics in biomedical research. Nature 507:181–189
2. Chen JD, Chen D, Xie Y et al (2013) Progress of microfluidics for biology and medicine. Micro Nano Lett 5:66–80
3. Manage DP, Lauzon J, Atrazev A et al (2013) An enclosed in-gel PCR amplification cassette with multi-target, multi-sample detection for platform molecular diagnostics. Lab Chip 13:2576–2584
4. Manage DP, Lauzon J, Atrazhev A et al (2013) A novel method for sample delivery and testing of whole blood: gel strip PCR for point of care (POC) molecular diagnostics. Lab Chip 13: 4011–4014
5. Manage DP, Lauzon J, Zahariadis G et al (2013) Storing self-contained gel capillary cassettes for POC medical diagnostics. Lab Chip 13: 4087–4095
6. Manage DP, Ma L, Lauzon J et al (2014) Genotyping single nucleotide polymorphisms with an automated and self-contained PCR cassette. J Mol Diagn 16:550–557

Chapter 16

Geno- and Phenotyping of Human Neutrophil Antigens

Angelika Reil and Jürgen Bux

Abstract

For typing of human neutrophil antigens (HNA) usually genotyping techniques are used, except for HNA-2, which—due to a gene expression defect—requires phenotyping. For genotyping, several techniques have been described. Most reference laboratories use variations of the polymerase chain reaction (PCR) for antigen typing which showed good results in international quality assessment exercises. The granulocyte immunofluorescence test has been the gold standard technique for phenotyping for all HNA antigens except for HNA-3a and -3b phenotyping. The expression of the latter antigens on neutrophils is often better shown by the use of the granulocyte agglutination test.

Key words Genotyping, Phenotyping, Antigens, HNA, Neutrophils, Granulocytes, PMN

1 Introduction

Typing of human neutrophil antigens (HNA) is essential for confirmation of alloantibody specificities and therefore for diagnosis of alloimmune neutropenias such as neonatal alloimmune neutropenia (NIN). Since neutrophils are short lived and fragile cells which start autolysis soon after blood withdrawal, HNA typing nowadays is mainly performed using genotyping. In addition, good typing sera are rare and monoclonal antibodies for phenotyping are not available for many HNA antigens. On the other hand, genotyping is not applicable for all neutrophil antigens. Genotyping of HNA-3 became possible quite recently when the molecular background was elucidated in 2010 [1]. Typing of HNA-2 is still only possible by phenotyping as HNA-2-negative individuals possess the encoding gene but do not present the antigen on the neutrophil surface due to an expression defect [2]. For reliable phenotypes, typing should be performed soon after blood withdrawal and more than one typing serum or antibody should be used. The gold standard for HNA phenotyping is still the granulocyte immunofluorescence test (GIFT) either using microscopy or flow cytometry for evaluation [3]. However, there is one exception: since

Peter Bugert (ed.), *Molecular Typing of Blood Cell Antigens*, Methods in Molecular Biology, vol. 1310,
DOI 10.1007/978-1-4939-2690-9_16, © Springer Science+Business Media New York 2015

HNA-3 antibodies are strong agglutinins, the detection of the HNA-3a and -3b antigens on neutrophils succeeds often better when the granulocyte agglutination test (GAT) is used [4].

Here we describe methods for phenotyping based on established procedures with some modifications [5–8]. Genotyping showed in quality assessment exercises to deliver reliable results. However, for genotyping a number of different techniques have been developed [9–14]. Most reference laboratories, however, use variations of the polymerase chain reaction. The molecular basis of the HNA-3, -4, and -5 antigens consists of point mutations in the *SLC44A2, ITGAM,* and *ITGAL* genes, respectively. Concerning the HNA-1 antigens, the situation is more complicated. Four antigens, HNA-1a, -1b, -1c, and -1d, corresponding to three common alleles of the *FCGR3B* gene have been described [15]. It means that there is no one-to-one relation between antigen and allele. The three *FCGR3B* alleles differ in six nucleotides and five amino acids. Other rare alleles have been described in several population studies but alloimmunization to the corresponding gene products has not been reported so far. In rare cases (0.1 % of Europeans), individuals show a lack of the *FCGR3B* gene. These individuals do not express any of the HNA-1 antigens. At last, *FCGR3B* genotyping is hampered by the existence of the highly homologous *FCGR3A* gene. To exclude unintended amplification of the *FCGR3A* gene, at least one primer of each primer pair must be *FCGR3B* specific.

2 Materials

Prepare all solutions using ultrapure water and analytical grade reagents.

2.1 Cell Preparation

1. PBS buffer w/o Ca^{2+}/Mg^{2+} (10× PBS; Gibco BRL cat.-no. 14200-067).
2. Density gradient: Ficoll-Paque™ PLUS(GE Healthcare, Uppsala, Sweden).
3. Dextran, average M_w 500,000 for preparation of GAT neutrophils (Roth, Karlsruhe, Germany, code 9219.1).
4. Dextran sulfate sodium salt, average M_w 500,000 for preparation of GIFT/monoclonal antibody-specific immobilization of granulocyte antigen (MAIGA) neutrophils (Sigma-Aldrich, Taufkirchen, Germany, code D8906).
5. Dextran solution: 5 % Dextran/dextran sulfate in PBS buffer w/o Ca^{2+}/Mg^{2+}, adjust pH to 7.0–7.4 and filter through a 0.2 μm sterile filter. Make aliquots and store at 4 °C.
6. EDTA solution: 5 % EDTA in water.

7. Paraformaldehyde (PFA) solution: 400 mg PFA in 10 mL PBS buffer w/o Ca^{2+}/Mg^{2+}, add 300 μL 3 N NaOH and dissolve at 56 °C in a water bath. Adjust pH to 7.0–7.4 with 3 N HCl. Store at 4 °C in a tube wrapped with aluminum foil (*see* **Note 1**).
8. Hemolysis buffer: Weigh 8.3 g NH_4Cl, 1 g $KHCO_3$, and 0.037 g Na_2-EDTA. Add water to a volume of 1 L. Adjust pH to 7.0–7.4.

2.2 Granulocyte Agglutination Test

1. Terasaki plates (Greiner Bio-One, Frickenhausen, Germany, code 659180).
2. Paraffin oil.
3. Hamilton dispenser.
4. Inverted microscope.

2.3 Granulocyte Immunofluorescence Test

1. PS microplates, U-shape (Greiner Bio-One, code 650101).
2. Staining antibodies: Rabbit anti-human IgG-FITC, rabbit anti-human IgM-FITC (Dako, Hamburg, Germany, code F0315 and F0316, respectively).
3. Glycerol solution for microscopy: Dilute one part anhydrous glycerol with three parts of PBS buffer w/o Ca^{2+}/Mg^{2+}.
4. Fluorescence microscope or flow cytometer equipped with a 100 W Hg vapor lamp.

2.4 Monoclonal Antibody-Specific Immobilization of Granulocyte Antigen Assay

1. ELISA plates: Nunc MaxiSorp®, flat-bottom (Thermo Fisher Scientific, Roskilde, Denmark, code NC9229197).
2. Coating buffer: Weigh 0.3975 g Na_2CO_3, 0.7325 g $KHCO_3$, and 0.05 g NaN_3. Add water to a volume of 250 mL. Adjust pH to 9.6 (*see* **Note 2**).
3. Coating antibody: Goat anti-mouse IgG (Dianova, Hamburg, Germany, code 115-005-071), dilute 1:500 with coating buffer.
4. Bovine serum albumin (BSA) solution 22 % (Bio-Rad, Dreieich, Germany), dilute with PBS to 2 or 0.2 %, respectively.
5. Monoclonal antibodies for immobilization: For CD16b clones DJ130c (HNA-1a, -1c) (Acris Antibodies, Herford, Germany, code AM01321PU-N), 3G8 (HNA-1b) (Beckman Coulter, Krefeld, Germany, code IM0813), and LNK16 (HNA-1d) (GeneTex, Irvine, CA, USA, code GTX74720); for CD177 (HNA-2) clone MEM-166 (Acris Antibodies, code SM2003S); for CD11b (HNA-4a) clone Bear-1 (Acris Antibodies, code AM00640PU-N); for CD11a (HNA-5a) clone 25.3.1 (Beckman Coulter, code IM0157).

6. Peroxidase-labeled goat anti-human IgG, Fcγ fragment specific (Dianova, code 109-035-098), dilute 1:5,000 with TRIS wash buffer/BSA 0.2 %.
7. Substrate: o-Phenylendiamin (OPD) (Dako, Glostrup, Denmark, code S2045): Dissolve one tablet OPD in 3 mL water and add 1.25 μL H_2O_2 30 %. Prepare directly before use.
8. Lysis buffer: Weigh 2.4 g Tris base, 8.76 g NaCl, 1.86 g EDTA and add 9.5 mL Triton X-100. Add water to a volume of 1 L.
9. Protease inhibitors: 0.1 M Pefabloc SC (Merck, code 1.24839), 0.001 M Leupeptin hemisulfate (Applichem, Darmstadt, Germany, code A2183) in 0.9 % NaCl. Add 30 μL Pefabloc SC and 20 μL Leupeptin solution per 950 μL lysis buffer directly before use.
10. Tris wash buffer: Dissolve 1.21 g Tris base and 72.5 mg $CaCl_2 \times 2H_2O$ in 0.9 % NaCl. Add 9.5 mL Triton X-100 and 4.5 mL Tween 20. Add 0.9 % NaCl to final volume of 1 L. Adjust pH to 7.0–7.4.
11. Tris wash buffer/BSA 0.2 %: Dilute 22 % BSA with Tris wash buffer 1:100.
12. Blocking reagent: Add 0.05 % Tween 20 to PBS.
13. 0.5 M H_2SO_4.
14. Microplate reader.

2.5 Genotyping Using PCR-SSP

1. 10 pmol/μL primers (Table 1) (Eurofins Genomics, Ebersberg, Germany).
2. HotStart Taq Polymerase (BioThermStar, Genecraft, Lüdinghausen, Germany).
3. dNTP mix 10 mM each.
4. Gel electrophoresis: Prepare 1.5 % agarose (Roth, code 297.2) gel in TBE buffer (Serva, Heidelberg, Germany, code 42557.01).
5. PCR tubes.
6. Thermocycler (GeneAmp PCR System 2700, Applied Biosystems, Weiterstadt, Germany).
7. Electrophoresis chamber.

3 Methods

Carry out all procedures at room temperature unless otherwise specified. Perform all centrifugation steps for cell suspensions with low brake.

Table 1
Primers for PCR-SSP

	Allele/antigen	Primer sequences (*S* sense, *AS* antisense)
1	*FCGR3B**01/HNA-1a	S: 5′-CAGTGGTTTCACAATGAGAA-3′ AS: 5′-ATGGACTTCTAGCTGCAC-3′
2	*FCGR3B**02/HNA-1b, -1d	S: 5′-CAATGGTACAGCGTGCTT-3′ AS: 5′-ACTGTCGTTGACTGTGTCAG-3′
3	*FCGR3B**03/HNA-1b, -1c	S: 5′-CAATGGTACAGCGTGCTT-3′ AS: 5′-ACTGTCGTTGACTGTGTCAT-3′
4	*SLC44A2**461G/HNA-3a	S: 5′-AGTGGCTGAGGTGCTTCG-3′ AS: 5′-GTGCGCCAATATCCTCACTTG-3′
5	*SLC44A2**461A/HNA-3b	S: 5′-GAGTGGCTGAGGTGCTTCA-3′ AS: 5′-GTGCGCCAATATCCTCACTTG-3′
6	*ITGAM**230G/HNA-4a	S: 5′-TCATGCGAGCCCATCCG-3′ AS: 5′-ACAAGGAGGTCTGACGGTG-3′
7	*ITGAM**230A/HNA-4bw	S: 5′-TCATGCGAGCCCATCCA-3′ AS: 5′-ACAAGGAGGTCTGACGGTG-3′
8	*ITGAL**2372G/HNA-5a	S: 5′-AGGTTGAGGCAGGAGAATGG-3′ AS: 5′-CAGTTAGACGCAGGGCTC-3′
9	*ITGAL**2372C/HNA-5bw	S: 5′-AGGTTGAGGCAGGAGAATGG-3′ AS: 5′-CAGTTAGACGCAGGGCTG-3′
	Int. control *HGH*	S: 5′-CAGTGCCTTCCCAACCATTCCCTTA-3′ AS: 5′-ATCCACTCACGGATTTCTGTTGTGTTTC-3′

3.1 Preparation of Neutrophils for GAT

1. Mix 3 mL EDTA-anticoagulated blood, 1 mL 5 % dextran, and 300 μL 5 % EDTA. Close the test tube with plastic film and incubate for 30 min at 37 °C at an angle of 45°.
2. Transfer the dextran plasma (supernatant) gently onto 2.5 mL Ficoll in a new test tube and centrifuge for 20 min at 310×*g*.
3. Obtain 1 mL plasma and spin down for later adjustment of the neutrophil suspension.
4. Discard the remaining supernatant and add 2 mL hemolysis buffer to the pellet.
5. Incubate for 5 min on melting ice.
6. Fill the tube with PBS buffer and spin down for 5 min at 140×*g*.
7. Discard the supernatant, resuspend the pellet with PBS buffer, and repeat the last step.
8. Discard the supernatant, resuspend the pellet with autologous plasma mentioned above, and adjust neutrophil concentration at 5,000 cells/μL with autologous plasma.

3.2 Preparation of Granulocytes for GIFT and MAIGA

1. Mix 10 mL EDTA-anticoagulated blood and 2.5 mL 5 % dextran. Close the test tube with plastic film and incubate for 30 min at 37 °C at an angle of 45°.
2. Transfer the dextran plasma (supernatant) gently onto 2.5 mL Ficoll in a new test tube and centrifuge for 20 min at 310 × *g*.
3. Discard the remaining supernatant and add 2 mL hemolysis buffer to the pellet.
4. Incubate for 5 min on melting ice.
5. Fill the tube with PBS buffer and spin down for 5 min at 140 × *g*.
6. Discard the supernatant, resuspend the pellet with PBS buffer, and repeat washing twice.
7. Discard the supernatant, resuspend the pellet with 1.5 mL PBS buffer, and add 0.5 mL PFA solution. Incubate exactly for 5 min in the dark.
8. Fill the tube with PBS buffer and spin down for 5 min at 140 × *g*.
9. Discard the supernatant, resuspend the pellet with PBS buffer, and repeat washing twice.
10. Discard the supernatant, resuspend the pellet with PBS buffer, and adjust neutrophil concentration at 5,000 cells/μL with PBS buffer.

3.3 Granulocyte Agglutination Test

To prevent evaporation during incubation, pipette one drop of paraffin oil into each well of a terasaki plate (60 well). Perform all tests in duplicate.

1. Pipette 2 μL granulocyte suspension (cell concentration 5×10^3 /μL) per well for each HNA-specific antiserum.
2. Add 6 μL HNA-specific antiserum to the neutrophils.
3. Incubate for 2 h at 37 °C and evaluate using an inverted microscope (*see* **Note 3**, Fig. 1).

3.4 Granulocyte Immunofluorescence Test

1. Pipette 40 μL granulocyte suspension (PFA-fixed, cell concentration 5×10^3/μL) per well for each HNA-specific antiserum (U-well microplate).
2. Add 40 μL HNA-specific antiserum to the neutrophils and mix manually.
3. Incubate for 30 min at 37 °C and mix again after 15 min.
4. Wash the cells three times with PBS buffer: Add 200 μL PBS buffer, and spin down for 1 min at 275 × *g*. Discard the supernatant and resuspend the cells using a shaking machine.
5. Add 40 μL anti-IgG-FITC (diluted 1:50 with PBS buffer) to each well and mix manually.

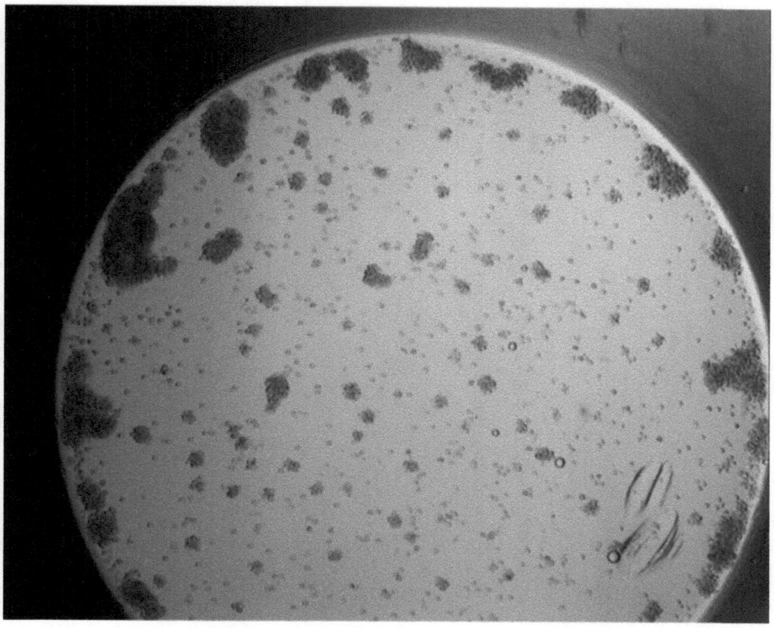

Fig. 1 Granulocyte agglutination test: Positive reaction with anti-HNA-3a typing serum

6. Incubate for 30 min in the dark and mix again after 15 min.
7. Wash the cells three times with PBS buffer.
8. For microscopic endpoint, resuspend the pellet with 50 μL glycerol solution and transfer to a microscope slide and cover. Store the slides in the dark for at least 15 min to allow the neutrophils to adhere. Evaluate using a fluorescence microscope with a 100 W Hg vapor lamp.
9. For flow cytometric endpoint, resuspend the pellet with 100 μL PBS (Fig. 2).

3.5 Monoclonal Antibody-Specific Immobilization of Granulocyte Antigens Assay

When the ambient air temperature is above 25 °C, perform the test in an air-conditioned room.

1. Coat the microtiter plates with 100 μL goat anti-mouse IgG (dilution 1:5,000 in coating buffer) in each well. Cover the plate and incubate for at least 12 h at 2–8 °C. One hour before plates are required on the day of testing, discard coating solution and fill the wells with 200–300 μL PBS/0.2 % BSA to block the plate. Incubate for 1 h at 2–8 °C. Wash the plate five times with PBS/0.05 % Tween 20 before use. Blot top face of microplate dry in between washes by placing on absorbent tissue.
2. Pipette 200 μL granulocyte suspension (PFA-fixed, cell concentration $5 \times 10^3/\mu L$) per well for each HNA-specific

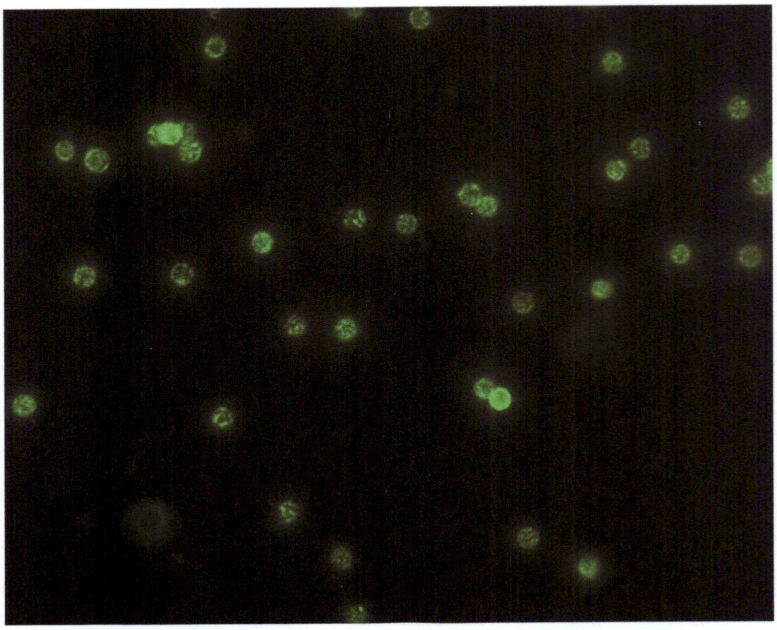

Fig. 2 Granulocyte immunofluorescence test: Positive reaction with anti-HNA-1a typing serum

antiserum in an U-well microplate, spin down for 1 min at 275 × *g*, discard the supernatant, and resuspend with 100 μL PBS/0.2 % BSA.

3. Add 50 μL HNA-specific antiserum to the neutrophils, mix manually, and incubate for 30 min at 37 °C.
4. Wash the cells with 50 μL PBS/0.2 % BSA, and spin down for 1 min at 275 × *g*. Discard the supernatant and resuspend the cells with 50 μL PBS/2 % BSA.
5. Add 10 μL of the respective monoclonal antibody (0.02 mg/mL) and incubate for 30 min at 37 °C.
6. Wash the cells three times with 150 μL PBS/0.2 % BSA, then resuspend the pellets with 100 μL lysis buffer containing protease inhibitors, and transfer to 1.5 mL microfuge tubes.
7. Lysis: Incubate for 30 min at 2–8 °C.
8. In the meanwhile prepare another set of microfuge tubes. For each test aliquot 180 μL Tris wash buffer/0.2 % BSA into the tubes and store at 2–8 °C.
9. Centrifuge the cell lysates at maximum speed in a microcentrifuge (14,000 × *g* approx.) for 30 min at 4 °C. Pipette 70 μL of the supernatant in the new tube containing 180 μL Tris wash buffer/0.2 % BSA.

10. Transfer 100 μL diluted granulocyte lysate, in duplicate, to the pre-coated and blocked F-well microplate. Add 100 μL Tris wash buffer/0.2 % BSA to 2 pre-coated wells (=reagent blank). Incubate at 4 °C for 90 min.
11. Wash the plate five times with PBS/0.05 % Tween 20. Blot top face of microplate dry in between washes by placing on absorbent tissue.
12. Add 100 μL diluted (1:5,000) peroxidase-labeled anti-human IgG to each well and incubate at 4 °C for 120 min.
13. Wash the plate five times with PBS/0.05 % Tween 20. Blot top face of microplate dry in between washes by placing on absorbent tissue.
14. Add 100 μL substrate solution to each well and incubate for 15 min at room temperature in the dark.
15. Stop the reaction by adding 100 μL 0.5 M H_2SO_4. Read the absorbance at 492 nm (for dual-wavelength ELISA readers a reference filter between 620 and 650 is suitable) within 1 h (*see* **Note 4**).

3.6 Genotyping with PCR-SSP

1. Prepare genomic DNA from anticoagulated blood and adjust concentration to 50 ng/μL.
2. Nine primer pairs (Table 1) are needed for complete HNA genotyping.
3. Use the pipetting scheme given in Table 2 to set up the PCR.

Table 2
Pipetting scheme to set up the PCR-SSP for HNA genotyping

		HNA-1, -3	HNA-4, -5
	Primer pair	1, 2, 3, 4, 5	6, 7, 8, 9
Reagent	Initial conc.		
PCR buffer	10×	2.0 μL	2.0 μL
dNTP mix	10 mM	0.4 μL	0.4 μL
Primer I	10 pmol/μL	1.0 μL	1.0 μL
Primer II	10 pmol/μL	1.0 μL	1.0 μL
HGH primer I	1.25 pmol/μL	1.0 μL	0.8 μL
HGH primer II	1.25 pmol/μL	1.0 μL	0.8 μL
Distilled water		11.4 μL	11.8 μL
Taq polymerase	5 U/μL	0.2 μL	0.2 μL
DNA	50 ng/μL	2.0 μL	2.0 μL

Table 3
Thermocycling program for PCR-SSP

	HNA-1	HNA-3, -4, -5
Initial denaturation	95 °C, 10 min	
Cycles	35 cycles: 95 °C, 30 s 59 °C, 1 min 72 °C, 30 s	10 cycles: 95 °C, 30 s 64 °C, 40 s 72 °C, 30 s 20 cycles: 95 °C, 30 s 61 °C, 40 s 72 °C, 30 s
Final elongation	72 °C, 5 min	72 °C, 5 min
Product sizes	FCGR3B*01: 141 bp FCGR3B*01: 157 bp	SLC44A2: 291/292 bp ITGAM: 249 bp ITGAL: 283 bp

4. Thermocycling is performed using the program given in Table 3.
5. Analyze PCR products by electrophoretic separation on a 1.5 % agarose gel stained with ethidium bromide (*see* **Note 5**).

4 Notes

1. The solution is sensitive to light and stable for 2 weeks maximum.
2. The buffer is stable for 2 weeks at 4 °C. Leave one aliquot at 4 °C for current use and store remaining aliquots at –20 °C.
3. If results are questionable or very weak, incubation may be extended to monitor changes or progress.
4. Positive reaction: OD >0.3 or at least double OD of negative control. The negative control should not exceed OD 0.2.
5. The product size of the internal control (HGH) is 439 bp. If there is only a weak reaction with the *SLC44A2**461G (HNA-3a) primer pair: in rare cases, there is a point mutation at position 457 (C457T) influencing primer binding. Up to now, the mutation was detected only in the *SLC44A2**461G allele [16].

References

1. Greinacher A, Wesche J, Hammer E, Fürll B, Völker U, Reil A, Bux J (2010) Characterization of the human neutrophil alloantigen (HNA) 3a. Nat Med 16:45–48
2. Kissel K, Scheffler S, Kerowgan M, Bux J (2000) Molecular basis of NB1 (HNA-2a, CD177) deficiency. Blood 99:4231–4233
3. Lucas G, Porcelijn L, Fung YL, Green F, Reil A, Hopkins M, Green A, de Haas M, Bux J (2013) External quality assessment of human neutrophil antigen (HNA)-specific antibody detection and HNA genotyping from 2000 to 2012. Vox Sang 105:259–269
4. Bux J, Chapman J (1997) Report on the second international granulocyte serology workshop. Transfusion 37:977–983
5. Böyum A (1968) A one-stage procedure for isolation of granulocytes and lymphocytes from human blood. Scand J Clin Lab Invest Suppl 97:51–76
6. Verheugt FW, von dem Borne AE, Décary F, Engelfriet CP (1977) The detection of granulocyte alloantibodies with an indirect immunofluorescence test. Br J Haematol 36: 533–544
7. Jiang A, Lalezari P (1975) A micro-technique for detection of leukocyte agglutinins. J Immunol Methods 7:103–108
8. Bux J, Kober B, Kiefel V, Mueller-Eckhardt C (1993) Analysis of granulocyte-reactive antibodies using an immunoassay based upon monoclonal antibody-specific immobilization of granulocyte antigens (MAIGA). Transfus Med 3:157–162
9. Bux J, Stein EL, Santoso S, Mueller-Eckhardt C (1995) NA gene frequencies in the German population, determined by polymerase chain reaction with sequence-specific primers. Transfusion 35:54–57
10. Bux J, Stein EL, Bierling P, Fromont P, Clay M, Stroncek D, Santoso S (1997) Characterization of a new alloantigen (SH) on the human neutrophil Fc gamma receptor IIIb. Blood 89:1027–1034
11. Steffensen R, Gülen T, Varming K, Jersild C (1999) FcgammaRIIIB polymorphism: evidence that NA1/NA2 and SH are located in two closely linked loci and that the SH allele is linked to the NA1 allele in the Danish population. Transfusion 39:593–598
12. Sachs UJ, Chavakis T, Fung L, Lohrenz A, Bux J, Reil A, Ruf A, Santoso S (2004) Human alloantibody anti-Mart interferes with Mac-1-dependent leukocyte adhesion. Blood 104: 727–734
13. Sachs UJ, Reil A, Bauer C, Bux J, Bein G, Santoso S (2005) Genotyping of human neutrophil antigen-5a (Ond). Transfus Med 15:115–117
14. Reil A, Wesche J, Greinacher A, Bux J (2011) Geno- and phenotyping and immunogenicity of HNA-3. Transfusion 51:18–24
15. Reil A, Sachs UJ, Siahanidou T, Flesch BK, Bux J (2013) HNA-1d: a new human neutrophil antigen located on Fcγ receptor IIIb associated with neonatal immune neutropenia. Transfusion 53:2145–2151
16. Flesch BK, Reil A, Bux J (2011) Genetic variation of the HNA-3a encoding gene. Transfusion 51:2391–2397

Chapter 17

Allelic Discrimination by TaqMan-PCR for Genotyping of Human Neutrophil Antigens

Rudi Steffensen, John Baech, and Kaspar R. Nielsen

Abstract

Neutrophil antigens are implicated in a variety of clinical conditions, including neonatal immune neutropenia, transfusion-related acute lung injury, refractoriness to granulocyte transfusions, febrile transfusion reactions, and autoimmune neutropenia. In this report, we describe simultaneous genotyping of human neutrophil antigens (HNA)-1, -3, -4, and -5 using PCR with allele-specific TaqMan probes and end-point fluorescence detection, which is a robust, rapid, and reproducible method, allowing for high-throughput genotyping.

Key words Human neutrophil antigen, Genotyping, Real-time PCR, TaqMan, HNA

1 Introduction

The current HNA nomenclature defines eight antigens that are assigned to five antigen groups, where seven antigens have been characterized on the molecular level. In this report, we describe the genotyping of HNA epitopes, which is routinely performed in most laboratories due to their clinical significance as part of an investigation of antibodies against neutrophil antigens that are involved in a variety of clinical conditions, such as immune neutropenia, transfusion-related acute lung injury, and febrile transfusion reactions [1–3].

The HNA-1 antigens are encoded by the Fc gamma receptor IIIb (*FCGR3B)* gene, which consists of five exons within 699 bp encoding 233 amino acids. cDNA analysis of this gene revealed five single-nucleotide polymorphisms (SNPs) in nucleotides (nts) 141 (rs403016), 147 (rs447536), 227 (rs448740), 277 (rs428888), and 349 (rs2290834) that are associated with the HNA-1a and HNA-1b antigens [4]. An additional SNP at nt position 266 (rs52820103) in the allele encoding HNA-1b defines the HNA-1c antigen [5]. As a result, three alleles exist on the FCGGR3 locus: FCGR3B*01 (HNA-1a), FCGR3B*02 (HNA-1b), and

Peter Bugert (ed.), *Molecular Typing of Blood Cell Antigens*, Methods in Molecular Biology, vol. 1310,
DOI 10.1007/978-1-4939-2690-9_17, © Springer Science+Business Media New York 2015

Table 1
Interpretation of the five single-nucleotide substitution in the HNA 1 system compared with FCGR3A

	Old nt ID	147	227	266	277	349
Allele	New nt ID	114	194	233	244	316
FCGR3B*01	HNA-1a	C	A	C	G	G
FCGR3B*02	HNA-1b	T	G	C	A	A
FCGR3B*03	HNA-1c	T	G	A	A	A
FCGR3B*04	HNA-1a	C	A	C	G	A
FCGR3B*05	HNA-1b	T	G	C	G	A
FCGR3A		C	G	C	G	A

FCGR3B*03 (HNA-1c). HNA-1 genotyping is complicated by the existence of the highly homologous *FCGR3A* gene because FCGR3B*01 and FCGR3A are identical at nts 141, 147, and 277, whereas FCGR3B*02 and FCGR3A are identical at nts 227 and 349 (Table 1) [4, 5]. These are the nucleotide positions according to the old system described in 1989, but the adapted numbers according to the NCBI database entry (NM_000570.4) are 114 (147), 194 (227), 233 (266), 244 (277), and 316 (349) [6]. In addition to two new alleles, FCGR3B*04 and FCGR3B*05 were recently defined as variations of the HNA-1a and HNA-1b antigen system, respectively, by the granulocyte immunology workshops.

HNA-3, -4, and -5 are biallelic antigens, which are encoded from the choline transporter-like protein-2 (*SLC44A2*) gene, the integrin alpha M (*ITGAM*) gene, and the integrin alpha L (*ITGAL*) gene, respectively (Table 2) [1, 7, 8].

Because the HNA-1, -3, -4, and -5 antigens are identified as SNPs, they can be detected by TaqMan-based genotyping assays using two TaqMan probes labeled with two different reporter dyes, FAM or VIC, at the 5′ end and a non-fluorescent quencher attached to a minor groove binder (MGB-NQF) at the 3′ end to increase the stability and specificity of probe hybridization [9]. The two TaqMan probes are used in the same PCR mix, allowing single-tube genotyping for each biallelic system. During the primer extension phase of PCR, the 5′–3′ exonuclease activity of Taq polymerase cleaves and releases the reporter dye from bound probes, which results in an increase in fluorescence. At the end of the PCR, the emission intensity of each fluorophore is measured and allele determination can be made.

TaqMan assays offer the advantages of using standardized reagents and thermal cycling protocols. Moreover, there is the obvious advance in an extensive assays-by-design service. These procedures, coupled with automated systems that employ real-time

Table 2
Primers and MGB probes used in real-time PCR for HNA-1 genotyping

Nucleotide change	SNP ID	Primers	Probes
nt 147/114	rs447536	for 5′-CCTGGCACTTCAGAG TCACA-3′ rev 5′-CCTGGAG CCTCAATGGTACAG-3′	5′-VIC-CTGTCCTTCTC GAGCAC-MGB-NFQ-3′ 5′-FAM-TGTCCTTCT CAAGCAC-MGB-NFQ-3′
nt 227/194	rs448740	for 5′-CCTGAGGACAATTC CACACAGT-3′ rev 5′-CGA GGCCTGGCTTGAGA-3′	5′-VIC-CACAATGAGAA CCTCA-MGB-NFQ-3′ 5′-FAM-CACAATGAGA GCCTCA-MGB-NFQ-3′
nt 266/233	rs52820103	for 5′-GCACCTGTACTCT CCACTGT-3′ rev 5′-AGC CAGGCCTCGAGCTA-3′	5′-VIC-CTTCATTGACGCT GCCAC-MGB-NFQ-3′ 5′-FAM-TTCATTGACG ATGCCAC-MGB-NFQ-3′
nt 277/244	rs428888	for 5′-GGCCTCGAGCTACT TCATTGAC-3′ rev 5′-GT TTGTCTGGCAC CTGTACTCT-3′	5′-VIC-CCACAGTCAACG ACAG-MGB-NFQ-3′ 5′-FAM-CCACAGTCGA CGACAG-MGB-NFQ-3′
nt 349/316	rs2290834	for 5′-AACCTCTCCACCC TCAGTGA-3′ rev 5′-GGTG ATTTTCCTCTTC CCCTTCATC-3′	5′-VIC-TAGAAGTCCATA TCGGTG-MGB-NFQ-3′ 5′-FAM-CTAGAAGTCCA TGTCGGTG-MGB-NFQ-3′

MGB-NFQ minor groove binder and non-fluorescent quencher

amplification and simultaneous detection in a closed system, have substantially reduced the possibility of false positive results because amplification products carry over contamination. The TaqMan SNP genotyping assay is an end-point detection system that can be used with 96- or 384-well plates. Thermal cycling can be performed on a standard PCR machine, and a real-time PCR instrument is required only for detection of increased fluorescence for genotype determination.

2 Materials

2.1 Genomic DNA Extraction

1. EDTA-stabilized peripheral blood sample (4 ml) stored at 4 °C until processing.
2. Maxwell 16 System Blood DNA Purification Kit (Promega, Madison, WI, USA).
3. NanoDrop ND-1000 spectrophotometer or similar spectrophotometer.

Table 3
Predesigned TaqMan assays used for HNA-3, -4, and -5 genotyping

System	Nucleotide change	SNP database ID	Assay ID
HNA-3	461G>A	rs2288904	C_25754090_10
HNA-4	328G>A	rs1143679	C_2847895_1_
HNA-5	2466G>C	rs2230433	C_11789692_10

2.2 TaqMan Allelic Discrimination Assay

1. All primers and predesigned TaqMan SNP Genotyping Assays used for PCR amplification were synthesized by and ordered from Applied Biosystems (Foster City, CA, USA) and are listed in Tables 2 and 3 [10].
2. TaqMan 2× Universal PCR master mix with UNG (Applied Biosystems, Foster City, CA, USA) stored at −20 °C.
3. Nuclease-free water.
4. DNA samples of a known genotype homozygous for the "a" and "b" alleles of the HNA system at a DNA concentration of 20–25 ng/μl.
5. MicroAmp optical 96-well or 384-well reaction plates (Applied Biosystems, Foster City, CA, USA).
6. MicroAmp Optical adhesive film (Applied Biosystems, Foster City, CA, USA).
7. GeneAmp PCR system 9700 Thermal cycler, Real-Time PCR System 7900HT or QuantStudio 12 K Flex (Applied Biosystems, Foster City, CA, USA).

3 Methods

3.1 Genomic DNA Extraction

1. Extract DNA from whole blood according to the manufacturers' instructions.
2. Measure the DNA concentration by using a NanoDrop ND-1000 spectrophotometer or a similar spectrophotometer.
3. Store purified DNA at −20 °C.

3.2 TaqMan Allelic Discrimination Assay

1. For each HNA system, prepare a reaction mix containing 2× Universal PCR master mix, 0.9 μM forward primer, 0.9 μM reverse primer, 0.2 μM VIC-labeled probe, 0.2 μM FAM-labeled probe, or 40× predesigned TaqMan SNP Genotyping Assays carried out in 5 μl using a 384-well plate or in 25 μl using a 96-well plate (*see* **Note 1**).

2. To each plate, add 1–2 μl of DNA samples at a concentration of 20–25 ng/μl, 1–2 μl of the "a" and "b" allele homozygous positive control samples, and 1–2 μl of nuclease-free water to provide "no-template" negative controls (NTCs).
3. Seal the plates with optical film.
4. Centrifuge the sealed plates at 900 ×*g* for 1 min (*see* **Note 2**).
5. Place the prepared assay plate in a PCR cycler under the following conditions: 50 °C for 2 min, 95 °C for 10 min, and 40 cycles of 95 °C for 15 s and 60 °C for 1 min, followed by incubation at 4 °C.

3.3 Result Interpretation

These directions assume the use of an ABI Prism 7900HT sequence detection system using SDS software version 2.3 or the QuantStudio 12 K Flex system QuantStudio 12 K Flex using software version 1.2.2.

1. Start the software program and create a new allelic discrimination 96- or 384-well plate.
2. Create two "detectors" (one for each probe, e.g., "1a" and "1b") and add these to a "marker" corresponding to the assay plate to be analyzed (e.g., HNA-1).
3. Select sample wells of the plate, assign the marker to the samples, and assign them as "Unknown." Select and assign the no-template control wells to designate them as "NTC" and select and assign the positive control wells as the genotypes of these samples.
4. Read the plates as a post-PCR run on a real-time system and save the raw data file.
5. View the results as a scatter graph and check that the no-template control wells and the positive control samples for both alleles have been amplified and correctly assigned by the software; an example is shown in Fig. 1.
6. Look at the clustering of the automatically assigned genotypes and check the raw spectra for any outlying or indeterminate results. If necessary, manually reassign any erroneous samples (*see* **Note 3** and Fig. 2).

4 Notes

1. The TaqMan 5′-nuclease assay will work on samples of varying quality or concentration; however, to ensure accurate pipetting, it is important to use a robot workstation, especially when working in a 384-well format, to ensure a good quality of DNA amplification.

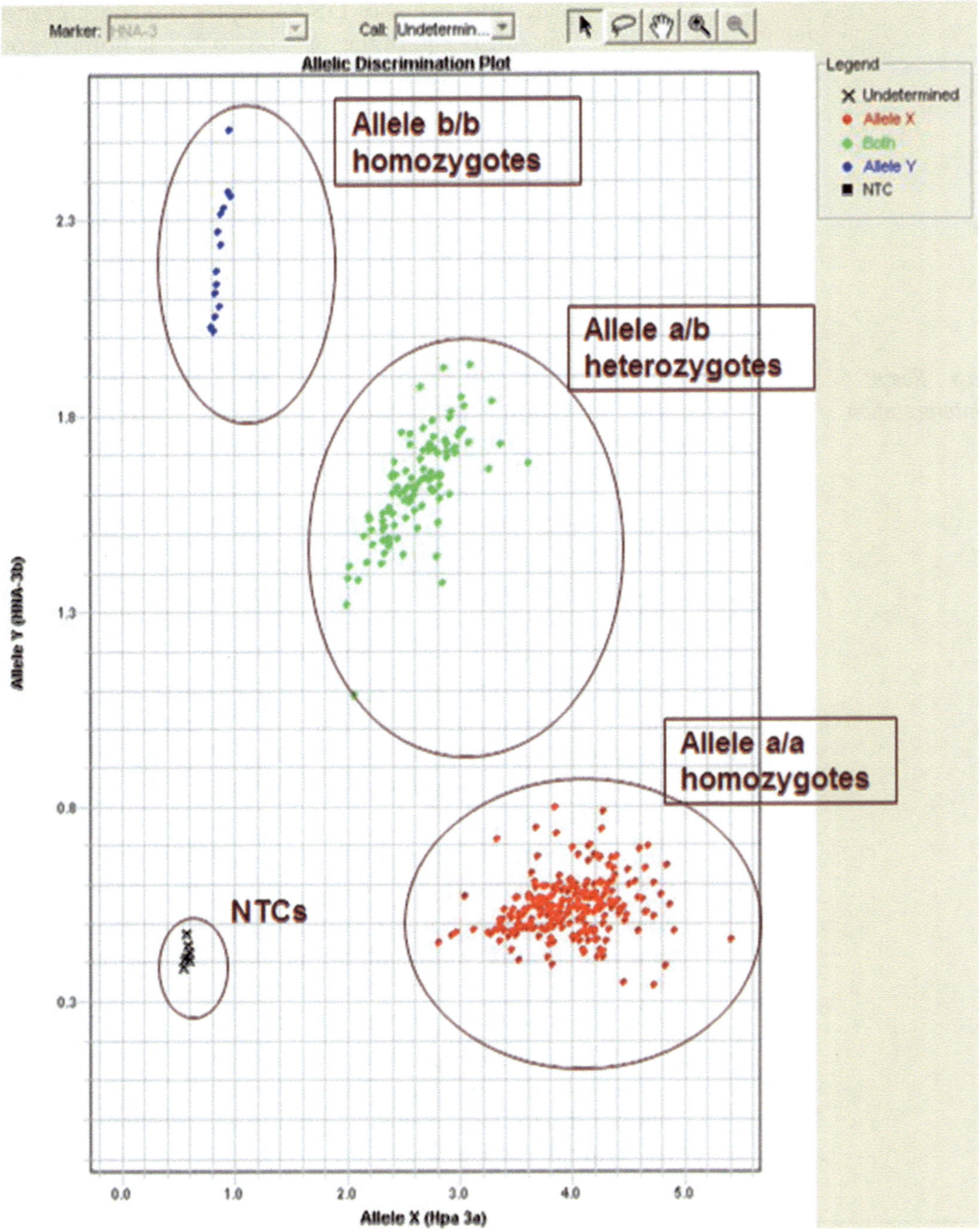

Fig. 1 Allelogram showing the HNA-3 genotyping distribution for 384-well samples after post-PCR assignment of three well-defined clusters and NTCs (*black crosses*) using the SDS software

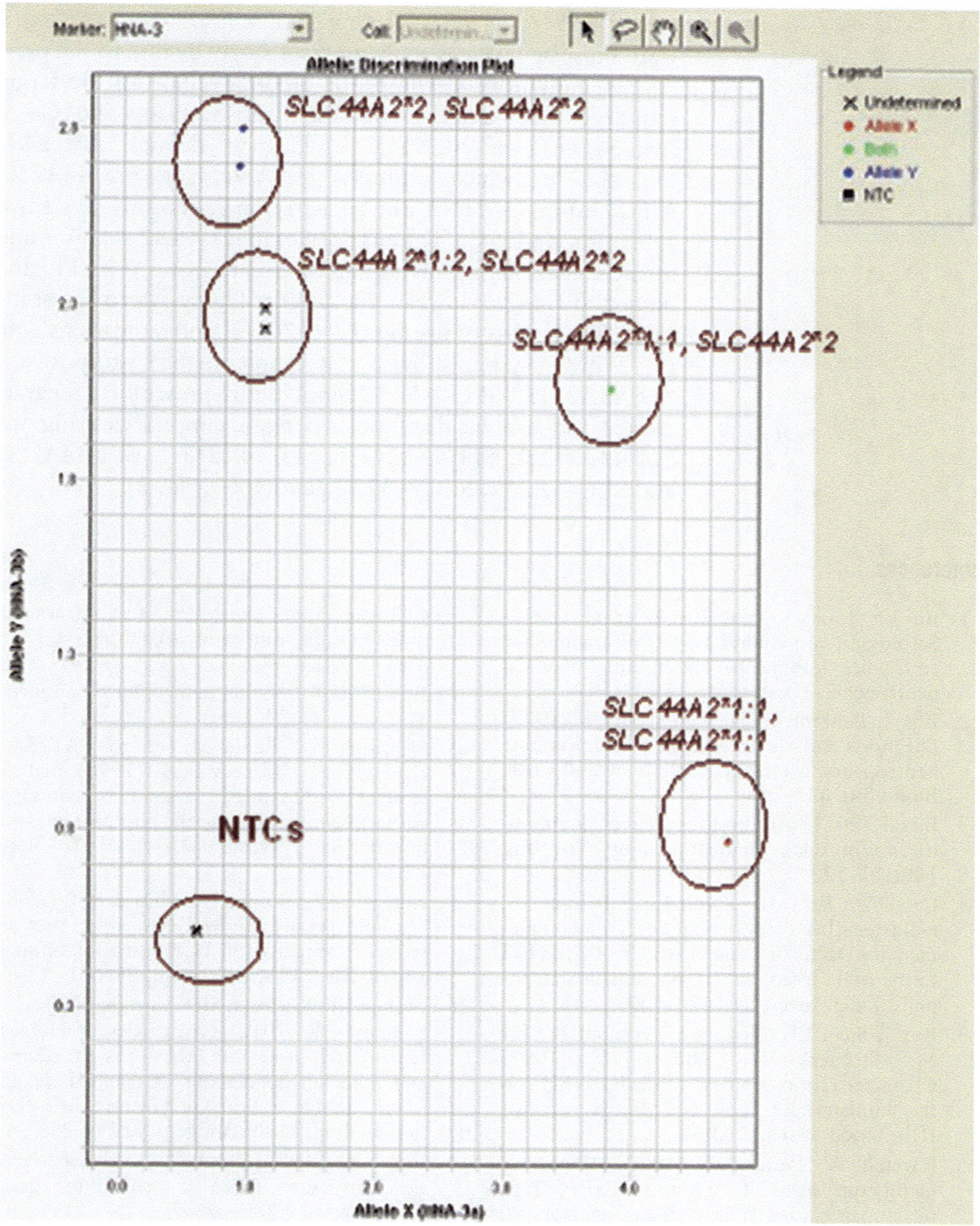

Fig. 2 TaqMan SNP genotyping results for the *SLC44A2* genotypes (rs2288904). The allelogram shows a typical TaqMan assay result with well-defined clusters. The *two dark-blue dots* are from two samples representing homozygous *SLC44A2*2, SLC44A2*2* samples, the *light-green dot* is a heterozygous *SLC44A2*1:1, SLC44A2*2* sample and the *red dot* represents a *SLC44A2*1:1, SLC44A2*1:1* sample. The *two black crosses* are from two samples carrying the rare *SLC44A2* 1:2, SLC44A2* 2* allelic combination

2. Centrifugation of the assay plates is important.
3. Care must be taken as outlying results may be due to the presence of mutations in the probe-binding region of the target sequence. A single-nucleotide substitution (461G>A; Arg154Gln) on the SLC44A2 gene defines the allele SLC44A2*1, which expresses HNA-3a, and SLC44A2*2, which expresses HNA-3b; an additional, recently described substitution (457C>T; Leu153Phe) inSLC44A2 that is found in the Caucasian population at a frequency of 1.0 % [11] and named SLC44A2*1:2 can impact genotyping systems in some cases. The results of testing the 457C>T polymorphisms with this TaqMan system showed that samples heterozygous for the SLC44A2*1:2; SLC44A2*2 genotype are present in a separate cluster and can be distinguished from samples carrying the SLC44A2*1:1, SLC44A2*1:1; SLC44A2*1:1, SLC44A2*2; and SLC44A2*2, SLC44A2*2 genotypes (Fig. 2).

References

1. Bux J, Jung KD, Kauth T et al (1992) Serological and clinical aspects of granulocyte antibodies leading to alloimmune neonatal neutropenia. Transfus Med 2:143–149
2. Bux J, Behrens G, Jäger G, Welte K (1997) Diagnosis and clinical course of autoimmune neutropenia in infancy: analysis of 240 cases. Blood 89:1027–1036
3. Bux J (2011) Antibody-mediated (immune) transfusion-related acute lung injury. Vox Sang 100:122–128
4. Ory PA, Clark MR, Kwoh EE, Clarkson SB, Goldstein IM (1989) Sequences of complementary DNAs that encode the NA1 and NA2 forms of Fc receptor III on human neutrophils. J Clin Invest 84:1688–1691
5. Bux J, Stein EL, Bierling P, Fromont P, Clay M, Stroncek D, Santoso S (1997) Characterization of a new alloantigen (SH) on the human neutrophil Fc gamma receptor IIIb. Blood 89:1027–1034
6. Ravetch JV, Perussia B (1989) Alternative membrane forms of Fc gamma RIII(CD16) on human natural killer cells and neutrophils. Cell type-specific expression of two genes that differ in single nucleotide substitutions. J Exp Med 170:481–497
7. Bux J (2008) Human neutrophil alloantigens. Vox Sang 94:277–285
8. Huizinga TWJ, Kleijer M, Tetteroo PAT, Roos D, von dem Borne AEGK (1990) Biallelic neutrophil NAantigen system is associated with a polymorphism on the phospho-inositol-linked Fcγ receptor III (CD16). Blood 75:213–217
9. Kutyavin IV, Afonina IA, Mills A et al (2000) 3′-minor groove binder-DNA probes increase sequence specificity at PCR extension temperatures. Nucleic Acids Res 28:655–661
10. Nielsen KR, Koelbaek MD, Varming K, Baech J, Steffensen R (2012) Frequencies of HNA-1, HNA-3, HNA-4, and HNA-5 in the Danish and Zambian populations determined using a novel TaqMan real time polymerase chain reaction method. Tissue Antigens 80:249–253
11. Flesch BK, Reil A, Bux J (2011) Genetic variation of the HNA-3a encoding gene. Transfusion 11:2391–2397

Chapter 18

Novel Approaches and Technologies in Molecular HLA Typing

Paul P.J. Dunn

Abstract

The invention of the Polymerase Chain Reaction (PCR) has revolutionized molecular biology enabling gene isolation and characterization in hours rather than days. Scientists working in transplant diagnostics have proven to be pioneers in adapting this molecular technique to the clinical needs of histocompatibility testing. This chapter describes a number of novel genotyping technologies which have been used to address the challenges posed by genetic diversity seen in the extensive polymorphism in HLA genes. These novel approaches include single-stranded and duplex conformational analyses, real-time PCR, microarray hybridization, RNA-based sequencing, and the present day Next Generation Sequencing. The chapter concludes with a brief look at a possible next, Next Generation Sequencing system.

Key words Human leukocyte antigens, HLA genotyping, Next generation sequencing

1 Introduction

The "Classical" Human Leukocyte Antigen system comprises six loci divided into class I (HLA-A, -B, and -C) and class II (HLA-DP, -DQ, and -DR). The principal function of these proteins is to present peptides which are derived from viral and intracellular proteins (class I function) or those derived from processing of pathogens and extracellular proteins (class II). Class I presented peptides are recognized by CD8+ cytotoxic lymphocytes and class II presented peptides by CD4+ T-helper cells [1]. HLA are the most polymorphic protein and genetic systems found in humans and represent a significant hurdle for successful allogeneic transplantation of an organ or stem cells [2, 3] and in stem cell banking and future applications [4].

Serological approaches were used for defining the tissue types, or HLA, in humans [5] but, since the development of the polymerase chain reaction (PCR) [6], DNA-based PCR methods have predominated in the tissue typing laboratory for HLA typing [7]. HLA typing techniques used by tissue typing laboratories need to

Peter Bugert (ed.), *Molecular Typing of Blood Cell Antigens*, Methods in Molecular Biology, vol. 1310,
DOI 10.1007/978-1-4939-2690-9_18, © Springer Science+Business Media New York 2015

be flexible to ensure typing of required loci at the appropriate levels of resolution. Most HLA typing (90 %) in a laboratory that supports transplant programs (solid organ and hematopoietic stem cell), transfusion support, autoimmune disease, and hypersensitive drug associations needs only to be at split specificity level or 2-digit level (e.g., HLA-A*02) rather than allele level which is 4 digits or more (e.g., HLA-A*02:01). HLA-A, HLA-B, and HLA-DRB1 are "routinely typed" for transplant patients and donors, but additional loci may need to be typed. For example, if a patient has been shown to have antibodies against HLA-C, or HLA-DQ or HLA-DP, then the appropriate locus needs to be typed for patient and potential donor.

The unceasing unraveling of the complexity of HLA polymorphism has spawned the adaption and development of new technologies used in tissue typing laboratories. Various techniques have been developed and modified in the post-PCR era, including PCR-sequence-specific primer (PCR-SSP) [8], PCR-sequence-specific oligonucleotide probe (PCR-SSOP) [9], PCR-sequencing-based typing (PCR-SBT) [10], oligonucleotide arrays [11], and, more recently, next generation sequencing (NGS) [12]. A comparison of these different technologies has been reviewed recently [13].

The complexity and expanse of HLA polymorphism has attracted laboratories to try many different molecular methods to achieve an HLA type. The unabating march of HLA polymorphism, mainly discovered through DNA sequencing, has revealed the inadequacies of many of these technologies. These methods must be robust and accurate, demonstrate reasonable throughput, and be cost effective. The purpose of this review chapter is to discuss novel approaches and technologies which have been applied to the science of HLA typing.

2 Conformational Analyses

DNA conformational analysis relies upon the sequence-dependent refolding of DNA after temperature denaturation. In PCR-Single Strand Conformation Polymorphism (PCR-SSCP), polymorphic exons are amplified then denatured and electrophoresed through a vertical polyacrylamide gel at 28 °C. Migrated DNA bands are revealed by silver staining and compared to the migration of known or reference alleles [14]. This method has a size limitation, only effective in analyzing one exon at a time. In a variation of this method [15], the HLA-DRB1 alleles in a sample were separated using a denaturing gel. Amplified HLA-DRB1 exon 2 was electrophoresed across the top of an entire vertical polyacrylamide gel maintained at 60 °C which contained a perpendicular gradient of 0–80 % denaturant, denaturant being 7 M urea and 40 % formamide. Silver staining the gel revealed DNA. The DRB1 alleles separate at a given concentration of denaturants which was confirmed by excising the DNA from acrylamide and DNA sequencing. Size limitations and throughput are the major drawbacks of this method and the concentration of denaturant for allele separation has to be determined.

Reference strand-mediated conformational analysis (RSCA) is a double-stranded DNA conformational method for high-resolution typing class I and II genes using native polyacrylamide gels [16–18]. In this method, amplified unknown sample (e.g., exon 2, class II, or exons 2 and 3, class I) is mixed with dye-labeled amplified reference allele (same locus), the mixture is heated to 95 °C, and the strands are allowed to reanneal in a thermal cycler. The resultant mixture of homo- and heteroduplexes is separated by electrophoresis through a native polyacrylamide gel system with a laser to detect fluorescence. Homoduplexes migrate faster through the gel than heteroduplexes, and only fluorescent duplexes are observed. With fluorescently labeled DNA standards run in the gel, it is possible to accurately type the samples at the allele level. At the time, this appeared to be a simple method for allele-level HLA typing but as more and more alleles were discovered, their RSCA characterization required more and more reference alleles. Also, the limit on amplicon size being 900 bp restricted the number of exons for analysis, and the inconsistent separation of duplexes in the newer high-throughput capillary electrophoresis machines meant that this technology disappeared from use almost as quickly as it had appeared. Such conformational analysis is probably more suited to less polymorphic systems.

Thorsby's group described a variation on heteroduplex separation of HLA-A alleles using denaturing High Performance Liquid Chromatography (dHPLC) [19]. This method also used a reference allele (A*01:01), but the allele required several mutant nucleotides to be introduced to enable allele separation. In this process the sample is amplified (e.g., exons 2 and 3 of HLA-A) with biotin attached to one primer [19]. One strand of denatured amplicon was captured on streptavidin-coated beads and mixed with the reference allele, heated to 95 °C, and then cooled to 65 °C followed by 4 °C. Heteroduplexes formed between the sample and reference alleles were separated on the WAVE™ DNA Fragment Analysis System (Transgenomic Inc, San Jose, CA, USA). Heteroduplexes were then reamplified prior to HLA typing by sequencing [19]. Although an elegant technique the addition of extra equipment plus low throughput and size limitation in gene analysis meant that the technology has not really been used for HLA typing. My laboratory also attempted separation of amplified class I HLA alleles, but the WAVE™ analysis produced very broad overlapping peaks and it was not possible to separate alleles (Day S and Dunn PPJ 2000, personal communication).

3 Real-Time PCR Technology

Real-time PCR has advantages over conventional PCR in increased sensitivity and the ability to quantify target nucleic acids. A number of real-time PCR techniques have been employed in HLA typing.

The "Taqman" assay (Fig. 1) is useful for interrogating individual SNPs. An oligonucleotide probe is designed for a specific SNP and this probe has a reporter fluorophore at the 3′ end and a quencher at the 5′ end. When the oligonucleotide is intact, the reporter cannot fluoresce because of the close proximity of the quencher. Two primers, sense and antisense, are also used to amplify a short region of the DNA which encompasses the SNP and its probe.

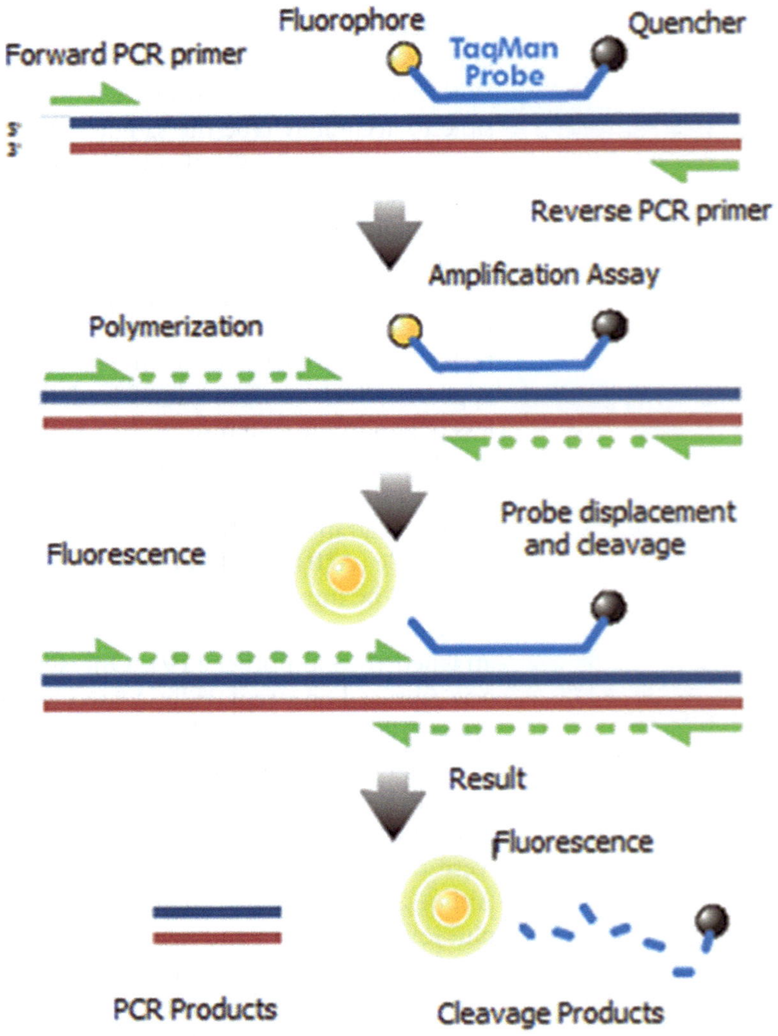

Fig. 1 The principles of the Taqman assay. The probe anneals to the informative SNP, if present

When PCR of this region of DNA occurs the polymerase copies DNA but when it reaches the probe nuclease activity inherent in the polymerase releases the probe nucleotide-by-nucleotide. The fluorophore is released enabling it to fluoresce as it is now not constrained by the quencher dye which is also released. The real-time machine detects the fluorescence. Taqman assays have been described in HLA typing but these are restricted to a specific work area in tissue typing, in identifying an HLA locus or its subtyping, such as HLA-B27 [20, 21] and DRB1*15:01 [22]. Although a very sensitive technique, the Taqman assay is not suited to routine HLA typing because it is not designed for the analysis of a large number of SNPs, does not have the throughput, and, using fluorescent probes, makes this an expensive technique. My laboratory does not use the Taqman assay for HLA typing but uses it for assessment of the Rhesus status of a fetus by genotyping free fetal DNA in mum's circulating blood—here a small number of SNPs are assayed and sensitivity is required to detect minute quantities of fetal DNA against a high maternal DNA background.

In contrast, High-Resolution Melting Assay (HRMA) utilizes a pair of amplification primers, sense and antisense, which are used to amplify a short region of DNA containing an informative SNP. A fluorescent dye is included in the PCR and when this is complete, the temperature is slowly increased to melt the DNA and displace fluorescent dye. Changes in the fluorescence intensity can be measured across small temperature increments. Using high-resolution melting curve analysis, the different SNPs or alleles or combination of alleles can be identified by the shape of their curve and the formation of clusters. The process measures the change in the melting curve when double-stranded DNA dissociates into single-stranded DNA as the temperature increases. While the DNA remains double stranded, the bound saturating dye fluoresces and as the DNA melts, this dye is displaced and the fluorescence decreases. A difference plot is constructed by subtracting each curve from a reference curve or the most abundant curve. The shape and clustering of the curves is the most important function and the instrument software can automatically calculate and cluster the samples into groups based on the melting profile and the differences between wild type and variants are clearly identified. HRMA analysis is a simple, cost-effective, fast, and robust technique. Figure 2 shows an example of an HRMA to genotype the *Kidd* blood group system, whose gene has one informative SNP and some rare nulls caused by SNPs (L Wall, NZBS, personal communication). HRMA has been applied in HLA typing in simple allelic systems such as for coeliac disease screening by HLA-DQA/DQB typing [23], HLA-B27 typing [24], B*57:01, and abacavir hypersensitivity [25]. Wittwer's group have also used HRMA to show HLA identity in a bone marrow transplant family study without HLA genotyping [26].

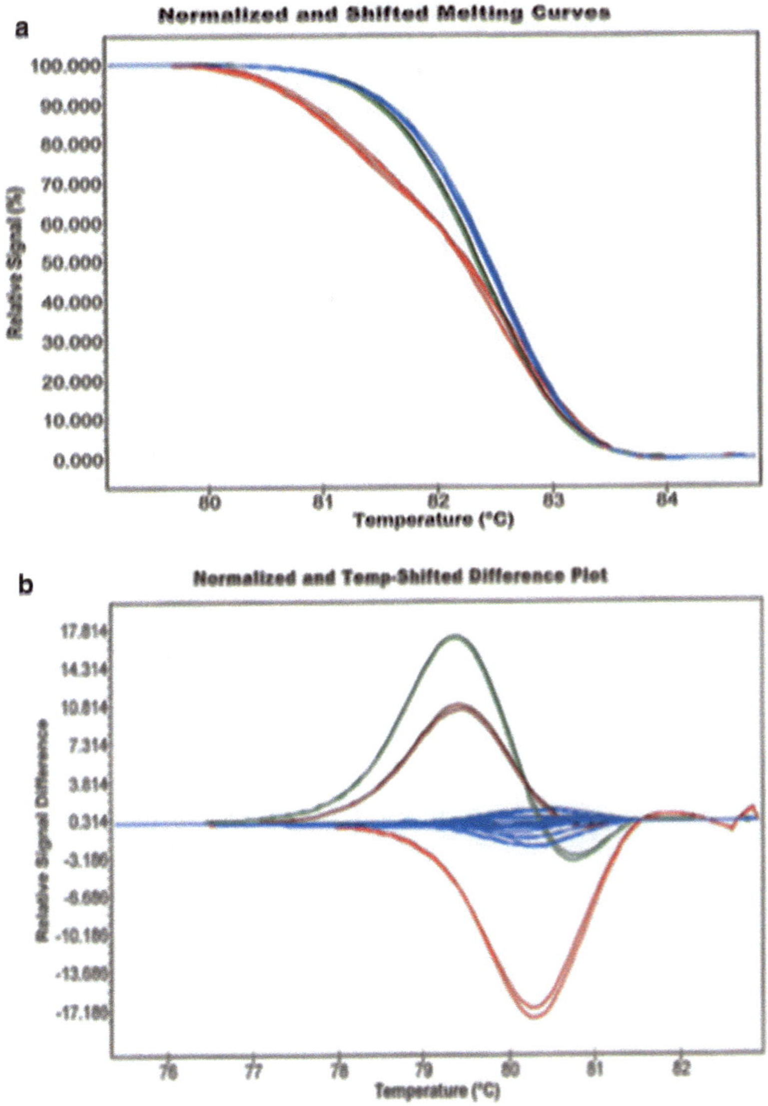

Fig. 2 (**a**) An example of a left shifted curve caused by a heteroduplex melting at a lower temperature (*red curves*). The wild type displays parallel curves (*blue curves*). (**b**) An example of a difference plot showing the homozygote (*red*), heteroduplex and wild type (*blue*) curve formed by the subtraction of each temperature increment from the reference (courtesy of Lorna Wall, Red Cell Reference Laboratory, NZBS)

By far the most innovative use of real-time PCR in HLA typing is a very simple one and is provided in a commercial kit with reagents and software developed and supported by Linkage Biosciences (Linkage Biosciences, San Francisco, USA). The LinkSeq™ kits, produced by Linkage Biosciences, have gained considerable momentum in HLA typing due to the ease of processing, and have significant advantages for deceased donor typing in solid organ transplantation, effectively replacing PCR-SSP as the technique of choice. The most suitable LinkSeq™ kits for solid organ applications will provide typing information for HLA-A, -B, -C, -DRB1/3/4/5, -DQA1/DQB1, -DPA1/DPB1 all on one plate in a 384-well format. Eleven HLA loci of a deceased donor have to be typed to ensure the potential recipient does not have any antibodies against the donor's HLA. Many tissue typing laboratories use Luminex technology for antibody screening which is a very effective and sensitive technology for identifying antibodies against all the "classical" HLA loci.

The LinkSeq™ kits have primers in each well for specific allele groups and an internal control primer pair, analogous to PCR-SSP. A DNA sample and DNA polymerase are added to a master mix containing PCR reagents and fluorescent dye. This solution is then dispensed into the 384-well plate. The kit design includes significant redundancy of the alleles across the various wells and also provides duplicate wells to help ensure a typing from each sample. Once the reagents are added, the plate is sealed and placed in the real-time PCR machine. The plate never has to be opened again which helps in eliminating contamination in a laboratory. After a conventional PCR, LinkSēq takes advantage of the fluorescent dye using melt curve technology to identify the amplicons produced from the PCR. The dye (SYBR Green) fluoresces when bound to double-stranded DNA, and stops fluorescing when released into solution. A melt curve is produced by looking at the change in the temperature as the solutions temperature is increased from 65 °C, where the amplicons will all be double stranded, to 95 °C at which point all the amplicons become single stranded and the SYBR Green is released into solution. Any particular amplicon will melt at the same temperature each time allowing the software to easily determine if a sample includes specific HLA alleles. Dedicated software called SureTyper™ looks for positive and negative reactions (Fig. 3). Each well in the test is multiplexed with an

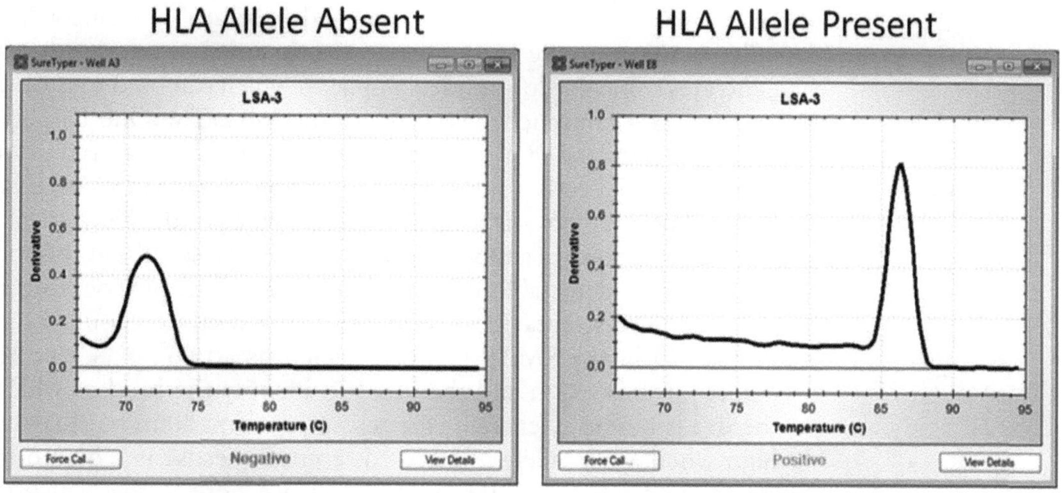

Fig. 3 HLA melt curve analysis (courtesy of Linkage Biosciences)

internal control amplicon that melts at a lower temperature than a positive HLA amplicon. The chemistry has been designed such that the internal control amplicon is absent when the HLA allele tested for in that well is present.

The software then analyzes the overall pattern of the wells and produces a low-intermediate resolution 11 locus HLA type in a matter of seconds with very little human interaction. The whole process from extracted DNA to complete HLA type is only 1.5 h (approximately)—such a quick method yielding the entire relevant donor HLA information in a time-critical process is indeed a revelation in the tissue typing world. It will be very interesting to see how the developers manage the rise in HLA polymorphisms.

4 Microarrays

If we define an array as "a display or ordered arrangement," then the Luminex platform with its differentially stained beads coated with arrays of oligonucleotides specifying particular HLA types represents the most popular microarray system in use in HLA typing. As more and more HLA alleles have been discovered [27], the PCR-SSOP technique has proved to be more adaptable than PCR-SSP and the Luminex platform utilizing bead array technology [28] is the current popular technology for "routine" testing in many tissue typing laboratories. There are 100 different colored polystyrene microspheres or beads used in Luminex kits and the analytes are measured in the xMAP platform (Luminex Corporation, Austin, Texas, USA), similar to a flow cytometer. Each bead can be differentiated by its unique spectral signature after excitation by a laser; therefore multiplexing is possible—up to 100 different assays can be performed per sample in 1 well of a 96-well plate. Similar to other PCR-SSOP techniques, HLA Typing by Luminex uses a biotinylated amplicon which is added to beads from the appropriate bead kit (locus-specific probes attached to beads). Immucor kits utilize an asymmetric PCR where one primer is in excess so that it generates some single-stranded amplicon which can bind to probes on the beads (Immucor, Norcross, GA, USA). The One Lambda kit uses a standard PCR so the amplicon must be denatured prior to adding to beads (one Lambda, Canoga Park, Los Angeles, USA). Specific hybridization is ensured by hybridization at elevated temperature in a thermal cycler. Beads with specifically bound amplicon are detectable by the addition of a dye, phycoerythrin, conjugated to streptavidin. Ninety-five samples plus a control can be assayed in the xMAP platform which uses two lasers, one to detect phycoerythrin and the other to identify the bead to which the dye is bound. Generally, the resolution is medium but may be high when a rare allele is detected. Some expertise is required in reviewing results, assessing beads which are close to the "cut off" between a positive and negative. High-resolution typing Luminex kits are also available and are finding increasing use. In today's Tissue Typing Laboratory Luminex is the predominant technology for routine HLA typing.

However, the complexity of the HLA system will soon see the demise of the Luminex XMAP 100, the 100 bead system, because there are insufficient beads especially for HLA-B. Luminex have now produced a 500-bead system which One Lambda are marketing as the LabScan 3D™ and their kits which will type the "Common well-defined Alleles" [29, 30] which should reduce/remove ambiguities. There are also high-resolution kits (XR™) which will compete with sequencing technologies such as Next Generation Sequencing, or NGS (*see* further).

Aside from Luminex, microarrays have been the "false dawn" of HLA typing—they have often promised to be a very useful technique but have not been adopted routinely. Generally, coated glass slides have been the surface of choice to which oligonucleotides are linked. Although there have been some reports of the use of oligonucleotide arrays specific for HLA typing [11, 31–35], this technology has not found widespread acceptance in the histocompatibility and immunogenetics field largely due to the cost. Attachment of oligonucleotide probes to a surface is usually achieved with a covalent linkage of a modified oligonucleotide, which is an expensive and inefficient process.

A novel method of attaching oligonucleotide probes to glass slides was described in 2001 and is based on simple electrostatic adsorption of oligonucleotides to a cationic glass surface [36]. This process is highly efficient with approximately 1/10th of the amount of oligonucleotide required compared with covalent linkage. No chemical modification is required. When a denatured amplicon is hybridized to the array, the probe and DNA form a unique nonhelical ribbon-like structure that still obeys Watson–Crick complementary base rules. The binding between the probe and amplicon is highly specific with single-nucleotide discrimination [36]. The number of probes required per array is optimized for the highest resolution, and the cis–trans linkage of SNPs in a heterozygous sample is ensured [37]. Another feature of the unique "ribbon-like" structure of the probe-amplicon structure is single-nucleotide discrimination with room temperature hybridization. Therefore, there is no requirement for complex washing/hybridization machinery which is a particularly attractive feature of this microarray system. In addition, HLA-A, HLA-B, and HLA-DRB1 can be amplified directly from only a drop of blood, with no requirement for DNA purification. This technology is being developed by GMS biotech (Tucson, AZ, USA), and microarrays (EZChip) using this technology for medium-resolution HLA-A, HLA-B, and HLA-DRB1 typing will be available late 2014 and are being tested in my laboratory. Dedicated software, "Ricimer," to convert hybridization signals into HLA strings is available from GMS biotech and is also being tested in my laboratory. Early results show the resolution matches Luminex SSOP typing, but at a fraction of the cost. The aim for this technology is to create an automated system using a series of cost-effective HLA microarrays for different loci and different levels of resolution.

5 RNA Sequencing-Based Typing

Sequencing-based typing (or SBT) genomic DNA, using dideoxy chain termination chemistry, has been in use for HLA typing for many years. The increasing numbers of alleles means that it is now a very laborious method to obtain an unambiguous HLA allele result—e.g., only two alleles at each locus.

An alternative method for conventional dideoxy sequencing utilizes RNA as the template. This method has been neglected because of general fears of working with RNA—it is unstable and prone to degradation by ubiquitous RNases, and unequal allele expression may mean preferential allele amplification prior to sequencing. Methods for HLA class I [38] and class II [39] sequencing using RNA have been published, but it is not accepted as a routine method for high-resolution typing. We carried out a small study on 64 blood samples and carried out RNA sequencing [40]. RNA was extracted using a small robot, cDNA synthesized, and HLA-A, HLA-B, HLA-DRB1, and HLA-DQB1 alleles amplified using locus-specific primers in exons 1 and 7 (class I) or exons 1 and 4 (class II), and the genes were sequenced by standard dideoxy chemistry. The results were concordant with the method used for genomic DNA HLA typing (either PCR-SSP or Luminex or SBT), and there was no evidence of allele dropout owing to reduced RNA levels [40]. What was striking was the smaller number of sequencing reactions that were performed to sequence a larger part of each HLA gene and to achieve the same result as with genomic DNA. Almost complete coding gene sequence for class I and exons 1–3 for class II could be achieved with 24 sequencing reactions or less (P. Dunn personal communication). Ambiguous sequencing combinations with this method are the same as you would observe for genomic DNA. An SNP overlooked in an intron by this method is only relevant if it affects expression through an effect on splicing.

6 Next Generation Sequencing

The complexity of HLA, especially the unceasing discovery of new alleles, poses a real challenge in HLA typing. However, for most applications in HLA typing it is not necessary to define the unambiguous alleles for each HLA locus as long as the technology employed defines no more than two split specificities per locus. DNA sequencing is employed for a stem cell patient and potentially matching unrelated donor when the HLA alleles do need to be identified unambiguously. For the last 20 years, the so-called Sanger sequencing (or dye-deoxynucleotide chain termination sequencing) has been employed in the HLA field [13, 41]. To achieve unambiguous allele typing, the alleles in each locus have to be amplified separately and each amplicon subjected to Sanger sequencing which makes this technique very laborious and relatively expensive in reagents. A new version of DNA sequencing called Next Generation Sequencing (NGS) has been developed following the publication of the nucleotide sequence of the whole human genome and has been gaining traction in the field of HLA typing since 2009 [42–45]. NGS technologies use different methods to separate HLA alleles followed by massively parallel sequencing and bioinformatics to compile and align sequences and to derive HLA type. Software which has been used for Sanger HLA SBT is currently being adapted for targeted HLA typing by NGS. NGS technology and techniques continue to evolve and below are described the latest popular versions of NGS as applied to HLA typing.

6.1 Illumina MiSeq

MiSeq uses sequencing-by-synthesis (SBS). Prior to SBS, sequencing libraries are created including the DNA/RNA to be sequenced, index barcodes for sample multiplexing, sequence adapters to initiate SBS, and flow cell adapters (complimentary oligonucleotide sequences attached to the flow cell allow the libraries to bind to the surface of the flow cell). Library preparation begins with fragmentation of the DNA using enzymes or mechanical shearing, followed by ligation of barcodes and adapters. One such method available from Illumina, Nextera™, simultaneously fragments and ligates adapters using a transposase. The libraries are immobilized on the flow cell and clonally amplified prior to SBS [46]. The whole process is shown in Fig. 4. In MiSeq HLA NGS the workflow starts with long range PCR of each HLA locus followed by amplicon fragmentation and the addition of adaptors enabling sequencing from the end of each fragment. Such "paired-end sequencing" enables phase-defined allele determination. MiSeq HLA NGS protocols have recently been described for exons 1–7 of HLA-A, -B, and -C (amplicon 3 kbp approximately) and 8 kbp of exons 2–5 of HLA-DRB1 [47]. A more comprehensive MiSeq HLA NGS method has recently been described [48] with amplicons spanning from the promoter to 3′UTR of HLA-A, -C, -B, -DRB1, -DQB1, and -DPB1. The largest amplicon is HLA-DPB1 (13,605 bp) and the smallest HLA-A (3,398 bp). Individual genes were sequenced using MiSeq after transposase-based library preparation. Paired-end sequences were compared to an HLA reference sequence.

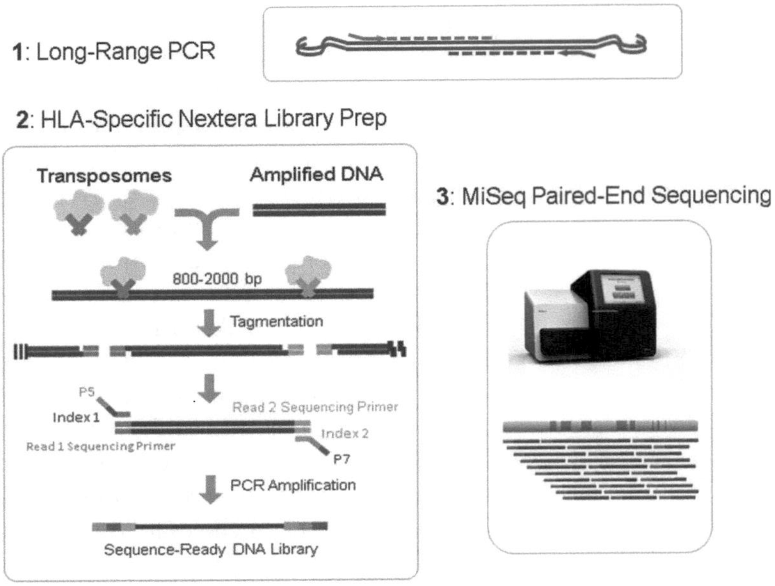

Fig. 4 Illumina's HLA NGS TrueSight Workflow (courtesy of Illumina)

6.2 Ion Torrent Personal Genome Machine (PGM)

PGM is a semiconductor sequencer which detects protons released as nucleotides are incorporated into a growing DNA strand [49]. DNA fragments with specific adaptor sequences are clonally amplified by emulsion PCR on the surface of 3 μm diameter beads called Ion Spheres. Beads plus template are loaded into proton sensing wells fabricated on a silicon wafer and sequencing is primed from specific part of the adaptor sequence. In the sequencing process each nucleotide is added individually; if one is incorporated the released proton is detected and a signal released. If there are two or more identical nucleotides, then the signal is increased proportional to the number of nucleotides. When a nucleotide is added to the chip which is not complementary to the template, there is no signal and the next nucleotide is added (Fig. 5).

In NGS HLA typing by PGM, a long range PCR strategy has been employed for the HLA-A, B, C, DRB1 genes to evaluate the scalability of the platform [45, 50]. Adaptors are ligated to size-selected, fragmented long range PCR amplicons. Adaptors contain sequences complementary to sequencing primers and also contain sequences enabling attachment of DNA to ion sphere. The adaptors have a third sequence motif or "barcode" which allows tracing of fragments (e.g., to sample or HLA locus or both). DNA fragments are mixed with ion spheres and oil under pressure and emulsion PCR performed with DNA and bead ratios fixed so that one DNA fragment binds to one bead in one micelle. After this clonal PCR DNA on beads is denatured allowing sequencing of the single-stranded library using the semiconductor chip. HLA NGS kits to type A, B, C, DRB1, DR3/4/5, DQA1, DQB1, DPA1,

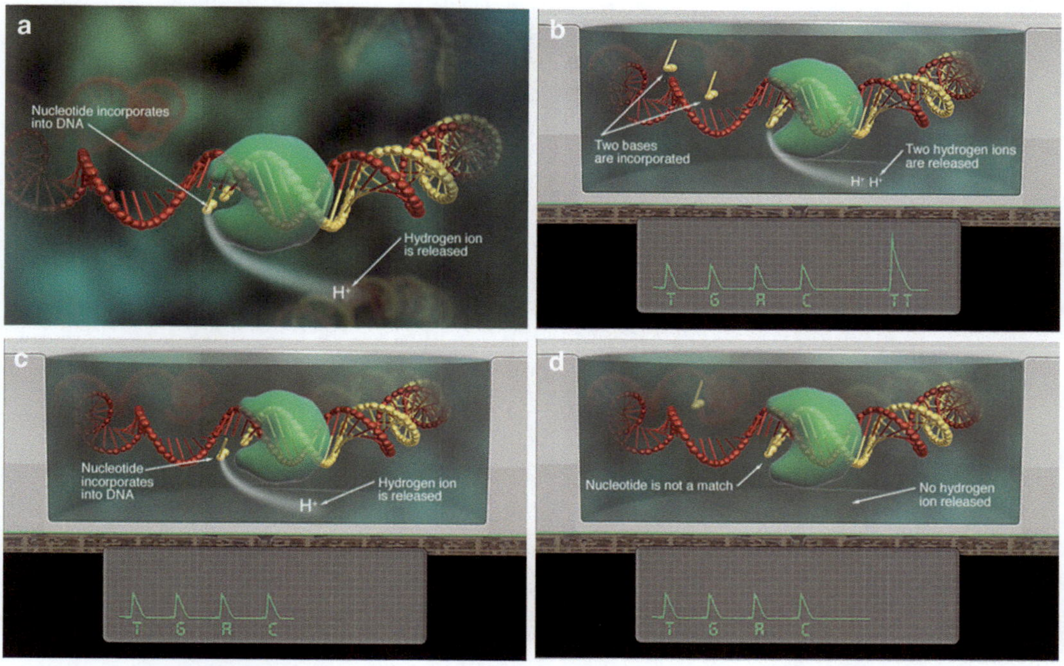

Fig. 5 Ion Torrent™ Technology directly translates chemically encoded information (A, C, G, T) into digital information (0, 1) on a semiconductor chip. (**a**) When a nucleotide is incorporated into a strand of DNA by a polymerase, a hydrogen ion is released. (**b**) If there are two identical bases on the DNA strand, the voltage will be double, and the chip will record two identical bases. (**c**) If a nucleotide, for example a C, is added to a DNA template and is then incorporated into a strand of DNA, a hydrogen ion will be released. The charge from that ion will change the pH of the solution, which can be detected by an ion sensor. (**d**) PGM™ sequencer then sequentially floods the chip with one nucleotide after another. If the next nucleotide that floods the chip is not a match, no voltage change will be recorded and no base will be called (courtesy of Life Technologies)

DPB1 will soon be available (end 2014/beginning 2015) and the emulsion PCR step will be replaced by clonal isothermal amplification (Inta Veldre, personal communication).

6.3 Pacific Biosciences

In Single Molecule Real-Time (SMRT®) Sequencing, DNA polymerase bound to DNA template is attached to the bottom of 50 nm-wide wells called zero-mode waveguides (ZMWs). Polymerase copies the template DNA in a reaction containing nucleotides which have a fluorescently labeled terminal phosphate. As a base is incorporated, a distinctive pulse of fluorescence is detected in real time. In a recent description of an HLA SMRT sequencing protocol [51], full-length HLA class I genes were barcoded and the PCR products were blunt-ended prior to the addition of SMRTbell™ adaptors. Barcoding means that the amplicons can be pooled and the addition of the SMRTbell™ adaptors means continuous sequencing enabling whole-allele genotyping. A similar HLA SMRT sequencing method has recently been described using barcodes attached to generic PCR primers and SMRT sequencing but also encompassing multiplexing of class II genes prior to sequencing ([52], Fig. 6).

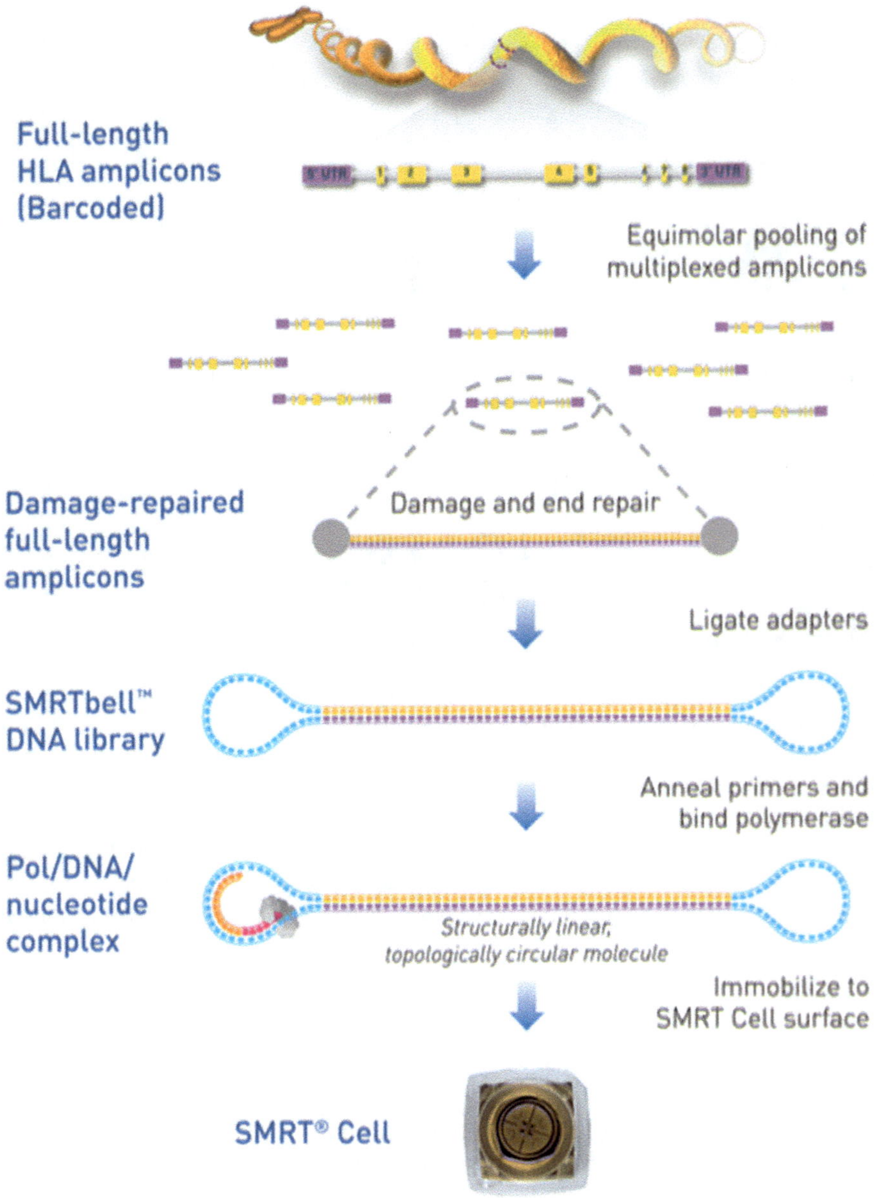

Fig. 6 Pacific Bioscience SMRT® HLA NGS workflow (courtesy of Pacific Biosciences)

7 The Future? Next, Next Generation Sequencing

An exciting application of genomics in medicine in the future is to extend the capabilities of point of care (POC) testing where a healthcare professional may be able to test a patient immediately and at their convenience (e.g., bedside). It is an exciting prospect, a handheld DNA sequencing device which will provide the patient's

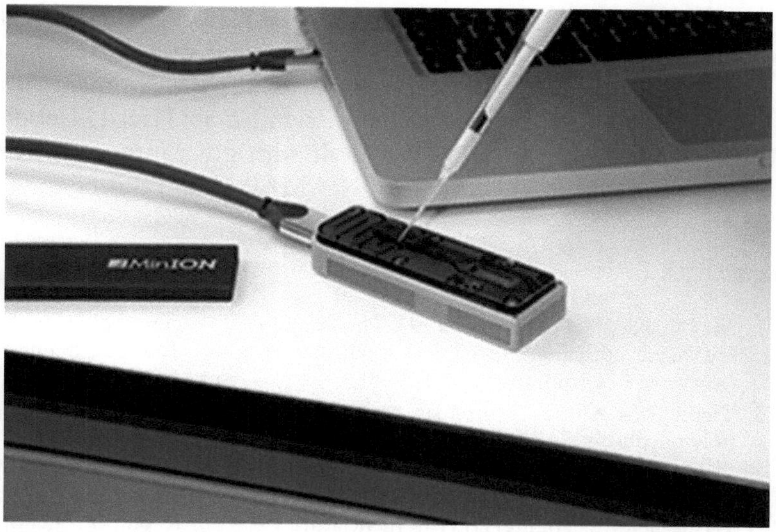

Fig. 7 The MinION™—a next, Next Generation Sequencing device (courtesy of Oxford Nanopore Technologies)

genomic DNA sequence in a matter of minutes with analysis of informative sequences.

Oxford Nanopore Technologies (Oxford, UK) have produced a handheld DNA sequencer (MinION™) which is currently being tested by a number of laboratories worldwide (Fig. 7). Oxford Nanopore technology utilizes an engineered protein nanopore, adapted so that the identity of DNA bases can be ascertained as they pass through the nanopore by measuring variations in an ionic current passing through the pore. A single-stranded DNA molecule is ratcheted through the nanopore by an enzyme attached to the nanopore.

The MinION™ device (Fig. 7) is a small instrument that is compatible with consumable flow cells containing the equipment needed to perform a single-molecule sensing experiment; a proprietary sensor chip, accompanying bespoke Application Specific Integrated Circuit (ASIC), and nanopores. MinION™ plugs directly into a laptop or desktop computer through a USB port.

Currently, several hundred participants (including this laboratory) in the MinION Access program (MAP) are working with the MinION system to explore how its features—including long read lengths, real-time digital data, portability and compressed workflows—might help to answer a range of biological questions.

Oxford Nanopore technology and philosophy is very attractive for the HLA typing laboratory as it is focused on delivering the simplest possible sample preparation and workflows. Early disclosures by participants in MAP indicate that the technology can process long read lengths presented to the system. Nanopore sensing technology was originally researched at Oxford University, UK, in the laboratory of Hagan Bayley and other institutions including Harvard University and the University of California, Santa Cruz [53–55]. However the development of the technology has been performed by scientists at Oxford Nanopore Technologies (Oxford UK). We await with great interest the results and feedback from the MinION™ MAP. Could this be the future of HLA typing?

References

1. McCluskey J, Peh CA (1999) The human leukocyte antigens and clinical medicine: an overview. Rev Immunogenet 1:3–20
2. Tiercy J-M (2002) Molecular basis of HLA polymorphism: implications in clinical transplantation. Transpl Immunol 9:173–180
3. Tait BD (2011) The ever expanding list of HLA alleles: changing HLA nomenclature its relevance to clinical transplantation. Transplant Rev 25:1–8
4. Taylor CJ, Bolton EM, Bradley AJ (2011) Immunological considerations for embryonic and induced pluripotent stem cell banking. Philos Trans Roy Soc B 366:2312–2322
5. Thorsby E (2009) A short history of HLA. Tissue Antigens 74:101–116
6. Saiki RK, Scharf S, Faloona F, Mullis KB, Horn GT, Erlich HA, Arnheim N (1988) Primer directed enzymatic amplification of DNA with a thermostable DNA polymerase. Science 239: 487–491
7. Middleton D (1999) History of DNA typing for the human MHC. Rev Immunogenet 1:135–156
8. Bunce M, O'Neill CM, Barnardo MC, Krausa P, Browning MJ, Morris PJ, Welsh KI (1995) Phototyping: comprehensive DNA typing for HLA-A, B, C, DRB1, DRB3, DRB4, DRB5 & DQB1 by PCR with 144 primer mixes utilizing sequence-specific primers (PCR-SSP). Tissue Antigens 46:355–367
9. Cao K, Chopek M, Fernandez-Vina M (1999) High and intermediate resolution DNA typing systems for class I HLA-A, -B, -C genes by hybridization with sequence-specific oligonucleotide probes (SSOP). Rev Immunogenet 1:177–208
10. Dunn PPJ, Day S, Williams S, Bendukidze N (2003) HLA sequencing as a tissue typing tool. In: Goulding N, Seward C (eds) Pediatric hematology. Humana Press, Totowa, NJ
11. Guo Z, Hood L, Petersdorf EW (1999) Oligonucleotide arrays for high resolution HLA typing. Rev Immunogenet 1:220–230
12. Holcomb CL, Höglund B, Anderson MW, Böhme I, Egholm M, Ferriola D et al (2011) A multi-site study using high resolution HLA genotyping by next generation sequencing. Tissue Antigens 77:206–217
13. Dunn PPJ (2011) HLA typing: techniques and technology, a critical appraisal. Int J Immunogenet 38:463–473
14. Wang H, Tokunaga K, Ishikawa Y, Tanaka H, Kashiwase K, Shibata Y, Juji T (1997) A high-resolution genotyping method for HLA-C alleles and possible shared HLA-C-B haplotypes between Japanese and Caucasians. Tissue Antigens 50:620–626
15. Knapp LA, Lehmann E, Hennes M, Eberle ME, Watkins DI (1997) High-resolution HLA-DRB typing using denaturing gradient gel electrophoresis and direct sequencing. Tissue Antigens 50:170–177
16. Arguello JR, Pay AL, McDermott A, Ross J, Dunn P, Avakian H, Little A-M, Goldman J, Madrigal JA (1997) Complementary strand analysis, a new approach for allelic separation in complex polyallelic genetic systems. Nucleic Acids Res 25:2236–2238
17. Arguello JR, Little A-M, Pay AL, Gallardo D, Rojas I, Marsh SG, Goldman JM, Madrigal JA (1998) Mutation detection and typing of polymorphic loci through double-strand conformation analysis. Nat Genet 18:192–194
18. Arguello JR, Madrigal JR (1999) HLA typing by reference strand mediated conformation analysis (RSCA). Rev Immunogenet 1:209–219
19. Etokebe GE, Opsahl M, Tveter AK, Lie BA, Thorsby E, Vartdal F, Spurkland A (2003) Physical separation of HLA-A alleles by denaturing high performance liquid chromatography. Tissue Antigens 61:443–450
20. Kuzio S, Hanguehard A, Morelle M, Ronsin C (2004) Rapid screening for HLA-B27 by a TaqMan-PCR assay using sequence-specific primers and a minor groove binder probe, a novel type of TaqMan trade mark probe. J Immunol Methods 287:179–186
21. Fan W, Huang L, Zhou Z, Zeng X, Li G, Deo P, Hi L, Li Y (2012) Rapid and reliable genotyping of HLA-B*27 in the Chinese Han population using a duplex real-time TaqMan PCR assay. Clin Biochem 45:106–111

22. Goris A, Walton A, Ban M, Dubois B, Compston A, Sawcer S (2008) A Taqman assay for high-throughput genotyping of the multiple sclerosis-associated HLA-DRB1*1501 allele. Tissue Antigens 72:401–403
23. Profaizer T, Eckels D, Delgado JC (2011) Coeliac disease and HLA typing using real time PCR with melting curve analysis. Tissue Antigens 78:31–37
24. Kim SY, Chang HE, Song SH, Park KU, Song J (2011) Rapid genotyping of HLA-B27 among Korean population by real time PCR melting curve analysis. Clin Chim Acta 412:1912–1917
25. Hammond E, Mamotte C, Nolan D, Mallal S (2007) HLA-B*5701 typing, evaluation of an allele-specific polymerase chain reaction melting assay. Tissue Antigens 70:58–61
26. Zhou L, Vandersteen J, Wang L, Fuller T, Taylor M, Palais B, Wittwer CT (2004) High resolution DNA melting curve analysis to establish HLA genotypic identity. Tissue Antigens 64:156–164
27. Holdsworth R, Hurley CK, Marsh SG, Lau M, Noreen HJ, Kempenich JH, Setterholm M, Maiers M (2009) The HLA dictionary 2008, a summary of HLA-A, -B, -C, -DRB1/3/4/5, and -DQB1 alleles and their association with serologically defined HLA-A, -B, -C, -DR, and -DQ antigens. Tissue Antigens 73:95–170
28. Dunbar SA (2006) Applications of Luminex xMAP technology for rapid, high-throughput multiplexed nucleic acid detection. Clin Chim Acta 363:71–82
29. Cano P, Klitz W, Mack SJ, Marsh SGE, Noreen H, Reed EF, Senitzer D, Setterholm M, Smith A, Fernandez-Vina M (2007) Common and well-documented HLA alleles, report of the Ad-Hoc committee of the american society for histocompatibility and immunogenetics. Hum Immunol 68:392–417
30. Mack SJ, Cano P, Hollenbach JA, He J, Hurley CK, Middleton D et al (2013) Common and well-documented HLA alleles, 2012 update to the CWD catalogue. Tissue Antigens 81:194–203
31. Guo Z, Gatterman MS, Hood L (2002) Oligonucleotide arrays for high-throughput SNPs detection in the MHC Class I Genes, HLA-B as a model system. Genome Res 12:447–457
32. Bang-Ce Y, Xiaohe C, Ye F, Songyang L, Bincheng Y, Peng Z (2005) Simultaneous genotyping of DRB1/3/4/5 loci by oligonucleotide microarray. J Mol Diagn 7:592–599
33. Palmisano GL, Delfino L, Fiore M, Longo A, Ferrara GB (2005) Single nucleotide polymorphisms detection based on DNA microarray technology, HLA as a model. Autoimmun Rev 4:510–514
34. Zhang F, Hu SW, Huang J, Wang H, Wen Z, Yongyao G, Wang S (2006) Development and clinical evaluation of oligonucleotide microarray for HLA-A, B genotyping. Pharmacogenomics 7:973–985
35. Lee KR, Park E, Moon SH, Kim JM, Kwon OJ, Kim MH, Sohn YH, Ko SY, Oh HB (2008) Development and clinical evaluation of a microarray for HLA-A and -DRB1 genotyping. Tissue Antigens 72:568–577
36. Lemeshko SV, Powdrill T, Belosludtsev YY, Hogan M (2001) Oligonucleotides form a duplex with non-helical properties on a positively-charged surface. Nucleic Acids Res 14:3051–3058
37. Feng C, Putonti C, Zhang M, Eggers R, Mitra R, Hogan M, Jayaraman K, Fofanov Y (2009) Ultraspecific probes for high throughput HLA typing. BMC Genomics 10:85
38. Santamaria P, Boyce-Jacino MT, Lindstrom AL, Barbosa JJ, Faras AJ, Rich SS (1992) HLA class II typing, direct sequencing of DRB, DQB and DQA genes. Hum Immunol 33:69–81
39. Santamaria P, Lindstrom AL, Boyce-Jacino MT, Myster SH, Barbosa JJ, Faras AJ, Rich SS (1993) HLA class I sequence-based typing. Hum Immunol 37:39–50
40. Theseira M, Dunn PPJ (2011) Sequencing based HLA typing using RNA. Genet Eng News 31:66–69
41. Sanger F, Nicklen S, Coulson AR (1977) DNA sequencing with chain-terminating inhibitors. Proc Natl Acad Sci U S A 74:5463–5467
42. Bentley G, Higuchi R, Hoglund B, Goodridge D, Sayer D, Trachtenberg EA, Erlich HA (2009) High resolution, high-throughput HLA genotyping by next-generation sequencing. Tissue Antigens 74:393–403
43. Gabriel C, Danzer M, Hackl C, Kopal G, Hufnagl P, Hofer K, Polin H, Stabentheiner S, Proll J (2009) Rapid high throughput human leukocyte antigen typing by massively parallel pyrosequencing for high resolution allele identification. Hum Immunol 70:960–964
44. De Santis D, Dinauer D, Duke J, Erlich HA, Holcomb CL, Lind C, Mackiewicz K, Monos D, Moudgil A, Norman P, Parham P, Sasson A, Allcock RJN (2012) 16th IHIW, Review of HLA typing by NGS. Int J Immunogenet 40:72–76
45. Gabriel C, Furst D, Fae I, Wenda S, Zollikofer C, Mytilineos J, Fischer G (2014) HLA typing by next-generation-sequencing – getting closer to reality. Tissue Antigens 83:65–75

46. Bentley DR, Balasubramanian S, Swerdlow HP, Smith GP, Milton J, Brown CG et al (2008) Accurate whole human genome sequencing using reversible terminator chemistry. Nature 456:53–59
47. Wang C, Krishnakumar S, Wilhelmy J, Babrzadeh F, Stepanyan L, Su LF et al (2012) High-throughput, high-fidelity HLA genotyping with deep sequencing. Proc Natl Acad Sci U S A 109:8676–8681
48. Hosomichi K, Jinam TA, Mitsunaga S, Nakaoka H, Inoue I (2013) Phase defined complete sequencing of the HLA genes by next generation sequencing. BMC Genomics 14:355
49. Rothberg JM, Hinz W, Rearick TM, Schultz J, Mileski W, Davey M et al (2011) An integrated semiconductor device enabling non-optical genome sequencing. Nature 475:348–352
50. Shiina T, Suzuki S, Ozaki Y, Taira H et al (2012) Super high resolution for single molecule-sequence-based typing of classical HLA loci at the 8-digit level using next generation sequencers. Tissue Antigens 80:305–316
51. Mayor N, Robinson J, McWhinnie A, Ranade S, Eng K, Bultitude WP, Midwinter W, Bowman B, Marks P, Braund H, Madrigal JA, Latham K, Marsh SGE (2014) Genomic DNA sequences of HLA class I alleles generated using multiplexed barcodes and SMRT DNA sequencing technology. Tissue Antigens 84: P155
52. Cahill N, Ameur A, Knutsson C, Orebrand U, Gyllensten U, Bengtsson M (2014) HLA typing by SMRT sequencing: advantages of full length HLA genotyping in clinical routine. Tissue Antigens 84:P196
53. Howorka S, Cheley S, Bayley H (2001) Sequence-specific detection of individual DNA strands using engineered nanopores. Nat Biotech 19:636–639
54. Stoddart D, Heron AJ, Mikhailova E, Maglia G, Bayley H (2009) Single-nucleotide discrimination in immobilized DNA oligonucleotides with a biological nanopore. Proc Natl Acad Sci U S A 106:7702–7707
55. Kasianowicz JJ, Brandin E, Branton D, Deamer DW (1996) Characterization of individual polynucleotide molecules using a membrane channel. Proc Natl Acad Sci U S A 93: 13770–13773

Chapter 19

Luminex-Based Methods in High-Resolution HLA Typing

Manuela Testi and Marco Andreani

Abstract

Luminex-based technology has been applied to discriminate between the different Human Leukocyte Antigens (HLA) alleles. The typing method consists in a reverse-SSO assay: Target DNA is PCR-amplified using biotinylated group-specific primers. A single PCR reaction is used for each HLA locus. The biotinylated PCR product is chemically denatured using a pH change and allowed to rehybridize to complementary DNA probes conjugated to microspheres. These beads are characterized by two internal fluorescent dyes that create a unique combination of color, make them identifiable. Washes are performed to eliminate any additional PCR product that does not exactly match the sequence detected by the probe. The biotinylated PCR product bound to the microsphere is labelled with streptavidin conjugated with R-phycoerythrin (SAPE). A flow analyzer identifies the fluorescent intensity SAPE on each microsphere. Software is used to assign positive or negative reactions based on the strength of the fluorescent signal. The assignment of the HLA typing is based on positive and negative probe reactions compared with published HLA gene sequences. Recently kits characterized by an extensive number of probes/beads designed to potentially reduce the number of ambiguities or to directly lead to an allele level typing, have been made available.

Key words HLA typing, Luminex, PCR-SSO, LABType®, High resolution

1 Introduction

Hematopoietic stem cell transplantation (HSCT) from volunteer unrelated donors can cure patients with malignant and non malignant hematological diseases who lack a suitable family member donor [1, 2]. The human MHC complex (HLA) includes the most polymorphic genes in the human genome [3]. The implications of this polymorphism in relation to transplantation and in particular, the knowledge that high-resolution DNA matching for Human Leukocyte Antigens (HLA) alleles is associated with higher rates of survival [4, 5], has led to the development of efficient methods for high-resolution typing. According to the international standards for histocompatibility, high-resolution typing is defined as the identification of HLA alleles that encode the same protein sequence within the antigen binding site of the molecule. HLA alleles must be identified at the level of resolution which defines the first and

Peter Bugert (ed.), *Molecular Typing of Blood Cell Antigens*, Methods in Molecular Biology, vol. 1310,
DOI 10.1007/978-1-4939-2690-9_19, © Springer Science+Business Media New York 2015

second fields according to WHO nomenclature, by resolving at least all ambiguities resulting from polymorphisms located within exons 2 and 3 for HLA class I loci, and exon 2 for HLA class II loci as well as those that encompass a null allele, wherever the polymorphism is located.

Luminex technology is based on a reverse sequence specific oligonucleotide (SSO) method on a suspension array platform using color-coded microspheres as a solid support to immobilize oligonucleotide probes. The target DNA is amplified by polymerase chain reaction (PCR) and then hybridized with the bead probe array. The entire process takes place in a single well of a 96-well PCR plate; thus, 96 samples can be processed at one time.

For each HLA locus, a series of fluorescently coded microspheres are used. Each bead is coupled with one or more probes able to hybridize with the biotin-labelled complementary product of amplification. After this step, the hybridization may be quantified by measuring the fluorescence signal originating from fluorescently (SAPE) labelled, biotinylated amplicons, captured on the beads being detected by a flow analyzer, the LABScan™ 100. In the last decade, the Luminex-based method for low resolution HLA typing has been well established. Of particular interest is the use of "specialty probe" technology that allows resolution of CIS/TRANS ambiguities, otherwise requiring an additional assay(s) when using conventional SSO methods. In order to obtain high-resolution (second field) HLA typing level, further reverse SSO Luminex-based kits have been subsequently developed.

At present, two approaches are commercially available, the differences consisting in the amplification and denaturation steps. One of these systems, the OneLambda LABType®High Definition System is described in detail in this chapter. The LABType® tests are able to resolve ambiguities, often eliminating the need for further testing by SBT. For HLA class I, the highest level of resolution is reached by combining LABType® SSO class I HLA-A, B, and C kits with the Exon 4–7 supplement kit. For class II, LABType® HD class II DRB1, LABType® class II DQA1/DQB1, and LABType® class II DPA1/DPB1 typing kits are available.

2 Materials

2.1 Specimens

1. Genomic DNA (*see* **Notes 1** and **2**).
2. Controls: samples with known HLA typing as positive controls (*see* **Note 3**); DNA-free sterile water as negative control.

2.2 Reagents

1. LABType® SSO Typing kits: LABType HD class I HLA-A, LABType HD class I HLA-B, LABType HD class I HLA-C, LABType SSO Exon 4–7 Supplement, LABType HD class II

Table 1
Reagents in the LABType® kits and storage temperatures

Reagent	Storage temperature
Locus-Specific Primer Set	−80 to −20 °C
Primer Set D-Mix	−80 to −20 °C
Denaturation buffer	Room temperature
Neutralization buffer	Room temperature
Hybridization buffer	Room temperature
Bead Mixtures	Unopened: −80 to −20 °C; opened: 2–8 °C
Wash buffer	Room temperature
SAPE buffer	Unopened: −80 to −20 °C; opened: 2–8 °C

DRB1, LABType class II DQA1/DQB1, LABType class II DPA1/DPB1. The reagents included in the different kits and the storage temperatures for each of them are specified in Table 1.

2. Taq DNA Polymerase 5 U/μL. Storage: −80 to −20 °C.
3. Stock SAPE solution (100×). Storage: +2 to 8 °C (*see* **Note 4**).
4. Luminex Sheath fluid. Storage: room temperature.
5. Luminex Calibrator beads. Storage: +2 to 8 °C.
6. Luminex Control beads. Storage: +2 to 8 °C.
7. Sterile distilled water. Storage: room temperature.
8. 70 % ethanol. Storage: room temperature.
9. 20 % bleach. Storage: room temperature.

2.3 Equipment

1. LABScan100 (Luminex®100) Flow Analyzer.
2. Luminex® XY platform.
3. Luminex® SDS.
4. Microcentrifuge.
5. 96-well microplate centrifuge.
6. Thermocycler (ABI 9700 or equivalent).
7. Vortex mixer with adjustable speed.
8. Cooling block or crushed ice.
9. 1.5 mL Eppendorf microfuge tubes.
10. 10 mL Falcon tubes.

11. 96-well, 0.2 mL thin-walled PCR tray, and PCR tray holders.
12. Tray seal.
13. PCR Pad.
14. Adjustable single and multichannel pipets and tips (Gilson or equivalent).
15. 96-well 250 μL V bottom polystyrene microplate.

3 Methods

3.1 PCR Amplification

The primers for HLA-A, -B, -C in OneLambda HD kits, as well as the primers in DQA1/DQB1 and DPA1/DPB1 kits usually give a locus specific product covering exons 2 and 3. LABType SSO Exon 4–7 Supplement primers amplify exons 4–5 for HLA-A and -B, and exons 4–7 for locus C. Primers for HLA-DRB1give a product covering exon2.

1. In the Luminex HD worksheet (Fig. 1) fill out the fields relative to the identification of the kits in use (Lot, Exp. Date) and the tray layout with the DNA identification numbers in the same order the samples will be placed in the PCR plate.
2. Table 2 is used to calculate the amplification volumes based on the number of samples to be run (add one extra sample for each row to take into account reagent loss during pipetting). Add the value calculations to the appropriate table in the Luminex HD worksheet.
3. Turn on the PCR cycler to warm up heated lid (*see* **Note 5**).
4. Thaw the Amplification Primers and D-Mix of the appropriate HLA kit.
5. Vortex D-mix and Amplification Primers for 15 s; pulse centrifuge briefly.
6. Mix the previously calculated volumes of D-mix and primers in a 1.5 mL Eppendorf tube. Keep on ice until use.
7. Pipette 2 μL of each DNA sample into the corresponding well of a 96-well PCR microplate and 2 μL of sterile distilled water in the well of the negative control (*see* **Note 6**).
8. Add the appropriate volume of Taq DNA polymerase to the D-mix/primers mixtures and vortex.
9. Add 18 μL of the amplification mixture to each well containing a DNA sample.
10. Seal the plate, vortex briefly and brief centrifugation.
11. Load the PCR plate in the thermocycler with PCR pad and run the LABType® PCR program (Table 3).
12. Remove the PCR plate and store tray in −20 °C or proceed immediately to the denaturation/neutralization step (*see* **Note 7**).

Luminex HD worksheet

Date: **Technician Name:** **Multibatch:**

Kits:

Locus	Lot	Exp.date	ID Batch
HLA-A HD			
HLA-B HD			
HLA-C HD			
EXON 1E47			
HLA DRB1 HD			
HLA-DQA1/DQB1			
HLA-DPA1/DPB1			

Plate layout:

	1	2	3	4	5	6	7	8	9	10	11	12
A												
B												
C												
D												
E												
F												
G												
H												

PCR set up: LABType amplification mixture

Locus	N. of samples	D-mix (μL)	Amplification primer (μL)	Taq Polym. (μL)
HLA-A HD				
HLA-B HD				
HLA-C HD				
EXON 1E47				
DRB1 HD				
HLA-DQA1-DQB1				
HLA-DPA1-DPB1				

Hybridization volumes:

Locus	N. of samples	Hybridization buffer (μL)	Beads (μL)
HLA-A HD			
HLA-B HD			
HLA-C HD			
EXON 1E47			
DRB1 HD			
HLA-DQA1-DQB1			
HLA-DPA1-DPB1			

SAPE volumes:

N. of samples	SAPE buffer (μL)	SAPE (μL)

Fig. 1 The Luminex HD work sheet

3.2 Denaturation/ Neutralization

The amplicons are denatured using a pH change to make a single strand of DNA. Then a neutralization step occurs in order to prepare the PCR product for hybridization with multiple probes specific for nucleotide sequences. The positivity/negativity of each probe for each sample creates a reaction pattern that is used to define the HLA alleles.

Table 2
LABType® amplification mixture

No. of reactions (sample/loci)	D-mix (μL)	Amplification primer (μL)	Taq polymerase (μL)
1	13.8	4	0.2
10	138.0	40	2.0
20	276.0	80	4.0
50	690.0	200	10.0
96	1,491.0	432	21.6

Table 3
LABType® PCR program

PCR step	Temperature (°C)	Time
Initial denaturation	96	3 min
Cycles (5×)	96 60 72	20 s 20 s 20 s
Cycles (30×)	96 60 72	10 s 15 s 20 s
Final extension	72	10 min
Hold	4	∞

1. Set the thermocycler for an indefinite hold at 60 °C.
2. Move reagents (except reconstituted 1× SAPE and SAPE buffer) from storage temperature to room temperature.
3. Before using amplification, let the PCR plate thaw to room temperature for 10–15 min.
4. Prepare a new 96-well PCR plate.
5. Using a multichannel pipette, dispense 2.5 μL of Denaturation Buffer into each well.
6. Transfer into the corresponding well, 5 μL of each amplified DNA sample according to the scheme, mix by pipetting up and down until the mixture color changes to dark pink; spin briefly.
7. Incubate at room temperature for 10 min.

8. Add 5 µL per well of Neutralization Buffer and mix by pipetting up and down until the mixture color changes to pale yellow. Seal the plate and vortex (*see* **Note 8**).
9. Place the plate on ice/cooling block.

3.3 Hybridization

After the denaturation/neutralization steps, the PCR products are incubated with a panel of microspheres coated with labelled oligonucleotides designed for the detection of different polymorphic sites. Different reaction patterns of these sites are specific for different HLA alleles or an allelic group.

1. Prepare the hybridization mixture according to the number of samples to be analyzed (Table 4). Add one extra sample for each row to take into account reagent loss during pipetting (*see* **Notes 9** and **10**).
2. Add the volume calculations to the appropriate table of the Luminex HD worksheet.
3. Add 38 µL of Hybridization Mixture to each well.
4. Seal the PCR plate and vortex thoroughly at low speed (*see* **Note 11**).
5. Put the tray into the pre-warmed (60 °C) thermocycler with PCR pad, close and tighten the lid.
6. Incubate for 15 min.
7. Place tray into a tray holder, remove the seal, quickly add 100 µL of Wash Buffer to each well and cover with a tray seal.
8. Centrifuge tray for 5 min at 1,300 × *g*.
9. Remove Wash Buffer (Quickly invert the tray, flicking off the Wash Buffer while holding the tray in a horizontal position. Gently pat on absorbent paper three times to remove any residual supernatant).
10. Repeat the Wash Step two more times for a total of three Wash Steps (*see* **Note 12**).

Table 4
Hybridization mixture volumes

Number of tests	Hybridization buffer (µL)	Bead mixture (µL)
1	34	4
10	340	40
20	680	80
50	1,700	200
96	3,264	384

3.4 Labelling

The microspheres are characterized by two internal fluorescent dyes. Hundred different dye combinations are created by the ratio of the two dyes. In this way, each microsphere is color coded and may be recognized by the flow analyzer (LABScan100™). Probes are conjugated to these microspheres. The probes are capable of hybridizing with the biotin-labelled complementary amplicons. The biotin-labelled amplicons are subsequently labelled with SAPE. Streptavidin binds to biotin and the R-phycoerythrin is excited and detected by the flow analyzer (LABScan100™).

1. During the third centrifugation step, prepare 1× SAPE Solution in a 10 mL Falcon tube.
2. Dilute the 100× SAPE reconstituted solution with SAPE Buffer.
3. Prepare the SAPE solution according to the number of samples to be analyzed (Table 5). Add one extra sample for each row to take into account reagent loss during pipetting.
4. Add the volume calculations to the appropriate table of the Luminex HD worksheet (*see* **Notes 13** and **14**).
5. After preparation of the SAPE Solution, the final 1× SAPE solution must be stored and protected from light. It is recommended to cover the Falcon tube with aluminum foil.
6. After the third Wash Step centrifugation and flick, add 50 μL of 1× SAPE Solution to each well.
7. Cover the tray with tray seal and vortex thoroughly at low speed.
8. Place the tray into the pre-warmed (60 °C) thermocycler with PCR pad on top of tray, close and tighten the lid.
9. Incubate for 5 min.
10. Place tray in tray holder, remove the seal, quickly add 100 μL of Wash Buffer to each well and cover with tray seal.
11. Centrifuge the tray for 5 min at 1,300 ×*g*.

Table 5
SAPE solution volumes

Number of tests	SAPE stock volume (μL)	SAPE buffer volume (μL)
1	0.5	49.5
10	5.0	495.0
20	10.0	990.0
50	25.0	2,475.0
96	48.0	4,752.0

12. Remove Wash Buffer (Quickly invert the tray, flicking off the Wash Buffer while holding the tray in a horizontal position. Gently pat on absorbent paper three times to remove any residual supernatant).
13. Add 70 μL of Wash Buffer to each well and gently mix by pipetting up and down with an 8-channel pipette, avoid the creation of air bubbles.
14. According to the sample scheme, transfer contents of each well to a reading plate by setting the pipette to 80 μL (since the final volume will be 80 μL).
15. Cover the reading plate with seal and aluminum foil. Keep tray in the dark at 2–8 °C for a maximum of 72 h, until placed in LABScan100™ for reading (*see* **Note 15**).

3.5 Analysis

Once hybridization occurs, the LABScan100™ will be used to quantify reactivity by measuring the fluorescence signal intensity originating from the SAPE (streptavidin R-phycoerythrin) labelled amplicons, captured by the probe conjugated beads. The LABScan instrument is a two laser system. It contains a red laser that excites the dyes within the microspheres and classifies them based on their mapped spectral emission and a green laser that is used to quantify the fluorescently labelled amplicons captured by the beads. Each probe mixture contains one or more oligonucleotides that react with all alleles within a specific HLA locus, thus serving as a positive control.

3.5.1 LABScan100™ Flow Analyzer Daily Setup

1. Before starting, monitor the waste and sheath fluid levels. If required, replace the sheath fluid and empty the waste container.
2. Turn on the LABScan100™. Turn on the computer, checking that the sheath delivery system is powered on.
3. The warm up of the system will automatically start. The process requires 1,800 s. When the laser status bar changes color from yellow to green, the instrument is ready for use.
4. Click on the “Prime” icon and select OK, to remove air bubbles in the lines.
5. Repeat the “Prime” the step three more times.
6. Click on the “Alcohol Flush” icon to remove air bubbles in the sample cuvette.
7. Click on “Eject” icon. Fill the reservoir with 70 % Ethanol. Click on OK.
8. Repeat the alcohol flush step two more times by selecting the “Alcohol Flush” icon and OK, allowing the alcohol flush to run, and selecting it one last time and allowing it to run.
9. Click on the “Wash” icon.

10. Click on the “Eject” icon. Fill the reservoir with Sheath fluid. Click OK.
11. Repeat the “Wash” step three more times by selecting the “Wash” icon and allowing the wash to run, repeat twice for a total of three additional washes (*see* **Note 16**).
12. To perform instrument calibration, place the Luminex Calibrator beads (CAL1 and CAL2) and Luminex Control beads (CON1 and CON2) at room temperature for at least 20 min.
13. Vortex CAL1, CAL2, CON1, and CON2 beads vigorously. Put five drops of each reagent in each of four wells of the calibration plate (e.g., A1, B1, C1, and D1).
14. In the maintenance menu click on “New CAL Target” to update or confirm the reagents lot number.
15. Select CAL1 to start the calibration of the red laser.
16. Repeat for CAL2 (green laser).
17. In the maintenance menu click on “NewCON Target” to update or confirm the reagents lot number.
18. Select CON1 to start the controls.
19. Repeat for CON2.
20. Wash four times.
21. Click on System Monitor—Diagnostics menu to verify calibration results (*see* **Notes 17** and **18**).

3.5.2 Data Acquisition

1. Once calibration has been carried out create a file name (new batch) for the samples to be run (example: locus_lot number_date). For multiple HLA loci, create a multibatch.
2. In the acquisition software, choose the correct template according to the product catalogue and lot number.
3. Create a patient list. Load samples IDs either manually, inserting the number of samples and clicking “Apply,” or electronically by using bar codes and bar-code readers, imported files, etc. Select “Save and load” (*see* **Note 19**).
4. Verify that the samples are loaded in the correct location as shown in the Plate Layout table or drag the highlighted square box to the desired well location. For a multi-batch, verify that each additional batch is in its desired location.
5. Load the reading plate and click the “Start” button to initiate the session.
6. After the end of the acquisition process, cover the reading plate with seal and wrap in aluminum foil. Keep tray in the dark at 2–8 °C until the session has been validated (*see* **Notes 20** and **21**).

7. The data output will be saved in a .csv file, containing the fluorescence values of each sample.
8. At the end of the run, wash the instrument three times with sheath fluid, sanitize once with 20 % bleach, and finish with three distilled water washes.
9. Turn off the Luminex instrument.

3.6 Interpretation of Results

Data analysis is performed by the software, HLA Fusion. First the analysis software classifies each bead by its fluorescence and then it measures the strength of the external fluorescent signal from the SAPE and assigns positive or negative reactions. Each microsphere mixture includes negative control microspheres and positive control microspheres for subtraction of nonspecific background signal and normalization of raw data to adjust for possible variation in sample quantity and reaction efficiency respectively. The mean fluorescence intensity (MFI) generated by the Luminex contains the FI for each probe per sample. The percent positive value is calculated as: [100 × (MFI probe *n* − MFI probe negative control)]/(MFI probe positive control − MFI probe negative control). The positive reaction is defined by the percent positive value being greater than the preset cutoff value for each specific probe, while a negative reaction is defined as the percent positive value being lower than the preset cutoff value. The assignment of the HLA typing is based on the reaction pattern compared to patterns associated with each HLA gene sequence. In order to obtain valid data, two parameters are taken into account: count (the total number of beads that have been acquired) and MFI. For each data acquisition: count should be above 100 and the MFI for the positive control probe is expected to be within the range 800–4,000 MFI, depending on the bead pool and lot (*see* **Note 22**).

1. Open HLA Fusion software.
2. Click the Folder icon. Browse to the location where the LABType HD files are stored on the system/network.
3. Choose and open the folder for a specific session. Select .csv output file and click the Open button; the associated samples are displayed in the Current Sample/Patient Details table.
4. Highlight the sessions to be analyzed and select the correct catalogue from pull-down list.
5. Click import to analyze the session.
6. For DPA1/DPB1 kits, find the session of .csvoutput files to be analyzed in the Luminex Raw Data section and click open.
7. Highlight the sessions to be analyzed and select the correct catalogue from pull-down list.
8. Click Import to analyze the session.

9. On the right side of the screen, in the section Navigator, click on the session to be analyzed.
10. The assay is considered valid when the Positive Control bead MFI results are greater than or equal to 800 and the Negative Control bead MFI results are less than or equal to 20.
11. Once opened, the completed analysis will be displayed, starting with the first sample.
12. The screen will show four quadrants: *Quadrant 1*: the upper left quadrant shows the OneLambda QC panel reactivity with the selected probe. Each bar represents a QC sample, and its height represents the normalized MFI reaction value. The cut-off line represents the One Lambda default cutoff value. Choose RXN (the Reaction Pattern tab), it will display the Positive reactions for each bead, (*X*-axis) versus every allele, (*Y*-axis) defined in the catalogue file. It is also possible to see the layout which maps the recognition sites of all probes in the bead mixture and highlights any probes that pick up any of two user-selected alleles for comparison. *Quadrant 2*: the upper right quadrant shows the probe reactivity of the samples analyzed. The Bead Tab displays the histogram for the currently selected bead. Each bar represents a sample. The bar height represents the normalized MFI reaction value for the selected bead with that sample. The cutoff line is located at the cutoff value for the current bead (values above this line are considered positive). Clicking the Raw tab will be displayed the Raw Data Table. Clicking the Bead Info tab will display the specificities each probe picks up as well as the probes recognition site. *Quadrant 3*: the lower left quadrant displays the reaction profile for the current sample against all beads in the analysis. Positive reactions are represented as red bars; negative reactions are represented as blue bars. *Quadrant 4*: the lower right quadrant displays the typing results for the current sample. In general, the typing results include possible results and user assignments for allele pairs, coded results, serological equivalency results, and other assignments, and various pairs tab assignments suggested by the software. You must make all final assignments by moving a suggested pair into the final assignment area or by typing in an allele pair.
13. If analysis gives a result that may be acceptable, click on "Assign" and move to the next sample.
14. A cutoff adjustment should be considered in the following cases: (a) no results match the sample reactions and the analysis doesn't result in an HLA assignment; (b) the analysis indicates a false reaction (negative or positive) for one or more specific beads; (c) the analysis shows a bead reaction normalized MFI close to the cutoff value.

15. To change the cutoff value of a specific bead, in quadrant two, click on the bead pull-down list and select the bead.
16. Click and hold to drag the horizontal cutoff bar up or down to a new cutoff setting.
17. If an adjustment results in clearly assigned alleles and the new assignment looks acceptable, click on “Assign” to assign the typing.
18. Continue until all samples for that locus have been analyzed and repeat for each locus.
19. Validate the results (*see* **Note 23**).

4 Notes

1. DNA samples must be resuspended in sterile water or 10 mM Tris–HCl, pH 8.0–9.0, at an optimal concentration of 20 ng/μL with a purity (260/280 ratio) of 1.65–1.8. If DNA concentration is less than 20 ng/μL, it may be possible to add a greater volume of genomic DNA, and subsequently decrease the D-Mix volume accordingly.
2. Heparin as an anticoagulant must be avoided as it interferes with Taq DNA polymerase activity resulting in PCR failure.
3. A positive control of a well-established HLA typing must be run each time the performance of a new shipment or lot must be documented.
4. The 100× SAPE stock solution must be reconstituted at least 2 h before use with 1 mL of distilled sterile water. After dilution, the expiry date will be of 6 months. It is recommended to aliquot the diluted reagent to avoid contamination, in dark tubes since 100× SAPE is light sensitive.
5. The thermocycler must have the following characteristics: presence of a heated lid and of an adjustable ramp speed. In the PCR program the ramp speed of the heating step must be set up to 1.0 °C/s, while the cooling step ramp speed must be set up to 1.5 °C/s.
6. When multiple samples are analyzed, the risk of samples being mix up is very high. To avoid errors, carefully check sample IDs and DNA locations while following the worksheet scheme.
7. After completion of the PCR program, it is recommended but not required, to verify sample amplification by running 2–5 μL of the PCR reaction in a 2.5 % agarose gel stained with ethidium bromide. All samples, except negative control, must show an amplification product band of the appropriate size.
8. If, after adding the Neutralization Buffer, the mixture color has not changed to yellow, add a supplementary 1–2 μL of

Neutralization Buffer until the mixture color changes to pale yellow.

9. The Hybridization Bead Mixture is light sensitive. Keep in dark before using.
10. Mix the beads very well before adding them to the Hybridization buffer.
11. Regulate the vortex speed to avoid liquid splashing onto the seal.
12. After the last wash, the buffer volume in the wells must be less than 10 μL. If more than 10 μL remains, repeat wash/centrifuge/flick steps.
13. SAPE Buffer is temperature sensitive. Store a +4 °C when not in use.
14. After the preparation, the final 1× SAPE Solution must be stored and protected from light. It is recommended to cover the tube with an aluminum foil.
15. After installation, the Luminex probe height must be adjusted to the plate being used.
16. For the LABScan 100 maintenance program, it is recommended to clean the Sample Probe weekly. Briefly, remove the sample probe and sonicate the narrow end for 2–3 min. Use a syringe to flush the sample probe with distilled water from the narrow end through the larger end. Replace the sample probe and readjust the sample probe height for the reading plates being used.
17. The calibration step must be performed at least weekly or any time the temperature delta cal is not correct. In addition, any time maintenance or adjustment of the instrument during operation is likely to have altered optical alignment, the calibration step must be performed.
18. To check calibration results, click on the Diagnostics menu of the System Monitoring. Green indicates pass and red indicates fail. In the last instance, repetition of the whole calibration process must be performed. If the problem persists, it is recommended to change the reagents using a new lot. In case of a new failure, call for instrument assistance.
19. The bar-code reader allows the user to quickly enter the sample identification numbers or accession numbers. The bar code is particularly useful when you have many samples to enter into the system. Use the code 128 bar code label type.
20. The data acquisition may be visualized in the Acquisition Details or Diagnostics Section. Make sure that the majority of the beads fall within the proper regions.

21. If a second acquisition session is required to control/confirm the results, centrifuge the reading plate at 1,300 × *g* for 5 min. Flick to remove the supernatant and resuspend the pellet in 70 μL of Wash Buffer per well. Pipet up and down to mix and repeat the reading process.
22. Significant reduction in the bead counts suggests bead loss during sample acquisition or during the assay. Significant reduction in the MFI for the positive control probe suggests inadequate sample quantity and/or quality, poor assay efficiency, or instrument failure. Both reductions can result in invalidation of the test results.
23. Each session must be validated by a second authorized operator, who would reanalyze each sample, its control, its results, and confirms its typing by clicking the "Confirm" button. After validation, the results may be printed in the preselected report.

References

1. Hansen JA, Petersdorf E, Martin PJ, Anasetti C (1997) Hematopoietic stem cell transplants from unrelated donors. Immunol Rev 157:141–51
2. Lee SJ, Klein J, Haagenson M et al (1997) High-resolution donor-recipient HLA matching contributes to the success of unrelated donor marrow transplantation. Blood 110:4576–83
3. The MHC sequencing consortium (1999) Complete sequence and genemap of a human major histocompatibility complex. Nature 401:921–923
4. Vandiedonck C, Knight JC (2009) The human major histocompatibility complex as a paradigm in genomics research. Brief Funct Genomic Proteomic 8:379–394
5. Park M, Seo JJ (2012) Role of HLA in hematopoietic stem cell transplantation. Bone Marrow Res. doi:10.1155/2012/680841

Chapter 20

In Silico HLA Typing Using Standard RNA-Seq Sequence Reads

Sebastian Boegel, Jelle Scholtalbers, Martin Löwer, Ugur Sahin, and John C. Castle

Abstract

Next-generation sequencing (NGS) enables high-throughput transcriptome profiling using the RNA-Seq assay, resulting in billions of short sequence reads. Worldwide adoption has been rapid: many laboratories worldwide generate transcriptome sequence reads daily. Here, we describe methods for obtaining a sample's human leukocyte antigen (HLA) class I and II types and HLA expression using standard NGS RNA-Seq sequence reads. We demonstrate the application using our algorithm, seq2HLA, and a publicly available RNA-Seq dataset from the Burkitt lymphoma cell line Raji.

Key words HLA type, HLA expression, NGS, RNA-Seq, Immunoinformatics, In silico

1 Introduction

Next-generation sequencing (NGS) platforms enable the generation of billions of sequence reads that unbiasedly sample the input nucleic acids. Several studies have described the use of NGS for high-throughput HLA genotyping using genomic and complementary DNA [1, 2]. These methods use specialized NGS protocols and primers designed to specifically amplify HLA alleles followed by amplicon sequencing using sequencing instruments that generate longer reads (≥150 nucleotides), including the Roche/454 GS FLX and IlluminaMiSeq instruments.

By contrast, gene expression profiling using whole-transcriptome sequencing, often called RNA-Seq, typically uses much shorter reads (<100 nucleotides) which are commonly generated by IlluminaHiSeq instruments. Adoption of the RNA-Seq platform has been rapid: as of 2014 May 19, clinical and research labs worldwide have deposited more than 22,000 human RNA-Seq profiles into public repositories such as NCBI's Sequence Read Archive (SRA). Profiled samples include, for example, cell lines

Peter Bugert (ed.), *Molecular Typing of Blood Cell Antigens*, Methods in Molecular Biology, vol. 1310,
DOI 10.1007/978-1-4939-2690-9_20, © Springer Science+Business Media New York 2015

after perturbations, primary tissues in healthy and disease states, and homogeneous cell types. Vast numbers of RNA-Seq profiles from tumor and normal tissues are publicly available from international consortia, such as ICGC [3], TCGA [4], and GTEx [5]. Given the plethora of RNA-Seq profiles available, we sought to develop an algorithm that can use standard RNA-Seq reads to determine both HLA type and HLA expression.

The main challenge in determining the HLA type from short RNA-Seq reads is the polymorphic nature of the HLA loci: exons 2 and 3 encode the peptide-binding groove of HLA class I molecules and contain the majority of the variation but nevertheless differ by fewer than 70 nucleotides, i.e., 13 % of the nucleotides of exons 2 and 3 [6]. This represents a challenge for mapping sequence reads to reconstruct HLA alleles. Furthermore, the single human reference genome (e.g., hg19) does not adequately reflect the highly polymorphic nature of the HLA loci in the human population, confounding read alignment to a standard reference. Moreover, using RNA rather than DNA has additional complications and benefits: the reads reflect both the HLA types (the sequence) and the HLA expression levels (the count). If an HLA locus is not expressed, it cannot be typed. At the same time, knowledge of the HLA expression can be extremely informative: for example, HLA downregulation is an established tumor escape mechanism.

Multiple algorithms have been recently developed to determine the HLA type directly from standard NGS data. HLAminer [7] uses a targeted de novo assembly technique to reconstruct the HLA genes and can be applied to whole-genome (WGS), whole-exome (WXS), and whole-transcriptome sequencing (RNA-Seq) data. ATHLATES [8] also assembles reads into contiguous sequences (contigs) and focuses on WXS reads to determine the HLA genotype. HLAforest [9] and PHLAT [10] use an alignment-based approach, mapping the sequencing reads against a HLA allele specific reference database. While HLAforest is intended to work with RNA-Seq reads, PHLAT accepts WXS, RNA-Seq, and Amplicon-Seq reads (Table 1) (*see* **Note 1**).

We have developed and continue to improve an algorithm, seq2HLA that uses RNA-Seq NGS sequence reads in conjunction with over 6,000 known HLA allele reference sequences [6]. It utilizes an alignment-based approach to determine the 4-digit HLA class I and class II types, a confidence score, zygosity, and locus-specific expression levels.

Here, we describe how to use our method, seq2HLA, to quickly and easily determine HLA class I and II types as well as HLA expression from a sample using standard next-generation sequencing RNA-Seq sequence reads (*see* **Note 2**). As an example, we demonstrate how to retrieve RNA-Seq sequence reads of the human Burkitt lymphoma cell lines Raji from NCBI SRA and determine the HLA type and HLA expression.

Table 1
Overview of available tools determining the HLA type directly from standard NGS data, ordered according to publication date

Name	Input	Strategy	Availability	Reference
HLAminer	WXS,RNA-Seq, WGS	Targeted read assembly, reciprocal BLAST	http://www.bcgsc.ca/platform/bioinfo/software/hlaminer	7
seq2HLA	RNA-Seq (WXS)	Alignment-based, bowtie	https://bitbucket.org/sebastian-boegel/seq2HLA/	6
ATHLATES	WXS	Alignment and assembly	Upon request	8
HLAforest	RNA-Seq (WXS)	Alignment-based, bowtie	https://code.google.com/p/hlaforest/	9
PHLAT	WXS,RNA-Seq, Amplicon-Seq	Alignment-based, bowtie2	https://sites.google.com/site/phlatfortype/	10

WXS whole-exome sequencing, *WGS* whole-genome sequencing, (*WXS*) those tools were designed for RNA-Seq, but can also be applied to WXS data

2 Materials

To determine the HLA type and expression of an RNA-Seq sample, seq2HLA and additional software tools must be installed on a computer (Fig. 1). Once everything described in the following chapter is set up, seq2HLA can be executed on NGS sequence datasets from publically available samples or from your own experiments (*see* Subheading 3).

2.1 Hardware

Seq2HLA was developed on SUSE Linux Enterprise Server 11 (x86_64). Running seq2HLA requires a computer with a POSIX environment, such as Linux or Mac OS. The computer should ideally have Internet access.

2.2 Software Dependencies

The software tool seq2HLA was written in the scripting language python. It uses the alignment algorithm bowtie [11] to map reads to the HLA allele references. For calculating confidence scores, the statistical programming language R is used. To run seq2HLA, the following tools and packages must be installed:

1. Python (https://www.python.org/download/): seq2HLA was developed using Python 2.6.8. We recommend using Python 2.6.8 or a newer 2.x version.
2. Python packages: biopython [12] and numpy (version 1.3.0). seq2HLA was developed with biopython version 1.58.

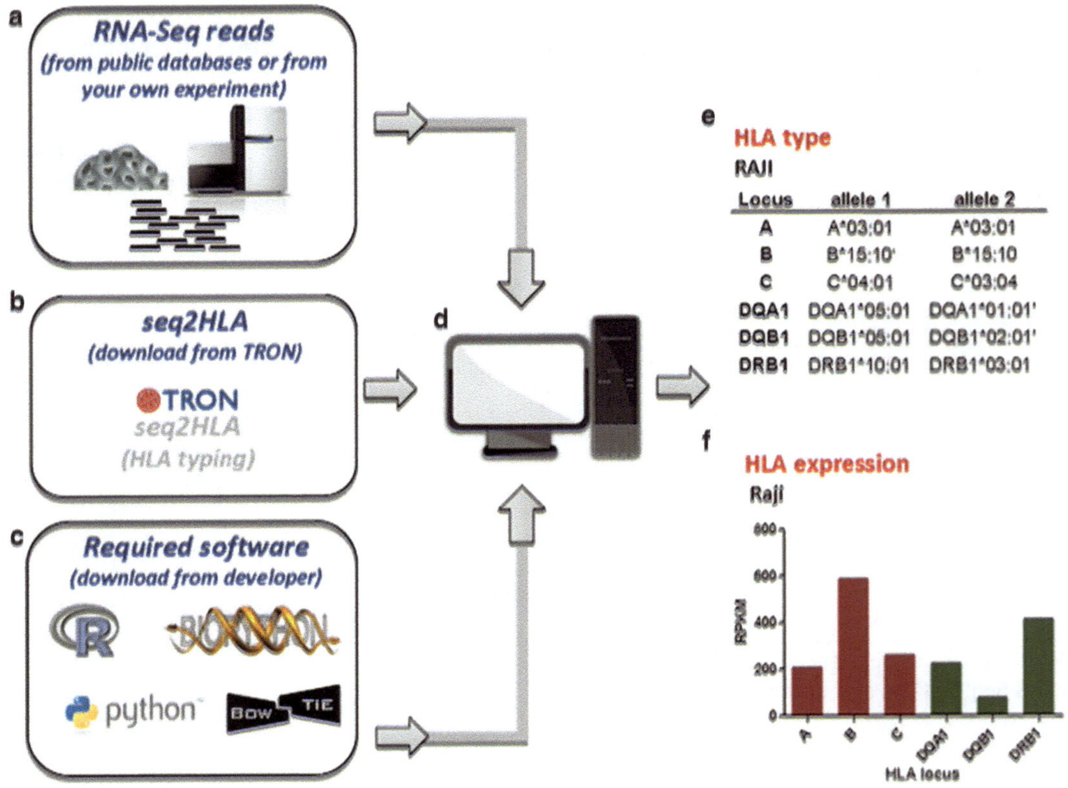

Fig. 1 Data integration and computational workflow. (**a**) RNA-Seq samples in fastq format are either retrieved from public databases (e.g., NCBI SRA) or from your own sequencing experiments. (**b**) Download the latest version of seq2HLA to your computer or server from the TRON homepage. (**c**) In order to run seq2HLA, download the following tools and packages from the website of the respective developer: programming language *Python*, *Biopython* and *numpy* (both *Python* packages), the statistical software *R*, and the alignment tool *bowtie*. (**d**) The RNA-Seq sample in fastq format are input to seq2HLA to determine the 4-digit HLA class I and class II type (**e**) as well as expression (**f**) of your sample

3. NGS read alignments: bowtie [11] version 1.0 or earlier. The environment must be able to execute bowtie by the command "bowtie".
4. R (http://www.r-project.org/): seq2HLA was developed and tested with R version 2.12.2 (2011-02-25).

2.3 Download seq2HLA

1. Download the latest version of seq2HLA from https://bitbucket.org/sebastian-boegel/seq2HLA to your computer (*see* **Note 3**).
2. Unzip the downloaded file using "gunzip". It is important that the bowtie index files remain located in the subfolder "references".

2.4 RNA-Seq Dataset

1. Seq2HLA is designed to run with standard paired-end RNA-Seq data as input. The file format can be uncompressed or gzip compressed fastq [13]. The fastq file format is the standard output format of many NGS instruments; it is also the most common file format used by NGS data repositories.
2. Here, we download paired-end RNA-Seq sequence reads from the human Burkitt lymphoma cell line Raji from the Sequence Read Archive (SRA), hosted by the National Center for Biotechnology Information (NCBI) (*see* **Note 4**).
3. To retrieve sequencing data stored at SRA, the program *sratoolkit* must be installed on your computer. It can be downloaded from http://eutils.ncbi.nih.gov/Traces/sra/?view=software. Let *</path/to/sratoolkit/>* denote the full path to your local copy of *sratoolkit*. The following command downloads the Raji RNA-Seq file with accession number SRR387401 in SRA format and splits this archive into two read files:/path/to/sratoolkit/bin/fastq-dump --split-3 SRR387401
4. Adding the option "--gzip" compresses the fastq files with gzip. Compression decreases disk space but increases runtime. Notwithstanding, seq2HLA accepts both uncompressed and compressed fastq files as input. The resultant files are the input to seq2HLA.

3 Methods

3.1 Running seq2HLA

1. Let */path/to/seq2HLA/* denote the full path to your local copy of seq2HLA. The standard usage of seq2HLA is: python/path/to/seq2HLA/seq2HLA.py -1<readfile1>-2<readfile2>-r "<runname>" [-p<int>] [-3<int>].
2. *readfile1* and *readfile2* can be uncompressed or gzipped fastq files. seq2HLA currently supports only paired-end reads.
3. *runname* should contain the path in with the output files should be stored and a prefix for the output file name, e.g., "/path/to/output/Raji".
4. *-p*: the number of parallel search threads for bowtie (optional, default 6).
5. *-3*: the number of nucleotides to trim from the low-quality end of each read (optional, default 0).
6. Using the paired-end fastq files of Raji as example and assuming that user has moved the files into the current directory, seq2HLA can be executed by the command:python /path/to/seq2HLA/seq2HLA.py -1 SRR387394_1.fastq -2 SRR387394_2.fastq –r "RAJI-SRR387394" (*see* **Note 5**).

3.2 Interpreting the Output

Results as well as intermediate steps are output to *stdout* (i.e., your console) and to text files in the working directory. The most important files are:

1. <*runname*>-ClassI.HLAgenotype2digits => 2 digit result of Class I.
2. <*runname*>-ClassII.HLAgenotype2digits => 2 digit result of Class II.
3. <*runname*>-ClassI.HLAgenotype4digits => 4 digit result of Class I.
4. <*runname*>-ClassII.HLAgenotype4digits => 4 digit result of Class II.
5. <*runname*>.ambiguity => reports typing ambiguities (more than one solution for an allele possible).
6. <*runname*>-ClassI.expression => expression of Class I alleles.
7. <*runname*>-ClassII.expression => expression of Class II alleles.
8. where <*runname*> denotes the name specified with "-r".

3.2.1 2-Digit Typing

1. *Seq2HLA* works by first determining the HLA groups, i.e., 2-digit resolution, as well as heterozygosity vs homozygosity for HLA class I (Table 2) and HLA class II (Table 3), as described in the original publication of seq2HLA [6].
2. In a second step, seq2HLA refines the calls by considering the number of reads assigned to any allele within the determined group and thus automatically assigning the 4-digit HLA types.
3. In the example of Raji, the HLA-A locus is predicted to be homozygous for HLA-A*03, as indicated by "hoz" in the prediction of the second allele. Given the significant confidence score (1.5E−06), it is likely that this locus is homozygous (Table 2).
4. In contrast, a large confidence score (large value) would indicate that this locus is likely not homozygous and instead HLA-A*23 might be the second allele. HLA-C is predicted to be heterozygous for HLA-C*04 and HLA-C*03 (Table 2).

Table 2
HLA class I type in 2-digit resolution for Raji stored in file RAJI-SRR387394-ClassI.HLAgenotype2digits

Locus	Allele 1	Confidence	Allele 2	Confidence
A	A*03	2.65E−12	hoz ("A*23")	1.5E−06
B	B*15	0	hoz ("B*35")	2.42E−05
C	C*04	1.52E−03	C*03	1.15E−02

Table 3
HLA class II type in 2-digit resolution for Raji stored in file RAJI-SRR387394-ClassII.HLAgenotype2digits

Locus	Allele 1	Confidence	Allele 2	Confidence
DQA1	DQA1*05	8.912E-04	DQA1*01	2.42E-01
DQB1	DQB1*05	8.86E-02	DQB1*02	2.42E-01
DRB1	DRB1*10	5.40E-02	DRB1*03	6.95E-02

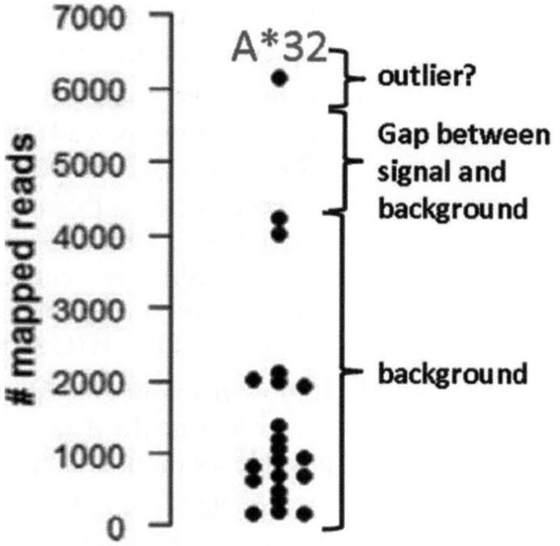

Fig. 2 Interpretation of the confidence score. The confidence score measures the gap between signal (i.e., reads mapping to the true HLA group) and noise (i.e., reads mapping to any other HLA group due to the polymorphic nature of HLA) by calculating the probability of the signal being an outlier given the distribution of mapped reads to each group resulting in a *p*-value (confidence score) indicating how good the separation between the true solution and the background is. (Figure adapted from ref. 6)

3.2.2 Interpreting the Confidence Score

1. The confidence score measures the gap between the signal (i.e., reads mapping to the true HLA group) and noise (i.e., reads mapping to any other HLA group due to the polymorphic nature of HLA).
2. The score is computed by calculating the probability of the signal being an outlier given the distribution of mapped reads to each group.
3. The outcome of this statistical test is a p-value (confidence score). A larger gap between the true solution and the background results in a clearer separation and thus a more confident typing result (Fig. 2).

3.2.3 4-Digit Typing

1. After the 2-digit typings (i.e., allele groups) are determined, the algorithm refines the typings to determine the 4-digit resolution, i.e., the actual protein which is presented on the surface. This is done by considering the distribution of reads mapped to any full digit resolution allele within an allele group.
2. For each allele group separately, the 95th percentile is determined to separate between the true signal (true allele) and noise (wrong alleles having reads due to their sequence similarity to the true allele).
3. After removing insignificant alleles based on read counts and confidence scores, the most likely 4-digit allele is reported. Due to the polymorphic nature of the HLA system, the allelic sequences within a group are very similar to each other.
4. Furthermore, the use of short reads increases the complexity of discrimination as reads may map to multiple alleles within a group (e.g., HLA-A*02), within a locus (e.g., HLA-B) or even between alleles of different loci. Thus, it is not always possible to determine a unique 4-digit solution. In these cases, the candidate list is further refined by filtering out alleles which do not appear in the pan-population allele frequency table provided by the NCBI dbMHC Anthropology Resources database [14].
5. If more than one solution is still possible, an ambiguity flag “’” is attached to the 4-digit type of the most likely allele and all possible solutions are reported in the file “<prefix>.ambiguity”.
6. In the Raji example, there are ambiguities at HLA-B*15 (Table 4) and at HLA-DQA1*01 and HLA-DQB1*02 (Table 5).
7. In those cases, it is helpful to look at possible solutions stored in the file “RAJI-SRR387394.ambiguity” (Fig. 3). This shows that HLA-B*15:10 and HLA-B*15:37 are equally likely and HLA-B*15:09 and HLA-B*15:18 are only slightly less significant.

Table 4
HLA class I type in 4-digit resolution for Raji stored in file RAJI-SRR387394-ClassI.HLAgenotype4digits

Locus	Allele 1	Confidence	Allele 2	Confidence
A	A*03:01	4.27E–12	A*03:01	1.50E–06
B	B*15:10′	0	B*15:10	2.42E–05
C	C*04:01	1.52E–03	C*03:04	1.15E–02

```
##########################################################################################
#Ambiguity:
#Based on the RNA-Seq reads and the dbMHC table, the following 4-digits alleles are possible:
B*15:18 4.083534e-11
B*15:10 0
B*15:09 7.948886e-08
B*15:37 0
#However, by taking into account the read data, the most probable 4-digit allele is:
B*15:10

##########################################################################################
#Ambiguity:
#Based on the RNA-Seq reads and the dbMHC table, the following 4-digits alleles are possible:
DQA1*01:04    0.2416226
DQA1*01:01    0.2416226
#However, by taking into account the read data, the most probable 4-digit allele is:
DQA1*01:01

##########################################################################################
#Ambiguity:
#Based on the RNA-Seq reads and the dbMHC table, the following 4-digits alleles are possible:
DQB1*02:02    0.2416419
DQB1*02:01    0.2416419
#However, by taking into account the read data, the most probable 4-digit allele is:
DQB1*02:01
```

Fig. 3 Reporting of ambiguities. Typing ambiguities are marked with a flag ("'") and all possible solutions are reported in the file RAJI-SRR387394.ambiguity

Table 5
HLA class I type in 4-digit resolution for Raji stored in file RAJI-SRR387394-ClassI.HLAgenotype4digits

Locus	Allele 1	Confidence	Allele 2	Confidence
DQA1	DQA1*05:01	8.92E−04	DQA1*01:01′	2.42E−01
DQB1	DQB1*05:01	8.86E−02	DQB1*02:01′	2.42E−01
DRB1	DRB1*10:01	5.40E−02	DRB1*03:01	6.95E−02

3.2.4 HLA Expression

1. Using RNA-Seq reads for HLA typing enables the determination of HLA expression. seq2HLA provides locus-specific expression values for HLA class I and HLA class II (Fig. 1f, Table 6), normalized according to "reads per kilobase of exon model per million mapped reads" (RPKM) [15].
2. RPKM normalizes the number of reads mapping to a transcript by the length of the transcript and the total number of generated reads in the experiment. In the downloaded Raji sample, HLA class I and class II (Table 6) molecules are expressed at 1,064 and 716 RPKM, respectively.
3. For comparison, we analyzed five human primary spleen (SRA: ERR315405, ERR315416, ERR315448, ERR315338,

Table 6
Locus-specific expression values for HLA class I and HLA class II for Raji. The values are output in the example files RAJI-SRR387394-ClassI. expression and RAJI-SRR387394-ClassII.expression

Locus	Expression [RPKM]
HLA class I	
A	210.38
B	590.62
C	263.53
HLA class II	
DQA1	77.14
DQB1	224.80
DRB1	414.46

ERR315473) and three human primary cerebral cortex RNA-Seq samples (SRA: ERR315477, ERR315432, ERR315455) from the Human Protein Atlas [16].

4. The determined HLA expression profile in the downloaded Raji sample is similar to that found in spleen, which is expected to contain high amounts of HLA molecules as part of the lymphatic system and much higher compared to the low HLA expression in cerebral cortex (Fig. 4).

4 Notes

1. Although seq2HLA is designed for RNA-Seq reads as input, it is also capable of determining HLA types from Whole-Exome Sequencing (WXS) datasets. RNA-Seq involves capturing the (spliced) mRNA using polyA selection, reverse transcription, amplification, and sequencing. In contrast, WXS comprises capturing exonic DNA. Small stretches of neighboring intronic sequences are also captured and sequenced. Those intronic nucleotides will count as mismatches when aligning the reads against the reference database of HLA allele transcripts. As previously shown by us [6], the number of allowed mismatches has a great influence in the mapping specificity when dealing with highly similar reference sequences. Nevertheless, ignoring the *p*-value as confidence score, the accuracy of the two-digit version of seq2HLA was found to be comparable to tools designed for WXS reads [10].

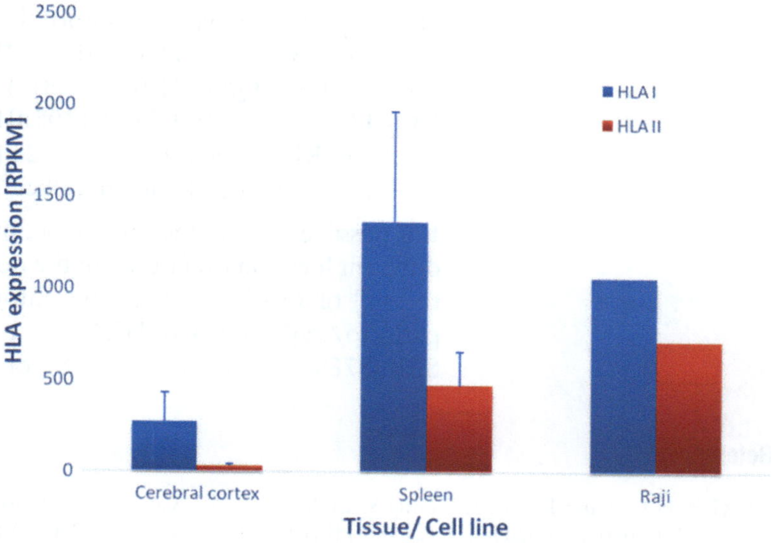

Fig. 4 Interpretation of RPKM expression values. In the downloaded Raji sample, HLA class I (*blue bars*) and HLA class II (*red bars*) molecules are both highly expressed. This becomes clear by comparing to HLA expression profiles of other tissues as reference. Spleen is expected to contain high amounts of HLA molecules as part of the lymphatic system and in contrast, brain is associated with very low HLA levels. The Raji HLA expression profile is similar to spleen and much higher than brain. Depicted is mean HLA class I expression (as sum of HLA-A, HLA-B, HLA-C), HLA class II expression (as sum of HLA-DQA1, HLA-DQB1, HLA-DRB1) and standard deviation of three cerebral cortex, five spleen, and one Raji RNA-Seq samples analyzed with seq2HLA

2. Using RNA reads in conjunction with over 6,000 known HLA allele reference sequences, seq2HLA incorporates genetics and expression, outputs HLA expression profiles and determines the HLA type based on expressed HLA transcripts. An allele can only typed if it is expressed. If the expression is too low, some ambiguities even on the 2-digit level cannot be resolved. This is particularly true when dealing with tumor samples: tumors frequently evolve to down regulate and even loose HLA expression as a tumor escape mechanism.

3. In addition to the publicly available downloadable software, seq2HLA is also an integrated tool in Galaxy. Galaxy is an open, web-based platform for analyzing biomedical data providing a plethora of tools without the need for installing them (http://galaxyproject.org) [17–19]. To obtain seq2HLA as Galaxy module, search for "seq2HLA" in the Galaxy toolshed (http://toolshed.g2.bx.psu.edu/) [20].

4. The reads are accessible using the run-ID SRR387394 at http://www.ncbi.nlm.nih.gov/sra/?term=SRR387394. The

HLA-type was previously reported as HLA-A*03:01, HLA-B*15:10, HLA-C*03:04, HLA-C*04:01 for HLA class I and HLA-DQA1*01:01, HLA-DQA1*05:01, HLA-DQB1*02:01, HLA-DQB1*05:01, HLA-DRB1*03:01, HLA-DQRB1*10:01 for class II [21] (http://www.ebi.ac.uk/cgi-bin/ipd/imgt/hla/fetch_cell.cgi?11295).

5. It is possible to store the output files produced by seq2HLA in a different location other than in the download by simply adding the full or relative path to the output folder, e.g., python /path/to/seq2HLA/seq2HLA.py -1 SRR387394_1.fastq -2 SRR387394_2.fastq –r "/path/to/output/RAJI-SRR387394".

References

1. Gabriel C, Fürst D, Faé I, Wenda S, Zollikofer C, Mytilineos J, Fischer GF (2014) HLA typing by next-generation sequencing – getting closer to reality. Tissue Antigens 83:65–75
2. de Santis D, Dinauer D, Duke J, Erlich HA, Holcomb CL, Lind C et al (2013) 16(th) IHIW. Review of HLA typing by NGS. Int J Immunogenet 40:72–76
3. Hudson TJ, Anderson W, Artez A, Barker AD, Bell C, Bernabé RR et al (2010) International network of cancer genome projects. Nature 464:993–998
4. Chang K, Creighton CJ, Davis C, Donehower L, Drummond J, Wheeler D et al (2013) The Cancer Genome Atlas Pan-Cancer analysis project. Nat Genet 45:1113–1120
5. The Genotype-Tissue Expression (GTEx) Project (2013) Nat Genet 45:580–585
6. Boegel S, Löwer M, Schäfer M, Bukur T, de Graaf J, Boisguérin V et al (2012) HLA typing from RNA-Seq sequence reads. Genome Med 4:102
7. Warren RL, Choe G, Freeman DJ, Castellarin M, Munro S, Moore R, Holt RA (2012) Derivation of HLA types from shotgun sequence datasets. Genome Med 4:95
8. Liu C, Yang X, Duffy B, Mohanakumar T, Mitra RD, Zody MC, Pfeifer JD (2013) ATHLATES: accurate typing of human leukocyte antigen through exome sequencing. Nucleic Acids Res 41:e142
9. Kim HJ, Pourmand N, Colombo G (2013) HLA haplotyping from RNA-seq data using hierarchical read weighting. PLoS One 8:e67885
10. Bai Y, Ni M, Cooper B, Wei Y, Fury W (2014) Inference of high resolution HLA types using genome-wide RNA or DNA sequencing reads. BMC Genomics 15:325
11. Langmead B, Trapnell C, Pop M, Salzberg SL (2009) Ultrafast and memory-efficient alignment of short DNA sequences to the human genome. Genome Biol 10:R25
12. Cock PJA, Antao T, Chang JT, Chapman BA, Cox CJ, Dalke A et al (2009) Biopython: freely available Python tools for computational molecular biology and bioinformatics. Bioinformatics 25:1422–1423
13. Cock PJA, Fields CJ, Goto N, Heuer ML, Rice PM (2010) The Sanger FASTQ file format for sequences with quality scores, and the Solexa/Illumina FASTQ variants. Nucleic Acids Res 38:1767–1771
14. Helmberg W, Dunivin R, Feolo M (2004) The reagent database at dbMHC. Tissue Antigens 63:142–148
15. Mortazavi A, Williams BA, McCue K, Schaeffer L, Wold B (2008) Mapping and quantifying mammaliantranscriptomes by RNA-Seq. Nat Methods 5:621–628
16. Uhlen M, Oksvold P, Fagerberg L, Lundberg E, Jonasson K, Forsberg M et al (2010) Towards a knowledge-based Human Protein Atlas. Nat Biotechnol 28:1248–1250
17. Giardine B, Riemer C, Hardison RC, Burhans R, Elnitski L, Shah P et al (2005) Galaxy: a platform for interactive large-scale genome analysis. Genome Res 15:1451–1455
18. Goecks J, Nekrutenko A, Taylor J (2010) Galaxy: a comprehensive approach for supporting accessible, reproducible, and transparent computational research in the life sciences. Genome Biol 11:R86
19. Blankenberg D, von Kuster G, Coraor N, Ananda G, Lazarus R, Mangan M et al (2010) Galaxy: a web-based genome analysis tool for experimentalists. Curr Protoc Mol Biol 19(10):1–21
20. Blankenberg D, von Kuster G, Bouvier E, Baker D, Afgan E, Stoler N et al (2014) Dissemination of scientific software with Galaxy ToolShed. Genome Biol 15:403
21. Robinson J, Halliwell JA, McWilliam H, Lopez R, Parham P, Marsh SGE (2012) The IMGT/HLA database. Nucleic Acids Res 41:D1222

INDEX

Peter Bugert (ed.), *Molecular Typing of Blood Cell Antigens*, Methods in Molecular Biology, vol. 1310, DOI 10.1007/978-1-4939-2690-9, © Springer Science+Business Media New York 2015

R

S

T

U

W